Endurance Sports Nutrition

SECOND EDITION

Suzanne Girard Eberle, MS, RD

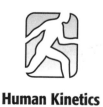

Human Kinetics

Library of Congress Cataloging-in-Publication Data

Eberle, Suzanne Girard, 1962-
   Endurance sports nutrition / Suzanne Girard Eberle. -- 2nd ed.
      p. cm.
   Includes bibliographical references and index.
   ISBN-13: 978-0-7360-6471-2 (soft cover)
   ISBN-10: 0-7360-6471-0 (soft cover)
   1. Athletes--Nutrition. I. Title.
   TX361.A8E39 2007
   613.2'024796--dc22

                                        2006036217

ISBN-10: 0-7360-6471-0
ISBN-13: 978-0-7360-6471-2

Acquisitions Editor: Jana Hunter; **Developmental Editor:** Anne Hall; **Assistant Editor:** Cory Weber; **Copyeditor:** Robert Replinger; **Proofreader:** Jim Burns; **Indexer:** Dan Connolly; **Permission Manager:** Carly Breeding; **Graphic Designer:** Nancy Rasmus; **Graphic Artist:** Sandra Meier; **Photo Manager:** Laura Fitch; **Cover Designer:** Keith Blomberg; **Photographers (cover):** Tom Roberts and Kelly Huff; **Art Manager:** Kelly Hendren; **Illustrators:** Craig Newsom, Kim Maxey, and Al Wilborn; **Printer:** United Graphics

Human Kinetics books are available at special discounts for bulk purchase. Special editions or book excerpts can also be created to specification. For details, contact the Special Sales Manager at Human Kinetics.

Printed in the United States of America   10 9 8 7 6 5 4 3 2 1

Human Kinetics
Web site: www.HumanKinetics.com

United States: Human Kinetics
P.O. Box 5076
Champaign, IL 61825-5076
800-747-4457
e-mail: humank@hkusa.com

Canada: Human Kinetics
475 Devonshire Road Unit 100
Windsor, ON N8Y 2L5
800-465-7301 (in Canada only)
e-mail: orders@hkcanada.com

Europe: Human Kinetics
107 Bradford Road
Stanningley
Leeds LS28 6AT, United Kingdom
+44 (0) 113 255 5665
e-mail: hk@hkeurope.com

Australia: Human Kinetics
57A Price Avenue
Lower Mitcham, South Australia 5062
08 8372 0999
e-mail: liaw@hkaustralia.com

New Zealand: Human Kinetics
Division of Sports Distributors NZ Ltd.
P.O. Box 300 226 Albany
North Shore City
Auckland
0064 9 448 1207
e-mail: info@humankinetics.co.nz

To the boys in my life,
John and Asa Babu

CONTENTS

Part II   Condition-Specific Nutrition Plans

PREFACE

I've got something that will help you be lean, strong, and full of energy—do you want some? It's simple, legal, and affordable—high-performance eating habits. As an endurance athlete who pursues such challenging feats as marathons, triathlons, and century bike rides, or desires to, you have to eat smart, not just on race or event days but also on all the days between them. The payoff is enormous. By eating smart, you set yourself up to perform better and enjoy your chosen endeavor more because you have greater energy to train, suffer fewer injuries, get sick less often, and recover more quickly. You'll also have an easier time reaching and maintaining a healthy weight.

If your goal is to complete an Ironman triathlon (swim 2.4 miles, or 3.8 kilometers); bike 112 miles, or 180 kilometers; and run 26.2 miles, or 42 kilometers), bike across your state, run 100 miles (160 kilometers) in less than a day (ultrarun), or some slightly saner version of a foot race such as your local marathon, climb a mountain, or complete an adventure race, you won't be able to succeed without knowing what to eat and drink while on the move. Equally important, however, is how you meet your fluid and fuel needs on a daily basis. Even if you're just starting out—running your first 10K road race, hiking along local trails, or thinking about trying a sprint triathlon—you can easily be knocked off track by frequent colds, nagging injuries, or the struggle just to get out the door. Paying more attention to what you eat from day to day will help you stay on course. No matter what your age, athletic ability, or goal—racing to a personal best or just wanting to finish—high-performance eating habits improve your chances of getting to the starting line and then crossing the finish line.

Besides genetics (which is out of our control), the essential planks of any endurance athlete's performance are training, mental preparation, nutrition, and rest and recovery. Because most active people don't have the time or the scientific background to keep up on the ever-evolving field of sports nutrition, I've done it for you. As a former elite runner (4:28 mile, 32:40 10K, member of three USA teams) and now a sports dietitian who runs, cycles, and climbs, I'm particularly qualified to guide you through the process. I've sorted through what the nutrition and exercise science professionals recommend, and I have translated that knowledge into what works in real life. To supplement my expertise and experience, I've included practical tips and tried-and-true nutritional strategies offered by some of the best endurance athletes in the country for getting the job done.

This sports nutrition book is unique in two aspects. First, it's not just another general sports nutrition book. It's specifically geared to the endurance athlete—the person who understands the saying "No guts, no story!" If you spend hours at a time training or competing, you have nutritional needs that differ from those of athletes in power, stop-and-go, or team sports. Part I of this book (chapters 1 through 8) delivers endurance-specific nutrition strategies that you can apply the next time you open the refrigerator door, head out to train, hear about the latest supplement, step on the scale, or panic, after signing up for an event, about how you're ever going to go that far or last that long. Even if your friends and family, coach, or teammates politely refer to you as nutritionally challenged, you will be ready to pursue smarter eating habits after reading these chapters.

In part II (chapters 9 through 16), I coach you through the unique nutritional challenges that endurance athletes must master so that they can go longer and longer, especially under challenging conditions such as altitude and extreme heat or cold. Regardless of your sport or activity—running, cycling, mountain-biking, triathlon, adventure racing, hiking, mountaineering, Nordic skiing, long-distance swimming, or rowing—your job is to go into an endurance event or race with a well-conceived nutritional game plan. Regardless of your goal—hoping just to finish or going farther and faster than ever before—your job is to monitor your food, fluid, and electrolyte needs while on the move. What bright athlete wouldn't want to have an endurance-minded nutrition coach by his or her side?

This book, then, is offered to you, the endurance athlete, as food for thought.

ACKNOWLEDGMENTS

Many thanks to acquisitions editor Jana Hunter and to developmental editor Anne Hall for making this an enjoyable endeavor the second time around.

I'm also grateful to the athletes who again shared their time and wisdom and to all those who continue to seek my advice. My gratitude also goes to my fellow sports dietitians around the world. This book wouldn't be nearly as comprehensive without their collective support. Last, to my brother Michael, my favorite cycling partner, and my husband John, my best friend and favorite running partner, I thank you for always being there.

PART I

Endurance-Specific Nutrition Strategies

1

Strengthening Your Nutritional Base

"I believe nutrition plays a huge role in the early years when you're 20 and 30. Why wait until you're 40? Younger athletes often get away with a poor diet because their strength levels are at their highest point. . . . If you've missed the opportunity to revamp your eating—it's never too late. Watch what you eat during the day and fuel up before, during, and after your training."

—Dave Scott, six-time winner of the Hawaii Ironman

Endurance athletes require different types and amounts of fluid and fuel than athletes in power or team sports do. If you think that you can eat like your buddies who play a pickup game a few days a week or if you think about your nutritional needs only on race day or if you want to lose weight, you're putting yourself at a real disadvantage. If you believe that only elite-level runners, cyclists, swimmers, rowers, triathletes, adventure racers, hikers, mountaineers, and backcountry and Nordic skiers benefit from paying attention to what they eat, think again. Whatever an athlete's age or athletic prowess, three factors figure prominently in his or her success: genetics, training, and nutrition. You can't do anything about your genetic makeup, so you can improve only by concentrating on the other two (along with getting adequate rest and working on your mental skills, too, of course).

Indeed, what you eat and how you train are inextricably linked. The people who are most successful at completing the endurance endeavors that they set out to do, like running a marathon or tackling a half Ironman, are those who consistently train smart. And the only way to do that is to eat smart, all the time. Whether you're highly competitive or just want to finish and live to tell about it, you won't truly excel unless you eat smart. That is, you must choose foods in optimal amounts that support what you're personally trying to accomplish that day, en route to your long-term goal. How else do you think that you can tackle an early morning swim workout, a full day at the office, and a long bike ride or run in the evening? More important, how do you think that you can get up the next day and do it all over again? And most important of all, how can you feel strong and confident, and enjoy every passing mile (or at least most of them) while you're doing it?

Eating a well-balanced, healthy diet doesn't guarantee success, but poor eating habits can literally stop you in your tracks or at least slow you down. The foods and fluids that you consume on a daily basis provide the fuel and nutrients that your body needs to perform day after day. Recurrent colds and illnesses, nagging injuries, and frequent poor training days signal that your nutrition program is out of sync with your training program. If you're a competitive athlete, you obviously must think about what to eat and drink on race day. But what about all the days that you're not racing? Even if you race every weekend—52 times a year—you still have 313 other days to think about!

Besides being good for you, the foods that you choose to eat from day to day must also taste good and be satisfying; otherwise, you won't want to eat them. The key is to follow an eating style that fulfills both these needs—high-performance nutritional foods that fuel your body (foods that you need) and foods that feed your mind (foods that you want). On top of that, unless you like to spend time in the kitchen or can afford to hire a personal chef, you probably want to figure out how to eat smart without spending too much time and energy.

Evaluating Your Daily Eating Habits

You may already know something about what constitutes a healthy training or day-to-day diet for an endurance athlete. Maybe you know a lot. Regardless, looking at what you're actually eating never hurts. Knowledge about a topic doesn't always translate into practice. Knowing what you are currently eating will help you answer for yourself the question I hear most often from fitness enthusiasts and athletes of all abilities: "What should I be eating?"

Review the New Food Pyramid

First, familiarize yourself with the recently updated MyPyramid (see figure 1.1), which you can use as a general guideline for building a smart, well-balanced sports diet. MyPyramid organizes foods by the nutrients that they contain into five major food groups: grains (complex carbohydrates); vegetables; fruit; milk; meat and beans; and a separate category for the modest amount of healthy fat (oils) that we need daily. It also reminds us to eat more of these high-performance (nutrient-dense) foundation foods and to limit

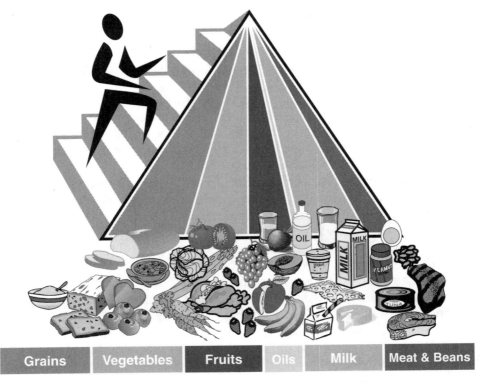

| Grains | Vegetables | Fruits | Oils | Milk | Meat & Beans |

Figure 1.1 High-performance eating habits require a balance of eating the foods you need and the foods you want. The food pyramid is a basic tool you can use to help assess your overall diet.

From the U.S. Department of Agriculture (USDA).

www.MyPyramid.gov

the extras that we may choose to top off our diets with, such as foods high in saturated or trans fat or added sugars, or foods that supply few or no nutrients, such as potato chips and alcohol. In addition, MyPyramid emphasizes that exercise and being fit is just as important as what we eat and, in fact, that how much you need to eat is particular to you and depends on how much you move. This is good news for endurance athletes: Those who move more get to eat more!

As you take a closer look at the food pyramid, you may wonder where some foods belong.

Grains group: all foods made from wheat, rice, oats, cornmeal, and barley and other whole grains, such as bread, pasta, oatmeal, breakfast cereals, tortillas, and grits; at least half of all grains consumed should be whole grains.

Vegetable group: all fresh, frozen, canned, and dried vegetables and vegetable juices.

Fruit group: all fresh, frozen, canned, and dried fruits and 100 percent fruit juices.

Oils: fats that are liquid at room temperature, such as canola, olive, peanut, corn, flaxseed, soybean, and sunflower oil; foods that are naturally high in oils like nuts, seeds, nut butters, flaxseed, olives, and avocados; fat supplied by fattier fish; and foods that are mainly oil such as mayonnaise, certain salad dressings, and soft (tub) margarine.

Milk group: all fluid milk products and foods made from milk that retain their calcium content, such as yogurt, cheese, and cottage cheese. Most choices should be low fat or fat free.

Meat and beans group: lean meat, poultry and fish, eggs, peanut butter, cooked dry beans (legumes), and tofu and other soy foods.

Extras (discretionary calories remaining after accounting for the calories needed for all food groups): coffee and tea, soda, fruit-flavored drinks, alcohol, cream cheese, butter and stick margarine, jam and jelly, nondairy creamer, condiments, sour cream, sugar, honey, maple syrup, pickles, sauces, gravy, bacon, fatty deli meats, hot dogs, sausage, french fries, onion rings, chips or crisps and snack foods, oil-popped popcorn, candy, chocolate, sherbet, gelatin desserts, high-fat ice cream and frozen yogurt, cookies, doughnuts, muffins, pastries, cakes, and pies.

Analyze One Day of Your Diet

Before you read any further, grab a pencil and get ready to look at your current eating habits. Take a few minutes to recall what you had to eat (and drink) yesterday from the time you arose until you went to bed. If yesterday was unusual, if, for example, you were ill or traveling, choose another day that you can recall. Now refer to figure 1.2, the personal food pyramid worksheet, and fill in the blanks by listing all the foods and beverages that you consumed from each food group in one day. For example, if you ate a standard size (large) bagel with cream cheese and orange juice for breakfast, you would write bagel in the grains group box, orange juice in the fruit group box, and cream cheese in the tip of the pyramid (extras).

Don't forget to include snacks, beverages, and foods that you ate on the run, such as the energy bar that you downed in the car on the way home following a workout or the cheese and crackers that you grabbed on the way through the kitchen. Be sure to record condiments or additions to food, such as the parmesan cheese (milk) that you covered your plate of spaghetti with or the olive oil (oils) in which you soaked your bread. Obviously, many of the foods that you eat will fit into more than one food group. A bean and cheese burrito, for example, would count in the grains group (tortilla, rice), the milk group (cheese), and the meat and beans group (beans). Count only the major ingredients in mixed foods.

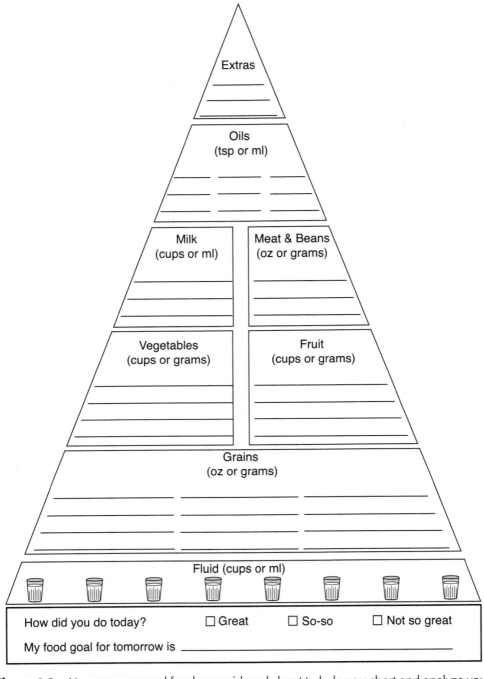

Figure 1.2 Use your personal food pyramid worksheet to help you chart and analyze your nutritional intake over a 24-hour period.

From S.G. Eberle, 2007, *Endurance sports nutrition*, 2nd ed. (Champaign, IL: Human Kinetics). Adapted from Sandy S. Miller, MS, RD, LD, *SMART Choices for Health*™ Copyright 1999, Providence Health System.

Next, estimate the amount that you ate by comparing it with what counts as one serving in each group (see table 1.1). For example, count the large bagel as four grains because the average bakery or grocery-store bagel weighs 4 ounces (112 grams), with one ounce (28 grams) of bread being equal to one serving. For the burrito, a good estimate would be two and one-half grains (small 6-inch, or 15-centimeter, tortilla; three-quarters cup of rice), one milk (one ounce of cheese), and two meat and beans (one-quarter cup of cooked dried beans is one serving; one-half cup would be two). Tally up the number of servings that you ate in each food group and put a circle around the number.

Keeping the particular needs of endurance athletes in mind, I've modified the food pyramid in a few ways. The modified base of my food pyramid emphasizes the importance of drinking a minimum of 8 to 10 glasses of fluid a day. Estimate your fluid intake by checking off one glass (as depicted at the base of the pyramid) for every cup (250 milliliters) of fluid that you consumed. Count water, fruit and vegetable juice, milk, sports drinks, other noncaffeinated beverages, and coffee and tea, but not alcoholic drinks (including beer). For more accurate tracking, write in the actual source of fluid under each water glass that you mark. I also place starchy vegetables (like potatoes, winter squash, corn, and green peas) in the grains group, and I put nuts and seeds in the oils category rather than thinking about them as a lean protein source. (One ounce, or 28 grams, of nuts provides 14 to 18 grams of fat and only 4 to 6 grams of protein.)

Granted, one day of tracking what you eat doesn't give you a complete picture of your eating habits. You may be pleasantly surprised at how well you're doing at meeting your nutrition needs, or you may be prompted to

Table 1.1   **What Counts As One Serving?**

Grains group	Single serving size
Bread	1 slice, 1 oz (28 g)
Tortilla	1 small flour, 1 corn
Roll, biscuit, or scone	1 small (2 in., or 5 cm, diameter)
Bagel	1 oz, 1 mini (2.5 in., or 6.5 cm, diameter)
Hamburger bun, English muffin	1/2
Ready-to-eat cereal	~1 cup
Pasta, rice	1/2 cup, cooked
Bulgur, millet, buckwheat, and so on	1/2 cup, cooked
Oatmeal	1/2 cup, cooked, 1 packet instant
Small crackers	2–7
Pancake	1 (4 in., or 10 cm)
Pretzels	1 oz
Popcorn	3 cups, popped

(continued)

Table 1.1 *(continued)*

Vegetable group	Single serving size
Leafy greens (lettuce, spinach, and so on)	2 cups raw, 1 cup cooked
Greens (collard, turnip, kale)	1 cup cooked
Raw or cooked vegetables	1 cup
Tomato or vegetable juice	1 cup
Spaghetti sauce	1 cup
Carrots	2 medium or 12 baby
Baked or boiled potato	1 medium
Mashed potatoes	1 cup
Sweet potato	1 large
Corn	1 cup or 1 large ear

Fruit group	Single serving size
Fruit	1 large piece
Banana	1 large (8 to 9 in. or 20 to 23 cm)
Applesauce	1 cup
Chopped, cooked, canned fruit	1 cup
Cantaloupe (rockmelon)	1/8 of medium
Grapefruit	1 medium
100% fruit juice	1 cup
Dried fruit	1/2 cup

Oils	Single serving size (count 5 grams of fat = 1 tsp)
Vegetable oils	count 1 tbsp as 3 tsp
Soft margarine (trans fat free)	count 1 tbsp as 2+ tsp
Mayonnaise	count 1 tbsp as 2+ tsp
Salad dressing	count 1 tbsp as 2+ tsp
Olives	count 8 large as 1 tsp
Avocado	count 1/2 medium as 3 tsp
Mixed nuts, peanuts, cashews, almonds	count 1 oz as 3 tsp
Sunflower seeds	count 1 oz as 3 tsp
Peanut butter	count 2 tbsp as 4 tsp

Milk group	Single serving size
Milk	1 cup (250 ml)
Yogurt	1 cup, 1 regular container
Hard cheese (cheddar, mozzarella, swiss, parmesan)	1 1/2 oz (42 g)
Shredded cheese	1/3 cup
Ricotta cheese	1/2 cup
Processed cheese	2 oz (56 g)
Cottage cheese	2 cups
Fat-free or low-fat frozen yogurt or ice cream	1 to 1 1/2 cup
Pudding made with milk	1 cup

Meat and beans group	Single serving size
Lean beef, pork, ham	1 oz, cooked
Chicken, turkey (without skin)	1 oz, cooked
Fish, shellfish	1 oz, cooked
Legumes (dried beans or peas, lentils)	1/4 cup, cooked
Baked, refried beans	1/4 cup
Hummus	2 tbsp
Tofu	1/4 cup (~2 oz, or 56 g)
Tempeh	1 oz, cooked
Roasted soybeans	1/4 cup
Egg	1
Peanut butter	1 tbsp

Examples of extras (discretionary calories)	
Regular soft drink	12 oz (350 ml) can = +155 cal
Wine	5 oz (150 ml) = + 115 cal
Beer	12 oz (350 ml) = +145 cal
Butter	1 tbsp = +100 cal
Cream cheese	1 tbsp = +50 cal
Cheese sauce	1/4 cup = +75 cal
Croissant	1 medium (2 oz) = +95 cal
French fries (chips)	1 medium order = +325 cal
Fried chicken (skin and batter)	3 wings = +335 cal

Note: Visit www.MyPyramid.gov for more information and examples of serving sizes.

rethink some of your current choices. Because both male and female endurance athletes come in all sizes and shapes, and because we participate in events ranging from running a 10K to cycling across the country, our fuel (caloric) needs vary widely.

Personalizing the Pyramid

Before you further analyze your one-day food intake, you'll need to estimate your individual calorie needs and determine the corresponding number of servings that you require from MyPyramid by completing the following sections. While doing this based on just one day is certainly beneficial, you'll learn even more by keeping a food journal.

To get a better handle on your typical eating habits, keep track of what you eat for three consecutive days (two weekdays and one weekend day) or, if you're really committed, for a full week. To understand what is most important nutrition-wise—to see the big picture, not a single food, day, or meal—track your choices (items and number of servings) on a personal food pyramid worksheet (refer back to figure 1.2). You'll be able to see patterns develop, such as how you might starve yourself during the week only to feast on weekends, or how you may be missing some key nutrients if you routinely skimp on certain food groups.

One of my clients, a health-conscious 20-year-old soccer player, came for a nutrition checkup before heading back to college. A vegetarian, she was worried that she wasn't getting enough protein to perform at her best and help her team return to the NCAA soccer tournament. After transcribing her food records for three days onto the pyramid, she saw for herself that she needed to boost her protein intake slightly by consuming more protein-rich foods such as eggs, beans, and tofu. But she was shocked to see that she hadn't eaten any vegetables in three days!

The value of using the food pyramid to guide your daily food choices is that you don't need to worry about tracking individual nutrients. Who has time to worry about the more than 40 nutrients that the body needs each day? Remember, each food group (and the oils) contains foods that are rich in a unique package of nutrients. Just by eating balanced meals most of the time, which contain a variety of foods from all five food groups and a modest amount of healthy fat, you will get all the nutrients that you need. Learning to achieve and maintain a balance between eating high-performance foods that you need and the extras that you want has other rewards too. You'll feel good, have plenty of energy to do what you want to do, and won't waste precious time and mental energy being preoccupied or obsessed with food. Last but not least, you won't need to worry about throwing your system off balance by taking supplements that can contain too much of certain nutrients and not enough of others.

A quick nutrition checkup using the pyramid can sometimes be particularly useful. Whenever you step up your training another notch, you'll want to bump up your diet too. Keeping nutrition records can be as useful as keeping a training log to determine what works and what doesn't. If you fall into a period of poor training days, look at both your diet and your training log. Poor food choices, such as skimping on carbohydrate or eating too few calories, can leave you feeling unusually tired and stale in a matter of days. On the other hand, failing to consume enough iron may not slow you down for a few weeks or a few months, but eventually you will feel the effects as your body's iron reserves become depleted. A constant battle with one injury after another may also be linked with poor eating habits. Athletes who routinely exercise with low muscle glycogen stores incur more injuries. Finally, if you're trimming calories to lose weight make sure that you don't trim nutrients by eliminating food groups. Keeping food records will help you be more aware of what you're eating and will help those trying to lose weight stick to a plan.

Estimate Your Daily Calorie Needs*

Determining how many calories you require on a daily basis is as much art as it is science. You don't need to begin counting calories. Simply estimating your calorie requirement can help you better understand your energy needs as an endurance athlete. Use this simple method to estimate the range of calories that you need daily. (Athletes desiring further information can use the more sophisticated method found in chapter 2.)

Less active: little or no purposeful exercise, such as when you're taking a break from training or recuperating from an injury or illness.

Body weight in pounds × 13.5 to 15 calories per pound (body mass in kilograms × 29 to 33 calories per kilogram) = _____ calories

Light to moderately active: approximately 45 to 60 minutes a day of purposeful exercise (moderate intensity), most days of the week.

Body weight in pounds × 16 to 20 calories per pound (body mass in kilograms × 36 to 44 calories per kilogram) = _____ calories

Very active: approximately 60 to 120 minutes a day of purposeful exercise (moderate intensity), most days of the week.

Body weight in pounds × 21 to 25 calories per pound (body mass in kilograms × 46 to 55 calories per kilogram) = _____ calories

Extremely active: training for an ultraendurance event, such as an Ironman triathlon or 100-mile (160-kilometer) ultrarun.

Body weight in pounds × 25 to 30 calories or more per pound (body mass in kilograms × 55 to 66 calories or more per kilogram) = _____ calories

---

*Note: Exercisers and athletes commonly overestimate their physical activity level. The high ends of the calorie ranges equate to consistently training or working out at moderate intensity or higher five or six days per week. Males should use the mid- to higher ends of the ranges and active females the lower- to mid ranges.

Translate Calories Into Daily Food Amounts

After you've estimated the number of calories that you need daily, use table 1.2 as a guide to translate your calories into the amounts of food that you need to eat to meet your nutrient needs and maintain your current weight. (Note that some endurance athletes may require more than 3,200 calories daily when racing or during periods of high-volume training.) Compare your circled values with the recommendations in table 1.2.

Analyzing Your Current Eating Style

Here are some points to consider as you look not only at your one-day food journal but also at what is really important—not any one food, meal, or even one day, but the big picture, or your typical food choices over the course of several days.

First, a smart sports diet is well balanced and conforms to the shape of the food pyramid. Does the personal pyramid that you just filled out look like a pyramid, or is it top-heavy or missing sections altogether? Do you build a strong base by eating wholesome, carbohydrate-rich foods, such as rice, whole grains, pasta, and whole-grain breads and cereals (as well as potatoes, sweet potatoes, and corn)? These foods provide complex carbohydrates, B vitamins, fiber, and numerous other nutrients while contributing little or no fat.

Carbohydrate provides the most readily available form of energy to fuel endurance exercise. Glycogen (stored carbohydrate), for example, is the primary fuel that your muscles rely on as you exercise more intensely. Your glycogen reserves also play a vital role in determining how long you can exercise. You need to consume a daily dose of carbohydrate-rich foods to replace the muscle glycogen that you use during exercise. Failing to do so can leave you feeling sluggish and tired, unable to maintain your normal training pace (or even get out the door). Eating foods such as bread, cereal, rice, and pasta, as well as ample amounts of other carbohydrate-rich foods like fruits and vegetables, legumes, and low-fat dairy foods, will ensure that approximately 60 percent of your total daily calories come from carbohydrate—the foundation of any serious endurance athlete's diet. Eating a high-carbohydrate diet every day, not just the night before an endurance endeavor, is the best way to maximize your glycogen stores and increase your ability to go fast and go long.

Moving on, do you eat enough fruits and vegetables? Nonfat and chockfull of nutrients such as vitamins A and C, fiber, and a host of health-promoting phytochemicals, fruits and vegetables are nature's vitamin pills. Do you average at least "5 A Day" or five cups a day? Fruits and vegetables are certainly much tastier and more fun to eat than a bunch of supplements.

As important as carbohydrates are, endurance athletes cannot live on carbs alone. In fact, many endurance athletes suffer from carbohydrate overload. Their diets are out of balance: too much carbohydrate and too little protein. As endurance athletes, our bodies require quality protein from the foods that we eat for numerous reasons: to build, maintain, and repair muscle fibers damaged

Table 1.2 Translating Calories Into Daily Food Amounts

Estimated calories (1 calorie = 4.18 kJ)	1,600 (6,690 kJ)	1,800 (7,525 kJ)	2,000 (8,360 kJ)	2,200 (9,200 kJ)	2,400 (10,030 kJ)	2,600 (10,870 kJ)	2,800 (11,700 kJ)	3,000 (12,540 kJ)	3,200 (13,375 kJ)
Fruits	1.5 cups	1.5 cups	2 cups	2 cups	2 cups	2 cups	2.5 cups	2.5 cups	2.5 cups
Vegetables	2 cups	2.5 cups	2.5 cups	3 cups	3 cups	3.5 cups	3.5 cups	4 cups	4 cups
Grain	5 oz-eq	6 oz-eq	6 oz-eq	7 oz-eq	8 oz-eq	9 oz-eq	10 oz-eq	10 oz-eq	10 oz-eq
Meat and beans	5 oz-eq	5 oz-eq	5.5 oz-eq	6 oz-eq	6.5 oz-eq	6.5 oz-eq	7 oz-eq	7 oz-eq	7 oz-eq
Milk*	3 cups	3 cups	3 cups	3 cups	3 cups	3 cups	3 cups	3 cups	3 cups
Oils	5 tsp	5 tsp	6 tsp	6 tsp	7 tsp	8 tsp	8 tsp	10 tsp	11 tsp
Extras (discretionary calories)**	132 (550 kJ)	195 (815 kJ)	267 (1,115 kJ)	290 (1,210 kJ)	362 (1,515 kJ)	410 (1,715 kJ)	426 (1,780 kJ)	512 (2,140 kJ)	648 (2,710 kJ)

*Teenagers, young athletes up to age 24, and women who are pregnant or breastfeeding need 3 or more servings a day (300 mg of calcium per serving) from the milk group.

**Obtain additional calories by choosing higher-calorie items from the five food groups, eating more servings of those foods and oils/fats, and enjoying more "extras." Athletes who eat a balanced diet and still have trouble meeting their daily energy needs can obtain additional calories from high-carbohydrate drinks, meal replacement beverages, and energy bars.

Data from the U.S. Department of Agriculture and the U.S. Department of Health and Human Services.

during daily exercise; to help injuries heal promptly; to make hemoglobin, which carries oxygen to exercising muscles; to form antibodies to fight off colds, infections, and other more serious diseases; to produce enzymes and hormones that help regulate critical energy processes in the body; and to help meet energy (caloric) needs in the latter stages of ultraendurance events. Up to 20 percent of your total daily calories should come from protein.

Lean meat, chicken, fish, eggs, legumes (black, kidney, pinto beans, and so on), peanut butter, and soy foods such as tofu, tempeh, and edamame supply protein and varying amounts of two other nutrients crucial to endurance athletes—iron and zinc. Low-fat dairy foods also supply high-quality protein as well as large doses of calcium, a nutrient needed for healthy nerves, muscles, and bones. How well are you doing at consuming enough protein daily from the meat and beans group and the milk group? Five to 7 ounces of meat (140 to 200 grams) or the equivalent, and 3 cups (750 milliliters) of milk a day or the equivalent covers the minimum needs of most endurance athletes. Athletes often go to one extreme or another when it comes to eating foods from these two groups. Some have little trouble exceeding their requirements, thanks to supersized burgers and pints of ice cream. Others, concerned about eating a meat-free diet or reducing their fat intake, skimp on or eliminate animal products with little regard to finding alternatives. In either case, the athlete is no longer eating a smart, well-balanced sports diet.

Fat, by the way, is an appropriate part of a healthy sports diet. Besides providing a concentrated dose of energy or calories, the fat supplied by the foods you eat has other important roles. Consuming fat enables your body to absorb and transport fat-soluble vitamins (A, D, E, and K) and ensures that you get an adequate amount of linoleic acid, an essential fatty acid (the body cannot make it) needed for growth and healthy skin and hair. Including enough fat also helps us feel satisfied so that we're not preoccupied with food or thinking about the next time that we can eat. A smart, well-balanced sports diet obtains at least 20 percent of its total calories from fat. If you're an elite swimmer, distance runner, triathlete, or cyclist who requires in excess of 4,000 calories a day, you may need to consume a greater percentage of your calories as fat to meet your high energy needs. How well are you doing at including enough healthy fat as vegetable oil, avocados, olives, or nuts (5 to 11 teaspoons, or 25 to 55 milliliters, a day covers most endurance athletes)?

The tip of the pyramid houses the extras—foods that supply more calories, unhealthy fat, or added sugar than they do nutrients, as well as foods that offer little in the way of nutrition at all, such as coffee and soda. These foods can round out a healthy diet and help you meet your energy requirements (discretionary calories). Go ahead and enjoy the taste, pleasure, and psychological boost that these foods provide. The question to ask yourself, however, is whether your extras routinely throw your diet (and your waistline) off balance by squeezing out healthier options from the five food groups. How do you tell? Your diet no longer resembles the triangular shape of the food pyramid.

Second, a healthy sports diet is full of variety. No single food, or food group for that matter, can supply the 40 or more nutrients that you need (see appendix B for vitamins and minerals needed for performance). Each food group contains foods that are particularly rich in a unique package of nutrients. Fruits and vegetables, for example, serve up mainly vitamins A, C, and fiber, whereas foods in the milk group supply protein, calcium, vitamin D (milk and yogurt), and riboflavin. You can get your calories from anywhere. Not so for nutrients. Eliminating entire groups of food puts you at risk for being low in certain essential nutrients needed for good health and optimal athletic performance. How well are you doing at eating from all five food groups on a daily basis?

Eating a varied diet also refers to eating many different foods from each of the five major food groups of the pyramid. If you always drink apple juice for breakfast and grab a banana for a snack, you've missed opportunities to boost your vitamin C intake, as well as experiment with other great-tasting foods rich in vitamin C, such as cantaloupe (rockmelon) and tangerine juice. (Apple juice provides no vitamin C unless it's been fortified, and bananas, although rich in potassium, carbohydrate, and fiber, provide minimal amounts of vitamin C.)

Keep in mind that some foods are nutritional powerhouses compared with others. Although you can certainly meet your carbohydrate needs by eating bagels, plates of spaghetti, and an energy bar or two, your health and performance (never mind your taste buds) would undoubtedly benefit from including more whole grains, such as kashi or oatmeal for breakfast, brown rice or couscous for dinner, and whole-wheat fig bars as a snack.

Taking a multivitamin can help ensure that you get an adequate intake of most nutrients, but it's no guarantee that the nutrients will be as well absorbed as those from food are. Supplements also don't supply all the health benefits, such as fiber, phytochemicals, and other yet undiscovered nutritional boosters, contained in food. What efforts do you typically make daily to eat a variety of foods from *within* each of the five food groups?

Moderation is the last key to a healthy sports diet. Endurance athletes are good at doing things in extreme and often struggle with eating in moderation. Many shun nutrient-rich foods because such foods also contain fat, or they continually rely on sugar and caffeine for a pickup instead of obtaining the energy that they need from real foods. No foods are good or bad for you; your overall diet is what counts. Eating a single food, a specific type of energy bar, for example, won't save an otherwise poor diet. At the same time, eating a bowl of premium high-fat ice cream or a fast-food meal won't erase all your healthier choices.

Look at your personal eating habits. Instead of eliminating foods or entire food groups, do you select healthier versions (less fat, sodium, calories, and so on) or work at incorporating alternatives into your diet? For example, if you choose not to eat dairy foods, do you replace milk with fortified soy or rice milk and eat plenty of dark green leafy vegetables to obtain calcium? If you're watching your weight or just trying to eat more healthfully, do you eat foods high in fat and added sugar, like chips or crisps and muffins, in smaller amounts or less frequently? Keep in mind with fat that you need to consider any significant amounts in your choices from all the food groups (for example, oatmeal versus a croissant? Grilled chicken breast or fried chicken?), as well as the oils and your extras.

For many athletes, performing a diet makeover or losing weight without skimping on good nutrition hinges on cutting out excess fat. A gram of fat supplies 9 calories (37 kilojoules) compared with the 4 calories (17 kilojoules) contained in a gram of protein or carbohydrate (a gram of alcohol supplies 7 calories, or 29 kilojoules). But this doesn't mean you should bypass a sandwich and a glass of low-fat milk to eat an entire box of fat-free cookies! Eating in moderation means that you strive to fit all foods into a healthy sports diet.

Reading Food Labels: Make Them Work for You

Being able to read and decipher the nutrition facts panels on food labels is the next best thing to having a personal sports dietitian accompany you to the grocery store. Read on for some tips on how to make food labels work for you (see figure 1.3).

1. Always start by checking the listed serving size. Compare it to the amount that you actually consume. Adjust the rest of the nutrition information contained on the label accordingly. For example, if you eat twice as much as the listed serving size, double all the values given. Use labels to compare similar food products because they generally have the same listed serving size.

2. Don't confuse *calories from fat* with *total fat* or percent of calories from fat. *Calories from fat* tells you the calories that you'll get from fat or, when compared to *calories*, how fatty a food is (in figure 1.3, a 1-cup serving provides 110 calories from fat, or about half of the 250 total calories supplied by this food). *Total fat* gives you the grams of fat in a serving (in this example, 1 cup provides 2 grams). If you're interested in determining the percentage of calories from fat, divide *calories from fat* by *calories* and multiply by 100 (in this example, 110 / 250 × 100 = 44 percent of calories from fat.)

3. Use *percent daily value* (% daily value, or % DV) to tell quickly whether a serving of food is high or low in nutrients. A low percent daily value (5 percent or less) means that the food provides a small amount or is a poor source of a nutrient, whereas a higher percent daily value means that it contributes a large amount (based on a 2,000-calorie diet). Check to see whether the food is a good source (at least 10 percent) or an excellent source (20 percent or more) of the nutrients that most endurance athletes need more of—fiber, vitamins A and C, calcium, and iron. Your goal is to select foods that together provide 100 percent or more of these nutrients (or average close to 100 percent over a few days). For nutrients that athletes need to eat in moderation, such as fat, saturated fat, cholesterol, and sodium, choose foods that together provide 100 percent or less of the daily value.

4. Check the ingredients list (required on most packaged foods) for information on ingredients that you may be trying to eat more of (whole wheat, for instance) and others that you want to avoid or limit for health,

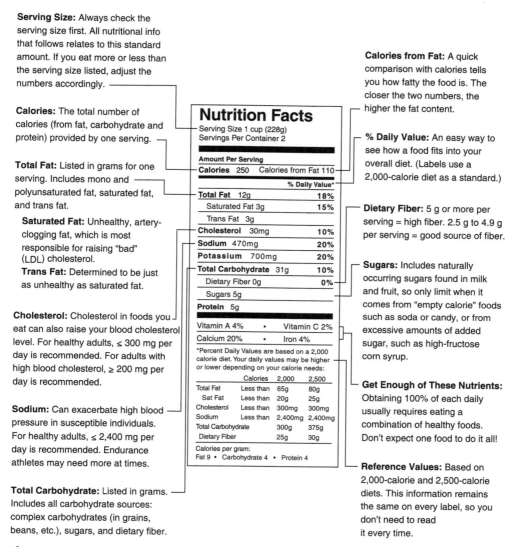

Serving Size: Always check the serving size first. All nutritional info that follows relates to this standard amount. If you eat more or less than the serving size listed, adjust the numbers accordingly.

Calories: The total number of calories (from fat, carbohydrate and protein) provided by one serving.

Total Fat: Listed in grams for one serving. Includes mono and polyunsaturated fat, saturated fat, and trans fat.

Saturated Fat: Unhealthy, artery-clogging fat, which is most responsible for raising "bad" (LDL) cholesterol.
Trans Fat: Determined to be just as unhealthy as saturated fat.

Cholesterol: Cholesterol in foods you eat can also raise your blood cholesterol level. For healthy adults, ≤ 300 mg per day is recommended. For adults with high blood cholesterol, ≥ 200 mg per day is recommended.

Sodium: Can exacerbate high blood pressure in susceptible individuals. For healthy adults, ≤ 2,400 mg per day is recommended. Endurance athletes may need more at times.

Total Carbohydrate: Listed in grams. Includes all carbohydrate sources: complex carbohydrates (in grains, beans, etc.), sugars, and dietary fiber.

Calories from Fat: A quick comparison with calories tells you how fatty the food is. The closer the two numbers, the higher the fat content.

% Daily Value: An easy way to see how a food fits into your overall diet. (Labels use a 2,000-calorie diet as a standard.)

Dietary Fiber: 5 g or more per serving = high fiber. 2.5 g to 4.9 g per serving = good source of fiber.

Sugars: Includes naturally occurring sugars found in milk and fruit, so only limit when it comes from "empty calorie" foods such as soda or candy, or from excessive amounts of added sugar, such as high-fructose corn syrup.

Get Enough of These Nutrients: Obtaining 100% of each daily usually requires eating a combination of healthy foods. Don't expect one food to do it all!

Reference Values: Based on 2,000-calorie and 2,500-calorie diets. This information remains the same on every label, so you don't need to read it every time.

Figure 1.3 Read food labels to choose high-performance foods that provide enough of the nutrients you need and limit those nutrients you need to consume in moderation.

religious, or other reasons. Labels list ingredients by weight from most to least and must now clearly indicate whether the food contains any of eight major allergens: milk, eggs, fish, shellfish, tree nuts, peanuts, wheat, or soybeans.

Building a Strong Diet:
Quick Fixes for Busy Endurance Athletes

You're not alone if your personal food pyramid doesn't quite measure up to the standard. Athletes of all abilities, from beginners to world class, shortchange their health and performance by not paying enough attention to their daily food choices (what to eat) and their typical eating patterns (how to eat). This section focuses on what to eat (see chapter 8 for advice on how to eat) and provides quick fixes for even the busiest or most nutritionally challenged endurance athlete. In other words, don't count calories. Instead, make your calories count! (See appendix B for a quick review of vitamins and minerals.)

Build a Firm Foundation: Eat More Whole Grains

Most athletes have little trouble racking up enough servings from the grains group. We like bread, cereal, rice, and pasta, and those foods tend to be affordable, easy to prepare, and readily available. In addition, serving sizes are modest and add up quickly. But consuming at least half of all the grains that we consume as whole grains is often another matter. The complex carbohydrates provided by foods in the grains group (as well as starchy vegetables, legumes, and low-fat milk and yogurt) feed your brain and replenish the glycogen used by working muscles and are superior to the carbohydrate provided by processed foods such as candy bars, snack items, desserts, and soft drinks. So, although it's wise to be discerning about the type and amount of carbohydrate that you eat (because all carbohydrates are not created equal), you don't need to be afraid of carbohydrate-rich foods or try to avoid them altogether. Whole grains supply more fiber, vitamin E, vitamin B_6, zinc, copper, manganese, and potassium than do refined grains. In addition, whole grains help fill you up, without filling you out.

The following are some quick fixes for eating more whole grains.

- Choose whole-wheat bread more often than you do white, wheat, multigrain, rye, or pumpernickel. Check the ingredients list and look for whole wheat (the key word is *whole*) as the first ingredient or at least the ingredient listed before any other flour. Try whole-wheat tortillas, bagels, pitas, and waffles too.

- Experiment with whole-wheat pasta or other whole grains, such as couscous, bulgur, kasha, quinoa, and brown rice. Look for prepackaged, quick-cooking (15 minutes or less) whole-grain mixes or premade salads featuring whole grains.

- Eat a whole-grain breakfast cereal (hot or cold) like oatmeal, Wheatena, Ralston, Roman Meal, Shredded Wheat, Grape Nuts, Cheerios, Wheaties, or Total. Bran cereals like Raisin Bran, All-Bran, or 100% Bran count too.

- Eat more whole-grain crackers and whole-grain crispbreads.

- Choose brown rice over white rice as often as you can.

- Substitute whole-wheat flour for half (or more) of the white flour when you bake at home.

Eat a Rainbow: Eat More Fruits and Vegetables

Remember, eliminating entire food groups or shortchanging yourself by barely squeezing in the recommended amounts every now and then can cause you, in the end, to run low on some essential nutrients. (Besides, if you aren't eating those wholesome foods, what are you filling up on?) When it comes to meeting daily quotas, fitness-minded people often come up short in the fruits and vegetables food groups.

As a rule of thumb, choose brightly colored fruits and vegetables to obtain the most nutrients, especially vitamins A and C. Think of the rainbow: red, orange, deep yellow, dark green, blue, and purple!

> ## Best Bets: Fruits and Vegetables
>
> High in vitamin A: apricots, cantaloupe, carrots, kale, collards, romaine lettuce, spinach, sweet potatoes, winter squash
>
> High in vitamin C: broccoli, cabbage, bell peppers, cantaloupe, grapefruit, kiwi, mangoes, oranges, spinach, strawberries, tomatoes
>
> High in fiber: apples, bananas, berries, carrots, cherries, dates, figs, pears, spinach, sweet potatoes

Here are some easy ways to consume more veggies:

- Drink tomato or vegetable juice. Keep individual-size cans or plastic bottles on hand.
- Include a cup (250 milliliters) of vegetable soup with lunch.
- Order vegetable-based soup as an appetizer instead of another pale green, nutrition-poor salad.
- Buy fresh, ready-to-eat varieties, such as bags of baby carrots and salad in a bag, or stop by the salad bar and pick up your precut favorites. These approaches are no more expensive than throwing away heads of slimy lettuce, wilted carrots, and mushy tomatoes. Keep your favorite low-fat salad dressing on hand for dipping and dressing salads.
- Keep frozen or canned vegetables on hand and toss them into whatever else you're heating up during the last few minutes—soup, spaghetti sauce, stew, casseroles, or mashed potatoes.
- Buy a vegetable steamer with an automatic timer, available at reasonable cost, or microwave your veggies. Either way of preparing vegetables takes only minutes.
- Bake a potato or sweet potato in the microwave. Add your favorite low-fat topping.
- Eat more of the ones that you like, especially if you eat vegetables at only one meal.
- Choose fast food with veggies—vegetarian pizza, Chinese stir-fry, vegetable curries, and so on.
- Always serve (or order) two vegetables at dinner.

- Learn to like vegetables that you hated as a kid, such as brussels sprouts, cauliflower, and squash. When you find yourself smiling and having a good time, simply take one bite (no more) of the veggie that you dislike. Do this at least a half dozen times, a few days to a week or more apart, and make sure that your brain is always dialed into a happy mode. After not experiencing misery or adverse reactions (like being sent to your room) several times, your brain may decide that this food isn't so bad after all.

The following tips can help you eat more fruit.

- Get a leg up by starting out the day right. Drink 100 percent fruit juice or add a piece of fruit to your morning meal. Try a banana, peach, or berries on cereal, pancakes, or waffles, or stir extra fruit into yogurt.
- Keep dried fruit such as raisins, dates, apples, cherries, or dried apricots stashed in your briefcase or desk drawer.
- Keep bananas in the refrigerator (only the skins turn black) so that they ripen more slowly.
- Purchase ready-to-eat fruit from the salad bar. You will be more likely to eat fruit if you don't have to prepare it first.
- Make or choose desserts that emphasize the fruit, such as fruit tarts or crustless pies.
- Buy frozen berries and use them as a topping for ice cream, frozen yogurt, plain cakes, or make fruit parfaits.

Best Bets: Iron

Animal Sources

Beef, pork, lamb, liver and other organ meats

Poultry (especially dark meat)

Fish and shellfish

Plant Sources

Dark leafy greens: spinach, beet, collard and turnip greens, Swiss chard

Tomato and prune juice

Dried fruit: apricots, raisins

Legumes: chickpeas; black, kidney, lima, navy, and pinto beans

Lentils

Soy foods: tofu, tempeh, textured vegetable protein, soy milk

Whole-grain and enriched breads and cereals (including hot cereals, such as oatmeal and Cream of Wheat)

Wheat germ

Go Lean With Protein: Eat Quality Sources of Meat and Beans

Eating enough lean, quality protein (or making sure that your day-to-day choices are lean) is another area where many endurance athletes, especially girls and women, shortchange themselves. We need ample amounts of protein, iron, and zinc to train and perform consistently at a high level. Iron is needed to form hemoglobin and myoglobin, the oxygen-carrying compounds in blood and muscles. If you don't have enough iron to produce new red blood cells, iron-deficiency anemia results, leaving you feeling fatigued and unable to perform at your best. Zinc is required to fight off infections and help wounds and injuries heal properly, including the cellular microdamage caused by logging an ambitious number of daily training miles.

Animal foods, such as red meat, dark poultry, and seafood, provide the most readily absorbable form of iron (heme iron) and zinc. Boost your absorption of nonheme iron from plant foods by eating a food rich in vitamin C at the same time. For example, have a glass of orange juice with your morning bowl of oatmeal. If you're eating enough protein, you are most likely getting enough zinc. Coffee and the tannins in tea (regular and decaffeinated) block the absorption of iron and zinc from foods, so drink these beverages between meals, not with them.

Try these simple strategies for choosing lean, quality protein-rich foods:

- To limit the fat that often accompanies meat, choose lean cuts (rounds and loins, such as tenderloin, sirloin, and round steak) and trim all visible fat. Choose the leanest ground beef that you can afford or substitute ground turkey breast instead. Buy boneless, skinless poultry or remove the skin.

- Use low-fat cooking methods, such as baking, broiling, and grilling. A 3-ounce (85-gram) serving of meat is only the size of a deck of cards.

- Eat more fish. Preparing fish takes only minutes. Or buy ready-to-eat shellfish, such as precooked shrimp. Just getting started or haven't liked fish in the past? Order fish when you dine away from home, from someone who is an expert at preparing it.

- Eat more beans. Keep several canned varieties on hand, buy beans from a salad bar to add to salads, or serve as a side dish instead of potatoes or rice. Choose soups made from beans or peas (minestrone, split pea, black bean, or lentil) and try meatless meals such as tacos or burritos stuffed with beans, vegetarian chili, or black beans with rice.

Best Bets: Zinc

Animal Sources

Shellfish: oysters, crab, shrimp, clams

Red meat: beef, pork, lamb, liver and other organ meats

Poultry

Fish

Dairy foods: milk, yogurt, cheese

Plant Sources

Legumes: chickpeas; kidney, lima, navy, and pinto beans; split peas

Lentils

Spinach

Soy foods: tofu, tempeh, textured vegetable protein

Peanut butter

Peanuts, cashews, Brazil nuts

Sunflower seeds

Whole-grain and enriched breakfast cereals, including oatmeal

Wheat germ

- Don't shy away from eggs. Inexpensive and easy to prepare, eggs provide high-quality protein. Most endurance athletes can afford to follow the American Heart Association guidelines and eat up to four eggs a week. Beyond that, use egg whites (toss the yolks) to get protein without the fat and cholesterol. Egg substitutes (such as Egg Beaters) provide another smart, easy option.

- Toss tofu (rich in high-quality protein and a good source of iron, magnesium, and zinc) into soups, stews, and lasagna, mash it with cottage cheese and seasonings to make a sandwich spread or dip, or blend it with lemon juice and salt for a baked-potato topping.

- Other time-savers include canned tuna (packed in water) or chicken, precubed meat for kebabs and stir-fries, precooked rotisserie chickens, frozen veggie burgers or garden burgers, and edamame (preboiled soybeans).

- Aim to include some protein at each meal. Don't eat your grains plain. Smear your bagel with peanut butter, toss baked beans over noodles, or throw seafood into your favorite sauce and pour it over pasta, rice, or couscous.

Get a Milk Mustache: Bone Up on Calcium

If the foods you choose to eat don't supply the calcium you need, your body will steal from the only source it has—your bones! To reduce the risk of osteoporosis, build for the future by optimizing your bone mass before you reach age 25. You can still build some bone up to age 35; after that, your goal becomes holding on to what you have. Because many endurance athletes hit their stride later in life, every day counts in consuming enough calcium.

If you choose not to drink milk or consume dairy foods, incorporate other calcium-rich foods into your daily diet. Aim for 1,000 milligrams a day (1,300 milligrams for younger athletes age 9 to 18 and 1,200 milligrams for adults over age 50). Determining how much calcium a food provides is easy. Check the nutrition facts section of the food label and add a zero to the percent daily value for calcium. For example, a food supplying 35 percent of the daily value provides 350 milligrams of calcium.

Here are some tips to help boost your calcium intake from low-fat, calcium rich foods:

- Drink milk whenever you can—any variety will do, but choose low-fat milk as often as you can. Drink low-fat milk shakes, fruit smoothies, lattes, and flavored milks (check the dairy case for chocolate and other varieties or stir in flavored syrups). Enjoy pudding or custard for dessert.

- Prepare foods such as hot chocolate, oatmeal, or tomato soup with low-fat milk rather than water.

- Snack on yogurt or use it to make a salad dressing or vegetable dip.

- Add a slice or two of low-fat cheese to a sandwich or burger, snack on low-fat string cheese or a slice of cheese pizza, and sprinkle low-fat Parmesan or mozzarella cheese on foods.

- Don't let less nutritious beverages, such as soda (diet and regular), coffee, tea, iced tea, lemonade, and fruit drinks, squeeze milk out of your diet.

- If you suffer from lactose intolerance, try drinking or eating a limited amount (one-half cup) of milk or ice cream at a time. Have it with a meal, not on an empty stomach. Experiment with lactose-reduced and lactose-free milk and milk products or take lactase tablets before you consume dairy foods. You can also substitute soy or rice milk (choose a brand fortified with calcium and vitamin D) for regular milk. Yogurt and natural-aged hard cheeses, such as cheddar and swiss, tend to produce fewer symptoms.

> ### Best Bets: Calcium*
>
> 1 cup (250 ml) of milk (nonfat, low fat, or whole)
>
> 1 cup of yogurt
>
> 1.5 oz (42 g) of cheese
>
> 2 cups of cottage cheese
>
> 1 1/2 cups of ice cream or frozen yogurt
>
> 1 cup of fortified soy or rice milk
>
> 1 cup of fortified orange juice
>
> 1 1/2 cups of cooked collards, turnip greens, or kale
>
> 3 cups of cooked broccoli
>
> 1 1/2 cups of baked beans
>
> 5 oz (140 g) of firm tofu (prepared with calcium sulfate)
>
> 1/2 cup of soy nuts
>
> 4 oz (112 g) of canned salmon with bones
>
> 1 3.75 oz can (105 g) of sardines with bones
>
> *Note: Contains at least 300 mg per serving.

- To boost your calcium intake beyond that contained in dairy foods, make sure that the tofu you consume is prepared with calcium sulfate (check the label) and add or substitute other calcium-fortified foods to your diet, such as calcium-fortified cereals, soy or rice milk, and orange juice. Eat plenty of dark green leafy vegetables such as kale, collard, and turnip greens, bok choy, and broccoli. (Don't count on the calcium in spinach because the body absorbs it poorly.)

The Oils Have It: Choose Healthy Fat Over Unhealthy Fat

As previously discussed, a smart sports diet contains a modest amount of fat. And just as all carbohydrates are not created equal, not all fats are the same. The goal is to include enough of the healthier fats and limit the unhealthy offenders—the saturated fats and trans fats. Fats that are liquid (or soft) at room temperature, like vegetable oils and tub margarine, tend to be healthier because they contain more monounsaturated fat and little or no saturated or trans fat. The same is true for the fat in nuts, seeds, avocados, olives, and fattier fish. Saturated and trans fat are the bad guys that tend to clog arteries, raise cholesterol levels, and lower the body's level of HDL, or good, cholesterol.

All fats are energy dense. They supply nine calories per gram (when looking at food labels, think of five grams of fat as being equal to a teaspoon), so only the most physically ambitious endurance athletes can get away with eating all the fat that they want. If you're trying to avoid eating fat altogether, though, your diet isn't healthy and it usually backfires. You eventually feel deprived and unsatisfied and can easily end up overeating (on high-fat foods or just in general) to compensate.

Here are some suggestions for improving on the types and amount of fat that you consume:

- Top salads with low-fat salad dressings or use low-fat dressings as a dip for vegetables.
- Switch to a liquid or soft (tub) margarine.
- Find a low-fat cheese and ice cream that you like.
- Read the nutrition facts panel and the ingredient list on items typically high in trans fats—store-bought baked goods, doughnuts, crackers, snack foods, and some cookies—and choose varieties free of trans fat or those that don't list partially hydrogenated oil as one of the first three ingredients.
- Eat fattier fish (rich in heart-healthy omega-3 fatty acids), like salmon, herring, sardines, striped bass, trout, halibut, or albacore tuna, at least twice a week.
- Limit saturated fats (which tend to be solid at room temperature) by removing fat visible on meat, by not eating chicken or turkey skin, by buying the leanest ground beef that you can afford, and by eating less of other major offenders, such as bacon, sausage, hot dogs, fatty deli meats, and ribs, or by eating them less frequently.
- Eat fried food (including french fries, fried fish sandwiches, and chicken nuggets) as infrequently as possible—save those foods for special occasions.
- Substitute a small handful of nuts for something less healthy (like chips or crisps, candy, or another energy bar) that you typically snack on.

Taste and Savor: Enjoy Your Extras

Who deserves to enjoy sweets, treats, and some extra fat and sugar more than endurance athletes putting in the miles? Occasional, even daily, indulgences are good for the body and spirit. After all, being a smart eater involves choosing foods that meet not just your daily nutritional or physical needs but also your emotional needs. In other words, food is not the enemy. Eating is supposed to be enjoyable and satisfying. Eating foods high in fat or sugar and otherwise low in nutrients does not cause active people to gain body fat or unwanted pounds. Excess calories from eating too much of those foods (and all other foods) is what contributes to weight gain. Extras become a problem only when those foods squeeze out healthier foods and fill you up with unnecessary empty calories.

On the other hand, the fact that you're working out doesn't mean that you can tune out and not pay any attention to what you eat. You are unlikely to be able to eat whatever food you want in whatever amount you want (or are served if you often dine away from home). Consuming too much fat or too much of the wrong kind of fat (saturated and trans fats), going overboard on cholesterol and sodium, or just eating more calories than you need to keep your weight in a healthy range increases your risk for heart disease, diabetes, and some cancers. That sort of diet is also unlikely to do much for your performance. So you're going to have to budget your extra calories and decide what luxuries to spend them on: more food from any food group, soft drinks, wine, beer, candy, desserts, solid fats like butter and cream cheese, or high-calorie versions of foods such as fried chicken, cheese sauce, and bacon.

The following are some tips for finding a balance when it comes to the extras in your diet:

- Snack on real food from the five food groups. Aim to put together snacks that include at least one food group (two is even better). Instead of plowing through a box of cookies, for example, enjoy a reasonable amount with a glass of milk. Better yet, on some occasions pour a bowl of your favorite cereal and add milk.

- Savor your favorites. Slow down and figure out what it is that you really crave or desire. Sit down, serve it on a plate, and consciously enjoy every bite. Rushing can leave you feeling unsatisfied and cause you to eat more than you really need, as can restricting or depriving yourself for as long as possible.

- Cut down on soft drinks and other caffeinated beverages. Drinking too much coffee, tea, and soft drinks fills you up and may temporarily perk you up, but that's it. Ask yourself whether what you really need is something to eat. Sustainable energy comes from the calories provided by foods and nutritious beverages. On top of that, you can only consume so much fluid, and water, low-fat milk, juice, and sports drinks (when appropriate) make far healthier choices.

- Make your own healthy soda by mixing 100 percent fruit juice and seltzer half and half.

- Answer a chocolate craving before it gets out of control—chocolate syrup drizzled on fruit, flavored hot chocolate made with low-fat milk, a couple of small chocolates, or a small piece of the real thing.

- On occasions when fun foods abound, such as buffets, parties, and holiday celebrations, choose one or two items that you really want, enjoy them, and move on. Spend your time and emotions connecting with people instead of worrying or feeling guilty about food.

Fill Up on Smart Fluids: Choose Water and Other Healthy Beverages

Before the advent of fruity juice concoctions, caffeinated beverages that take longer to make than to drink, and sports drinks full of ingredients that athletes don't need while exercising, there was water—pure, clear, calorie-free, fat-free water. Humble and unpretentious, water does yeoman's service in an athlete's body with barely a hint of recognition. Sure, you may crave it when you feel thirsty or curse the lack of it when you become dehydrated, but how much credit do you give water on a daily basis? (Look again at your personal food pyramid and see how many cups of water you actually drank.)

Water is the ultimate nutrient, especially for athletes. Roughly three-quarters of your body weight is water. Muscles are 70 to 75 percent water. Water is the medium in which the body conducts almost all its activities. Go a month without food and you can survive. Go a few days without water and you may not make it.

Working quietly behind the scenes, water has many functions.

- It helps digest food through saliva and stomach secretions.
- Water helps lubricate joints and cushion organs.
- It transports nutrients, hormones, and oxygen through the blood (of which water is the main ingredient) to working muscles and removes waste products such as carbon dioxide and lactic acid.

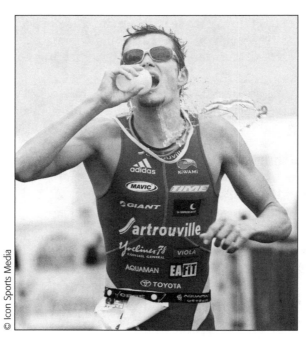

© Icon Sports Media

Olympian Frédéric Belaubre rehydrates on the move. Don't wait until race day to master this skill!

- In urine, water carries waste products out of the body.
- In sweat, it helps regulate body temperature during exercise by absorbing the heat generated by muscles and transporting it to the skin where it can evaporate. Under normal conditions, you lose a minimum of 8 cups (2 liters) of water a day through your skin, lungs, feces, and urine. You can easily sweat off several more cups every hour during exercise. Sweat losses of as little as 2 percent of your body weight—3 pounds (1.4 kilograms) for a 150-pound (68-kilogram) athlete—can impair your ability to perform athletic feats. How? Sweating reduces your blood volume, especially if you don't drink while exercising. This drop in blood volume will reduce your ability to take in and use oxygen, which decreases your endurance as well as your ability to handle the heat. Classic early signs of inadequate hydration (even when you're not exercising) include dizziness, light-headedness, headaches, loss of appetite, darkly colored urine, lack of energy, and fatigue.

Throughout the day during your typical routine or training diet, don't wait until your tongue sticks to the roof of your mouth to think about your fluid needs. Waiting until you're outright thirsty means that you've waited too long. Stay on top of your fluid needs by drinking a minimum of 8 to 10 cups (2.0 to 2.5 liters) of fluid a day, emphasizing healthy beverages such as water, 100 percent fruit juice or vegetable juice, low-fat milk, herbal tea, and, when appropriate (such as before, during, and immediately after exercise), sports drinks. To prevent kidney stones and reduce your risk of colon and bladder cancer, aim to drink at least 4 cups of water (half of your daily intake). Alcohol, soda, and other highly-caffeinated "energy drinks" aren't the best hydrating choices. Besides being nutrition zeros, alcohol and large doses of caffeine act as diuretics (they cause you to urinate), and the carbonation in fizzy beverages may cause you to drink less.

The following are some tips for increasing your fluid intake.

- Begin the day conscious of the need to stay hydrated. Drink an 8-ounce glass of water when you get up in the morning.
- If you take vitamins or other supplements, take them with a full glass of water, not just a few sips.
- Drink at least a cup of water or another healthy beverage with all your meals and snacks.
- For easy access, keep a jug of water on your desk or carry a water bottle with you when traveling or running errands.
- Hydrate before you head out to exercise by drinking water or a sports drink—aim for 2 cups during the two hours before exercise.
- Have a large glass of water along with your beer, wine, or other alcoholic drink. An added bonus is that you'll handle the alcohol better.
- Make your own healthy soda by mixing fruit juice and seltzer half and half.

2

Meeting Energy Needs of Distance Demands

"Breakfast is the most important meal of the day, especially for athletes and active people. A lot of your body's stored carbohydrate is burned up as you sleep, and that's energy your brain needs in order to have a productive morning."

—Chris Carmichael, Lance Armstrong's coach through seven consecutive Tour de France titles, on what is Armstrong's first critical feed zone

Consuming enough calories, or fuel, each day is key if you want to support and enhance your training and racing, or if you simply want to feel good while working out. But the more arduous the activity, the more important it becomes to consume the proper mix of the three energy-supplying nutrients—carbohydrate, fat, and protein. As you read in chapter 1, consistently eating well-balanced meals and snacks that contain a variety of foods will most likely supply all the nutrients and enough calories to perform prolonged bouts of exercise. This chapter will provide detailed information about obtaining the correct mix of fuel based on your training and competitive needs as an endurance athlete, which vary significantly from the needs of athletes involved in power or team sports.

This chapter is designed for the athlete who wants to look under the hood to understand how to prepare his or her body for future endurance endeavors. The fuel that you provide your body affects your workouts during the week and your races and endurance adventures on the weekend (as well as your overall health every day of the week). The type of exercise that you do also influences the fuel that your body uses. All of us have heard conflicting advice about eating for endurance activities. What you'll come to understand as the formula for athletic success is this: Carbohydrate makes up the backbone of a smart sports diet, but protein and fat play crucial roles too.

The Body's Fuel Sources

The foods that you eat provide the potential energy, or fuel, that your body needs in three forms: carbohydrate, fat, and protein. Your body can store some of these fuels in a form that offers your muscles an immediate source of energy (see table 2.1). Carbohydrates, such as sugar and starch, are readily broken down into glucose, the principal energy source of the body. Glucose can be used immediately, or it can be stored in the liver and muscles as glycogen. During exercise, muscle glycogen is converted back into glucose and can be used as fuel only by muscle fibers. The liver also converts its glycogen back into glucose and releases it directly into the bloodstream to maintain your blood sugar or blood glucose level. During exercise, your muscles pick up this glucose and use it in addition to their own private glycogen stores. Blood glucose also serves as the most significant source of energy for the brain at rest and during exercise. Your body constantly uses and replenishes its glycogen stores. The carbohydrate content of your diet and the type and amount of training that you undertake influence the size of your glycogen stores.

The capacity of your body to store muscle and liver glycogen, however, is limited to approximately 1,800 to 2,000 calories worth of energy, or enough fuel for approximately 90 to 120 minutes of continuous, vigorous activity. If you've ever hit the wall while exercising, you know what it feels like to deplete your muscle glycogen stores. As muscle glycogen runs low, blood glucose plays an increasingly greater role in meeting the energy demands of the body. To keep up with the high demand for glucose, the body can rapidly deplete its liver glycogen stores. If this happens, your blood glucose level dips too low and hypoglycemia (low blood sugar) results. As an athlete, you may be more familiar with the term *bonking*. Foods that you eat or drink during exercise that supply carbohydrate can help delay the depletion of muscle glycogen and prevent hypoglycemia.

Fat is the body's most concentrated source of energy, providing more than twice as much potential energy as carbohydrate or protein (nine calories per gram versus four calories per gram). During exercise, stored fat in the body (in the form of triglycerides in adipose or fat tissue) is broken down into fatty acids. These fatty acids are transported through the blood to muscles for fuel. This process occurs relatively slowly as compared with the mobilization of carbohydrate for fuel. Fat is also stored within muscle fibers, where it can be more easily accessed during exercise. Unlike your glycogen stores, which are limited, body fat is a virtually unlimited source of energy for athletes. Even

Table 2.1 Estimated Energy Stores in Humans

Energy source	Storage site	Approximate energy (kJ)
ATP–CP	Various tissues	5
Carbohydrate	Blood glucose	20
	Liver glycogen	400
	Muscle glycogen	1,500
Fat	Serum free fatty acids	7
	Serum triglycerides	75
	Muscle triglycerides	2,500
	Adipose tissue	80,000+
Protein	Muscle protein	30,000

Note: ATP–CP = adenosine triphosphate–creatine phosphate

those who are lean and mean have enough fat stored in muscle fibers and fat cells to supply up to 100,000 calories—enough for over 100 hours of marathon running!

Fat is a more efficient fuel per unit of weight than carbohydrate. Carbohydrate must be stored along with water. Our weight would double if we stored the same amount of energy as glycogen (plus the water that glycogen holds) that we store as body fat! Most of us have sufficient stores of fat, and the body readily converts and stores excess calories from any source (fat, carbohydrate, or protein) as body fat. But for fat to fuel exercise, sufficient oxygen must be simultaneously consumed. The second part of this chapter explains how your pace or intensity and the length of time that you exercise affect how you use fat for energy.

When it comes to protein, the body doesn't maintain any official stores for use as energy. Rather, it uses protein to build, maintain, and repair body tissues, as well as to synthesize important enzymes and hormones. Under ordinary circumstances, protein supplies only 5 percent of the body's need for energy. In drastic cases, such as rapid weight-loss diets, starvation, or the latter stages of endurance exercise when your glycogen stores become depleted, some amino acids (the building blocks of protein) within skeletal muscle can be converted into glucose to provide fuel for working muscles. The brain also needs a constant supply of glucose to keep functioning.

The Body's Energy Systems

Our ability to run, bicycle, ski, swim, and row hinges on the capacity of the body to extract energy from ingested food. As potential fuel sources, the carbohydrate, fat, and protein in the foods that you eat follow different metabolic paths in the body, but they all ultimately yield water, carbon dioxide, and a chemical energy called adenosine triphosphate (ATP). Think of ATP molecules

Sources of Fuel During Endurance Exercise

The key functions of carbohydrate, protein, and fat are summarized in the following sections.

Carbohydrate

- Provides an efficient source of energy—Because it requires less oxygen to burn than protein or fat does, carbohydrate is the body's most efficient fuel. Carbohydrate is vital during high-intensity exercise when the body cannot process enough oxygen to meet its needs.
- Fuels the brain and nervous system—When your carbohydrate stores run low, you become irritable, disoriented, and lethargic, and you may be incapable of concentrating or performing even simple tasks.
- Aids the metabolism of fat—To burn fat effectively, your body must break down a certain amount of carbohydrate. Because carbohydrate stores are limited compared to the fat reserves in the body, consuming a diet inadequate in carbohydrate essentially limits fat metabolism.
- Preserves proteins—Consuming adequate amounts of carbohydrate spares your body from using protein (from your muscles or your diet) as a source of energy. Using protein as a fuel is undesirable because you need adequate protein to grow, maintain, and repair body tissues, as well as synthesize hormones and enzymes.

Fat

- Provides a concentrated source of energy—Fat provides more than twice the potential energy that protein and carbohydrate do—nine calories per gram of fat versus four calories per gram of carbohydrate or protein.
- Helps fuel low- to moderate-intensity activity—At rest and during exercise, at or below 65 percent of your aerobic capacity, fat contributes 50 percent or more of the fuel that your muscles need.
- Aids endurance by sparing glycogen reserves—Generally, as the distance or time that you spend exercising increases and the intensity decreases, fat becomes more important as a fuel source. Because the body uses more fat during exercise, limited muscle and liver glycogen reserves are used at a slower rate, thereby delaying the onset of fatigue and prolonging the activity.

Protein

- Provides energy in late stages of prolonged exercise—When muscle glycogen stores fall, as may occur in the latter stages of endurance activities, the body breaks down amino acids found in skeletal muscle protein into glucose to supply up to 15 percent of the energy needed.
- Provides energy when daily diet is inadequate in total calories or carbohydrate—when the body is forced to rely on protein for fuel, leading to a loss of lean muscle tissue.

as high-energy compounds or batteries that store energy. Anytime you need energy—to breathe, to tie your shoes, or to cycle 100 miles (160 kilometers)—your body uses ATP molecules.

The body stores a small reserve of ATP and another high-energy compound called creatine phosphate (also called phosphocreatine) within muscles to power activity instantly. This reserve is sufficient to fuel several seconds of short, high-power, all-out efforts, such as when you lift weights or serve a tennis ball. When you perform exercise lasting beyond 10 seconds, however, your body requires an additional energy source for the continual resynthesis of ATP. Fat and glycogen represent the major energy sources that the body uses.

The second energy system that the body relies on is glycolysis, which is a series of biochemical reactions that don't require oxygen to convert the glycogen stored in muscles into useable energy. Carbohydrates are the only nutrient whose stored energy can be used to generate ATP anaerobically (without oxygen). This factor becomes important during high-intensity exercise of short duration. The anaerobic breakdown of muscle glycogen generates ATP (as well as lactic acid) rapidly for a short amount of time, and it serves as the primary fuel for all-out exercise lasting one to two minutes, such as running 800 meters. During anaerobic metabolism, every molecule of glucose burned yields two molecules of ATP.

As an endurance athlete interested in completing longer bouts of exercise, you rely predominantly on aerobic metabolism, or oxygen-requiring reactions, to generate a constant supply of ATP. Endurance and ultraendurance activities require the body to take in more oxygen (hence your relatively slower pace) so that carbohydrate and fat will be oxidized more completely and yield a more substantial amount of ATP. During aerobic metabolism, every molecule of glucose oxidized yields 36 ATP (as compared with only 2 ATP when broken down anaerobically). For example, during the first 20 minutes of moderately paced, less-than-all-out exercise, liver and muscle glycogen are broken down to glucose, and the ATP generated supplies about half the energy that the body requires. The breakdown of fat stores supplies the remainder of energy at this time.

Thank goodness for our ability to store fat. The complete oxidation of a triglyceride molecule yields 460 ATP! During light to moderate exercise, fat supplies about 50 percent of the energy required. The oxidation of fat gradually increases as moderately paced exercise continues past an hour or two and muscle glycogen stores become depleted. During prolonged exercise, the oxidation of fatty acid molecules can provide nearly 80 percent of the energy that the body needs. The complete breakdown of fatty acids, however, depends in part on the breakdown of carbohydrate. When carbohydrate levels (that is, glycogen and blood glucose) in the body fall, the ability of the body to break down fat for fuel also falls. So, as an endurance athlete, keep the science in mind and remember that fats burn in a carbohydrate flame.

If not enough carbohydrate and fat are present to meet energy needs, the body must turn to using protein for energy. Protein must first be converted into a form that can enter various metabolic pathways to produce ATP aerobically.

In some cases, amino acids can be broken down directly in muscles, and the by-products can be converted into glucose and used for energy. In other cases, amino acids are converted into intermediate products in the liver and then broken down through the same pathways as glucose to yield energy.

Energy Demands for Intensity and Duration

Don't fall into the mind trap that causes many athletes to think that we burn solely carbohydrate or solely fat during exercise. Your body uses a mixture of fuels during every activity that you do, from resting on the couch to sprinting for the finish line. How hard you work (the intensity) and how long you go (the duration) ultimately determine what proportion of fuels the body uses. At rest, you use more fat than carbohydrate (blood glucose) to meet your energy needs. During low-intensity exercise (at 25 percent of your maximal aerobic capacity) such as walking, fat continues to supply more than half the energy that you need. The body uses fat because adequate oxygen is available to break it down for use as fuel. As long as you consume enough calories and carbohydrate from day to day, your body won't have to resort to using protein to fuel everyday activities or exercise.

If the intensity of the exercise that you perform remains low to moderate (up to 65 percent of your maximal aerobic capacity), your body relies on a mixture of fat and carbohydrate (glycogen and blood glucose) as fuel. As you pick up the pace (increase the intensity above 70 percent of $\dot{V}O_2$max), you have trouble consuming enough oxygen to meet your needs. Your body responds by relying less on fat for energy, shifting instead to burning more glycogen (see figure 2.1). First, fat cannot be mobilized (broken down into free fatty acids and brought to the muscle from adipose tissue) or burned quickly enough to meet the energy demands of intense muscle contractions. Second, the burning, or oxidation, of carbohydrate for energy requires less oxygen than does the oxidation of fat, so carbohydrate becomes the preferred fuel whenever oxygen is a limiting factor. On top of that, as lactic acid accumulates (as a by-product of the breakdown of glycogen when enough oxygen isn't available), it further hinders the ability of muscles to burn fat. At times of high-intensity, all-out exercise (90 to 95 percent of aerobic capacity), your body relies essentially on glucose.

You've probably figured out by now that how long you go (duration) is inversely related to how fast you go (intensity). For example, no matter how talented you may be, your average speed in a marathon won't be as fast as it is during a 10K race. Fat becomes more important as a fuel source as the intensity of exercise decreases, which occurs as the distance or time that you exercise increases. The oxidation of fat, for example, contributes up to 70 percent of the energy needed during moderate-intensity exercise lasting four to six hours. As exercise continues and glycogen stores run low, the breakdown of fat supplies most of the energy needed. Because the burning or oxidation of fat supplies ATP at a significantly slower rate, however, you cannot maintain the same intensity or pace. Intensity becomes limited to approximately 60 percent or less of aerobic capacity, and only if some carbohydrate is still available.

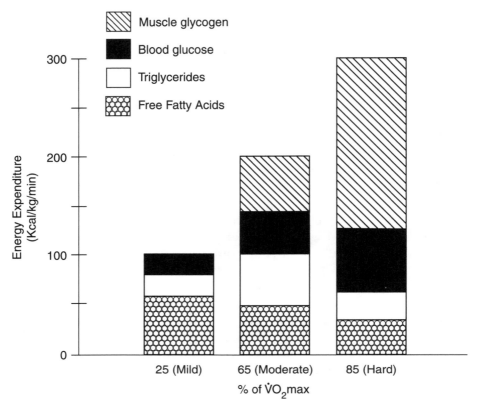

Figure 2.1 As exercise intensity increases, the body's dependence on carbohydrate for fuel (glycogen and blood glucose) increases.

Adapted, by permission, from J.A. Romijn et al., 1993, "Regulation of endogenous fat and carbohdrate metabolism in relation to exercise intensity and duration," *American Journal of Physiology - Endocrinology and Metabolism* 265(3): E387.

The limiting factor on performance, therefore, even during moderate-intensity exercise, remains the body's limited carbohydrate stores. No matter how ample your fat stores, after you deplete your muscle glycogen stores, you will experience fatigue to some degree and be unable to sustain your current pace. On top of that, your brain needs a constant supply of glucose. As previously mentioned, if you exhaust your liver glycogen stores and thus cannot maintain an adequate blood sugar level, your body simply shuts down. Remember, too, that a certain amount of carbohydrate breakdown is required for the complete burning of fat as fuel. The longer that you exercise past an hour, the more important an outside source of glucose (for example, sports drinks, energy gels, or other carbohydrate-rich foods) becomes to compensate for the depleted glycogen reserves of the body.

Endurance events, such as marathons and short-course triathlons, and ultraendurance events, such as the Race Across America, a 3,000-mile (4,800-kilometer) coast-to-coast cycling event, and 50- and 100-mile (80- and 160-kilometer) foot races, provide particularly challenging situations. Elite marathoners typically race at paces equivalent to 86 percent of $\dot{V}O_2$max. Marathoners who finish with times over three hours run at 65 percent of $\dot{V}O_2$max—exercise intense enough to require a substantial amount of glycogen for fuel. Glycogen depletion can also be a concern in ultraendurance cycling, such as the Race Across America, and multistage events like the Tour de France because these athletes generally cycle at an intensity greater than 70 percent of $\dot{V}O_2$max. Riders must constantly ingest carbohydrate-rich foods and beverages on a daily basis (before, during, and after their rides) to replenish their glycogen stores.

On the other hand, at the exercise intensities of most ultraendurance running events (less than 60 percent of $\dot{V}O_2$max), such as 50- and 100-mile running races, hypoglycemia, or bonking, is often more likely to occur than glycogen depletion is. Well-prepared ultraendurance runners may be very efficient at burning fat as fuel, but the brain still needs a constant supply of carbohydrate to function well. As a protective mechanism when muscle and liver glycogen levels run low, the brain shuts down the body until another source of carbohydrate comes along. (See chapter 4 for more on hitting the wall and bonking.)

What Is $\dot{V}O_2$max?

$\dot{V}O_2$max is a measurement of aerobic capacity—the ability of the body to take in, transport, and use oxygen. As you exercise more intensely, the rate at which you consume oxygen increases. At some point, however, your body reaches a limit on the amount of oxygen that it can consume, even if the intensity of the exercise continues to increase. This point is known as your maximal oxygen uptake, or $\dot{V}O_2$max. As an indicator of aerobic fitness, $\dot{V}O_2$max can predict which athletes will perform well in endurance activities, but it can't determine who will win the race!

Two other factors influence your performance in endurance activities: your ability to perform at a high percentage of your $\dot{V}O_2$max for a prolonged period (referred to as your lactate threshold) and your efficiency or skill at performing an exercise. Your lactate threshold is the exercise pace above which lactic acid begins to accumulate significantly in the blood. This occurs when glycogen and glucose are broken down rapidly because sufficient oxygen is unavailable (as occurs during anaerobic metabolism). By developing a higher lactate threshold, you can exercise more intensely without accumulating lactate—a distinct advantage because the buildup of lactate contributes to fatigue. By becoming more skilled or economical at performing an exercise, you need less oxygen to perform the same rate of work (that is, you work at a lower percentage of your maximal $\dot{V}O_2$max), which helps you conserve energy over the long run.

Supplying the Demands Efficiently

Endurance athletes vary tremendously in their energy needs depending on their size, gender, and the training program and sport that they engage in. Some athletes may at times need over 10,000 calories a day! Endurance athletes, in particular, can have trouble consuming enough calories to balance the energy demands of a rigorous training schedule. No magic foods or formulas exist, but all athletes can benefit from taking a closer look at the quantity and blend of carbohydrate, fat, and protein in their daily diet.

Carbohydrate Intake

Carbohydrate is critical for an endurance athlete. You can tap into the power of carbohydrate in four main ways:

1. By eating a carbohydrate-rich training diet
2. By taking advantage of the carbohydrate window immediately following exercise
3. By loading up on carbohydrate-rich foods for three days before long events and races
4. By consuming sports drinks, energy gels, and other carbohydrate-rich foods (if applicable) during exercise

Athletes who consistently eat a carbohydrate-rich diet have greater muscle glycogen stores to draw on during training and racing efforts. Remember, adequate muscle glycogen stores help delay the onset of fatigue as you pick up the pace or exercise more intensely (such as in a 10K running race or a sprint triathlon) or when you exercise longer than 90 to 120 minutes (such as a marathon or an Olympic or Ironman distance triathlon.) Another bonus is that workouts (and races) will seem easier to complete when you have enough glycogen on board to fuel the entire session.

For fitness enthusiasts working out consistently for an hour a day or those athletes training purposefully, eating a daily training diet approaching three to four grams of carbohydrate per pound of body weight (six to eight grams per kilogram) will speed your recovery from daily training bouts so that you can get out the door the next day. You'll also reduce your chance of being sidelined, because athletes who exercise with low muscle glycogen stores tend to incur more injuries. As discussed in chapter 1, breads, cereals, pasta, rice and other grains, fruit and vegetables, dried beans and lentils, and milk and yogurt are the best options for meeting your daily carbohydrate needs. Also useful are sports drinks and energy gels and bars, when used appropriately. Foods that contain a great deal of added sugar, such as cookies and other desserts, ice cream, frozen yogurt, candy, and soft drinks, supply carbohydrate but few nutrients. Eat these foods in moderate amounts to round out your carbohydrate intake.

Poor training days or unusual feelings of sluggishness are often caused by poor eating habits. Why? The effects of glycogen depletion are cumulative. Many exercisers and athletes start out the week strong only to feel as if they are running on fumes by Friday. If you don't replenish your glycogen stores on a daily basis, you run the risk of digging yourself into a hole. You'll be forced either to back off or to take time off to recover completely. By the way, planning rest days into your training schedule is a good idea. Rest gives your body time to replenish its glycogen stores, which takes about 20 hours.

Refueling after a workout is the last crucial step to getting the most out of your training. The first hour following exercise, a period known as the carbohydrate window, is the time when muscles are most receptive to replacing glycogen. Unfortunately, rather than eating, many athletes spend this time stretching, showering, and racing back to their desks, or traveling home in the car after running or riding their favorite trail. Furthermore, because exercise elevates your body temperature, which in turn depresses your appetite, you can't rely on feeling hungry to prompt proper refueling.

In the first 15 to 30 minutes after a workout, get in the habit of immediately consuming a recovery drink that supplies both fluid and carbohydrate, such as a sports drink, fruit juice, or a meal replacement beverage (even a soft drink in a pinch). Aim to consume at least half a gram of carbohydrate per pound (1 to 1.2 grams per kilogram) of body weight within the first 30 minutes following exercise, which equates to 50 to 100 grams for most athletes. Ease in carbohydrate-rich foods as soon as you can tolerate them. Popular choices include yogurt, fruit, a low-fat milk shake or smoothie, cereal, bagels, baked potatoes, and energy bars. Be sure that you're putting in carbohydrate, not fat. To determine the carbohydrate content of sports drinks and foods, check the nutrition facts panel on food labels. See appendix C for a list of high-carbohydrate foods.

In addition, numerous studies have shown that endurance athletes can enhance their performance during continuous exercise lasting longer than two hours by carbohydrate loading, or topping off, their glycogen stores. You can do this by boosting your carbohydrate intake to 4 to 5 grams per pound of body weight (8 to 10 grams per kilogram) for three days before the event or race. Athletes who have trouble eating enough carbohydrate can supplement their food intake with high-carbohydrate or meal-replacement beverages.

Last but not least, studies have shown that consuming beverages that contain carbohydrate (such as sports drinks) during moderately to vigorously paced exercise lasting longer than 60 to 90 minutes provides muscles with a ready supply of blood glucose for immediate energy, which further spares glycogen stores. Drinking a sports drink may also be valuable during intense anaerobic workouts lasting less than 60 minutes, such as hill repeats or interval sessions, when the body burns glycogen at a rapid rate.

Besides ensuring that you will perform better, consuming carbohydrate during exercise appears to boost the immune system by preventing precipitous dips in blood sugar. A low blood sugar level signals the body to release large quantities of stress hormones, particularly cortisol. Typically elevated after prolonged exercise, cortisol profoundly suppresses immune function. By taking in plenty of carbohydrate and keeping your blood sugar level steady during exercise, you will keep your cortisol levels significantly lower, which may provide just the edge that you need to keep a cold, sore throat, or the flu at bay.

The optimal concentration of carbohydrate-containing drinks intended for use during exercise appears to be 6 to 8 percent, the amount found in most commercially available sports drinks, such as Gatorade and PowerAde. (To determine the carbohydrate concentration of your favorite sports drink, divide the number of grams of carbohydrate in an 8-ounce, or 250-milliliter, serving

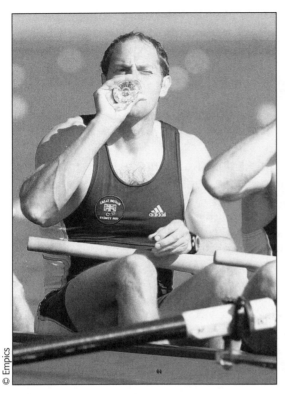

Sir Steve Redgrave, winner of five consecutive Olympic gold medals, is a master at being physically ready and mentally prepared.

by 250 and multiply by 100.) Fruit juice and soft drinks fall outside the established guidelines because they are more concentrated in carbohydrate (as well as low in sodium), which can delay their absorption from the stomach. With a carbohydrate concentration greater than 9 to 10 percent, water may actually be drawn into your gastrointestinal tract to dilute the excess carbohydrate, thereby robbing the blood and muscles of valuable water, and causing an upset stomach (or something worse). Drinking carbonated drinks during exercise may also upset your stomach. People respond in different ways to carbohydrate-based drinks and foods, however, so you may see some athletes consume juice and soda with no ill effects.

You may have noticed that sports drinks contain sodium and that some brands taste salty if you drink them when you're not exercising. Sports drinks include sodium for many reasons. Sodium helps speed the rate at which fluid and carbohydrate empty the stomach and are absorbed out of the intestinal tract—good news for working muscles and your brain, which needs a steady supply of glucose to keep functioning. The presence of sodium also makes you feel thirsty (stimulating you to drink), helps replace sodium lost in sweat, and helps you retain or hold on to the fluids that you ingest.

Fat Intake

Because endurance athletes rely increasingly on fat as an energy source during prolonged bouts of exercise, you may be tempted to eat a high-fat diet to improve your performance. Before you begin "fat loading" (well-designed studies have participants obtain at least 60 to 70 percent of energy or total calories from fat), look at the research. To date, studies reveal that endurance (also referred to as time-to-exhaustion) performance doesn't seem to be affected in any consistent manner after subjects followed a high-fat diet during an adaptation period lasting from two to seven weeks. Time to exhaustion in laboratory trials has been shown to increase (in one study), remain unchanged, or decrease, when subjects were on a prolonged high-fat diet as compared with a carbohydrate-rich diet. Consuming a high-fat diet beyond four weeks has been shown definitively to have a detrimental effect on endurance.

For example, in one study, trained cyclists improved their ability to adapt to and use fat as a fuel during exercise (increased fat oxidation) and were able to cycle longer. Their improved performance, however, was not statistically significant. In this case, after four weeks on a diet that obtained 85 percent of calories from fat, the trained cyclists rode 152 minutes (to exhaustion) compared with 147 minutes following an average or moderate carbohydrate diet (50 percent of calories from carbohydrate). Critics point out, however, that during the test the cyclists rode to exhaustion at an intensity low enough (63 percent of $\dot{V}O_2max$) to be fueled primarily by fat oxidation and not limited by glycogen depletion. In reality, most athletes train and certainly race at an intensity of 70 percent of their $\dot{V}O_2max$ or above, levels at which glycogen depletion is an increasingly limiting factor. Thus the attributed positive effect of fat loading as reported in the study isn't applicable for most endurance athletes.

On the other hand, ultraendurance athletes who perform at a relatively lower or submaximal intensity for long periods (greater than four hours) could possibly experience a greater benefit from fat loading. Enhanced ability to use fat as fuel would serve to spare the body's limited carbohydrate stores. Researchers continue to refine and test healthier and more realistic fat-loading protocols (e.g., six days followed by one day of restoring carbohydrate stores, with carbohydrate feedings during exercise). To date, studies have not shown statistically significant improvements in performance.

In general, though, fat loading, or following a high-fat diet that weighs in much above the recommended 30 percent of total daily calories, doesn't make sense for most endurance athletes. Such a diet squeezes carbohydrate out of the mix and lowers muscle glycogen stores, which reduces endurance and the ability to perform at high intensity. In the long term, eating a fat-rich diet could also increase the risk for heart disease and certain cancers. (Despite training heavily, the earlier mentioned competitive road cyclists saw their cholesterol levels rise while on the high-fat diet.) Don't forget that even lean athletes have more than enough body fat stored to fuel their endurance endeavors. If you want to improve your performance, focus on manipulating the way that you exercise or train, not the fat content of your diet. Aerobic or endurance exercise stimulates the body to use fat as an energy source. Highly trained endurance athletes are able to use more fat and less glycogen at the same absolute level of exercise compared with less fit athletes.

The news that merely eating more fat won't improve your performance in endurance events doesn't mean that you should shun all high-fat foods such as salad dressing, cheese, or an occasional bowl of ice cream. To perform at your best, you need muscles that have adapted to using both fat and carbohydrate as fuel. The metabolism of fat and carbohydrate requires different sets of enzymes. By training hard and long, you train your muscles to burn fat and spare glycogen during exercise. By eating a diet that contains adequate fat (approximately one-half gram per pound, or 1–1.2 grams per kilogram, of body weight), you also stimulate your muscles to make more of the enzymes necessary for fat metabolism. In other words, you support the efforts of your muscles to build extra cellular machinery for metabolizing fat.

Fat also provides more energy per pound of food. Eating an adequate amount of fat helps athletes obtain enough calories to fuel high-volume training, such as running 10 or more miles (16 or more kilometers) per day or participating in multiple training sessions throughout the day. Athletes who eat most of their calories from carbohydrate-rich foods (about 60 percent) still have plenty of leeway for some fat and, of course, protein. Besides, how much fun is a diet without some fat in it? Keep in mind though, that even athletes need to watch their intake of unhealthy fats, such as saturated fat and trans fats. (See the section in chapter 1 titled "The Oils Have It: Choose Healthy Fat Over Unhealthy Fat" on page 23.)

Athletes with high calorie needs often train quite successfully by consuming an adequate amount of carbohydrate (for example, 450 to 600 grams a day) and a relatively high percentage of fat calories (up to 35 percent of total calories). For example, an athlete who consumes 4,000 calories a day (50 percent derived from carbohydrate, 15 percent from protein, and 35 percent from fat) still receives a substantial amount of carbohydrate (500 grams). The calories provided by fat add up quickly and allow the athlete to do something other than train and eat all day. For instance, downing a stack of five pancakes with margarine and syrup is easier, and provides the same amount of calories, as eating 10 plain pancakes.

As for trying to improve your performance by supplementing with fat before or during exercise, little evidence exists for doing so. The fat in the foods that you eat (long-chain triglycerides) takes too long to be digested and absorbed to provide readily available energy during exercise, unless you're planning to be on the move all day. Dietary fat empties slowly from the stomach, and the fatty acids it provides typically don't appear in the bloodstream (as available energy for active muscles) until three to four hours after ingestion.

Medium-chain triglycerides (MCTs) represent another type of fat that could possibly enhance performance during endurance exercise. Unlike long-chain triglycerides, MCTs are rapidly broken down to fatty acids and directly absorbed into the bloodstream and liver. Theoretically, they could be delivered to muscles quickly enough to provide energy, thereby sparing muscle glycogen. MCTs are available as MCT oil, and some energy bars, sports drinks, and meal replacement beverages now contain MCTs.

When it comes to supplementing with MCTs during exercise, the research is inconclusive. Of studies looking at the effect of using a carbohydrate–MCT mixture (delivered by a sports drink) on time-trial performance, one has shown a positive benefit. After a long, low-intensity warm-up (two hours at 60% of $\dot{V}O_2max$), six endurance-trained cyclists immediately rode a simulated 25-mile (40-kilometer) cycling time trial. During the rides, the athletes consumed either a carbohydrate drink, an MCT solution, or a combined MCT–carbohydrate drink. The times recorded in the time trials in which the athletes consumed the MCT–carbohydrate drink were significantly faster (by 2.5 percent) than those turned in when they used carbohydrate alone. The riders turned in their worst performances when they drank the MCT (no-carbohydrate) beverage.

Other studies, however, have not been able to duplicate the positive effect of ingesting MCTs in conjunction with carbohydrate. In addition, some people will not be able to tolerate a large enough amount of MCTs (the riders in the study ingested 86 grams) to see a benefit. MCTs can cause cramping and diarrhea when consumed in amounts greater than 30 grams. (To learn more about MCTs, see chapter 5.)

Protein Intake

As much as you might like bagels and pasta, you can't live on carbohydrate alone if you are involved in endurance activities. Endurance exercise increases your need for protein. In fact, your daily protein requirement may be higher than that of strength and power athletes. Endurance athletes need protein to shore up the loss of amino acids oxidized during exercise and to repair exercise-induced muscle damage, especially the trauma that occurs during eccentric muscle work, such as downhill running. Protein typically supplies 5 percent or less of daily energy needs. During extreme bouts of prolonged exercise when glycogen stores run low, however, protein is used as fuel and may contribute as much as 15 percent of the energy needed. Dieting or failing to eat enough calories from day to day to match those burned during exercise, which may happen during periods of hard training, also raises daily protein needs.

Endurance athletes require .55 to .75 grams of protein per pound (1.2 to 1.7 grams of protein per kilogram). For example, a 120-pound (54-kilogram) athlete needs around 75 grams a day. A 150-pound (68-kilogram) athlete should get about 95 grams, and a 180-pound (82-kilogram) athlete needs about 115 grams. Competitive athletes involved in extremely intense training, such as Ironman triathletes, and growing teenage athletes may need as much as .8 to .9 grams of protein per pound (1.8 to 2.0 grams of protein per kilogram).

These quantities may sound like a lot, but most well-nourished athletes easily meet their protein needs. Consider this: If you eat two eggs and cereal with milk for breakfast, a tuna sandwich and yogurt for lunch, and grilled chicken with baked beans for dinner, you've devoured almost 100 grams of protein. Between-meal snacks can also provide protein, and vegetables, whole grains, nuts, and tofu and other soy products supply varying amounts as well. Another bonus of including some protein at every meal (and snacks, too) is that doing so helps stabilize your blood sugar level so that you feel full longer.

Branched-chain amino acids (BCAAs) are of particular interest to endurance athletes because of their potential role in enhancing mental strength and delaying fatigue during prolonged exercise. BCAAs, stored in muscle, can be converted into glucose and used as fuel during prolonged exercise. Normally, high levels of BCAAs help block the entry of tryptophan (another amino acid) into the brain, but during the latter stages of prolonged endurance exercise, BCAA levels may fall if they are used as energy to compensate for depleted glycogen stores. Consequently, tryptophan may have an easier time gaining entry to the brain, where it's converted into serotonin, a brain chemical that can induce sleepiness and fatigue.

Although supplementing with BCAAs during exercise to improve performance is sound in theory, the studies to date are limited. Adding BCAAs to sports drinks and other products doesn't appear to provide any additional benefits, nor does it appear to be detrimental, although large doses (most studies use 7 to 20 grams) can impair the absorption of water and contribute to stomach problems. Eating protein-rich foods, such as milk, yogurt, meat, poultry, and fish easily supplies the recommended daily dose (about three grams a day) of BCAAs. (To learn more about BCAAs, see chapter 5.)

Keep in mind that the goal is to maintain lean muscle tissue, not break it down during exercise for fuel! Beginning exercise with adequate glycogen stores and supplementing with carbohydrate (sports drinks, energy gels, and so forth) during prolonged exercise remains the best defense against fatigue and the breakdown of muscle tissue. Consuming protein-rich foods shortly after exercise (during the carbohydrate window or at your next meal, for example) promotes the rebuilding of muscle proteins and may help the body replenish its glycogen stores even more quickly.

High-Protein, Reduced-Carbohydrate Diets

Diets touting more protein (and fat) and less carbohydrate, such as the Atkins diet, continue to die a slow death. Nevertheless, some versions continue to remain popular among fitness buffs and athletes seeking to lose body fat and boost their performance. For instance, proponents of the 40–30–30 plan (40 percent carbohydrate, 30 percent protein, and 30 percent fat) shove carbohydrate aside and claim protein to be the most coveted nutrient for athletes. Carbohydrate is blamed for everything from unwanted weight to low energy levels. How can this be if glycogen (stored carbohydrate) is the body's preferred fuel during exercise, especially as you pick up the pace?

Take a closer look at this popular, but not necessarily beneficial diet. The 40–30–30 balance of nutrients supposedly keeps the correct balance between two hormones that the body produces, insulin and glucagon. Advocates reason that limiting the intake of carbohydrate keeps the body from producing too much insulin, while consuming protein boosts glucagon (a hormone that counteracts the effects of insulin) levels. This optimal insulin–glucagon balance supposedly maintains blood sugar levels better, improves endurance by increasing the use of fatty acids for fuel, and reduces body fat by increasing the use of stored fat. Incidentally, all the scientific jargon referred to in these diets about good and bad eicosanoids (hormonelike substances that regulate a variety of body functions) as being the key to all health and disease is unfounded and unproved by any published scientific research.

High-protein diets hinge on the theory that carbohydrate, not excess calories, does the damage. Eating high-carbohydrate foods, such as rice and potatoes, raises insulin levels. High insulin levels cause the body to store excess carbohydrate as fat instead of burning it for energy. The result is a feeling of lethargy and fatigue as the blood sugar level dips (insulin moves glucose out of the bloodstream) and a gain in weight as high insulin levels inhibit the ability of the body to access its fat stores. Eating protein, on the other hand, supposedly increases the level of glucagon, which directs the liver to release glucose, thereby replenishing the body's blood sugar supply. Lower insulin levels also promote the release of fatty acids from the fat cells of the body for use as energy.

Here is a look at the flip side of high-protein, low-carbohydrate diets. First, those who go too low in carbohydrate will pay the price. We have known since the 1930s that a high-carbohydrate diet enhances endurance during strenuous athletic events. As you've read in this chapter, consuming carbohydrate before, and especially during, exercise is crucial for endurance athletes. Eating carbohydrate-rich foods (for instance, an hour before exercise) does raise insulin levels and lower blood sugar levels, but this response is temporary. Most healthy, active people experience no negative effects on performance. Refilling glycogen stores following exercise is also simply smart science. Failing to do so will definitely hinder your ability to recover, and thus train, effectively.

Second, fat is an important source of energy, particularly at rest and during low-intensity exercise, and training promotes its increased use as a fuel source. The limited glycogen (stored carbohydrate) reserves of the body, however, remain the limiting fuel source during endurance exercise, even in marathons and ultraendurance events. In addition, the body shifts to burning carbohydrate, not fatty acids, as the pace increases or as exercise becomes more intense. The brain needs a steady supply of carbohydrate too. Seriously, who performs at their best when experiencing a headache and feeling grumpy and irritable? So, although terribly old-fashioned (and definitely unhip among those trying to sell you the latest "discovery"), carbohydrate is still king.

Remember, human sport physiology hasn't changed in the last 75 years. It still applies to all endurance athletes, from fast to slow. Furthermore, weight-loss or fad diets aimed at average people rarely work for active people, especially those serious about their athletic goals. Remember, you're eating to work out or train, not sit in a rocking chair. The ability to train smart and consistently leads to being fit. Fitness leads to leanness (a healthy weight that you can maintain without heroics), not the other way around.

Third, losing weight is about expending more calories than you consume. The total amount of calories burned during the day is what counts—not whether you burn fat or carbohydrate. (Otherwise, to lose weight, you could simply sleep more, an activity that burns few total calories, but a high percentage of fat calories.) Your body can pull from its fat stores at any time of day or night to compensate for the calories burned during exercise. Besides, if you consume too many calories from any source—carbohydrate, protein, or fat—your body will store the excess calories as body fat. As for high insulin levels causing people to become overweight, the reverse is more likely to be true. Being overweight drives insulin levels up. People have trouble regulating their blood sugar level and consequently feel hungrier, and thus more likely to overeat. Losing weight through a sound exercise program almost always brings insulin levels back down within the normal range.

By the way, it's not surprising that people can lose weight quickly on high-protein, low-carbohydrate diets because most provide too few calories for active people. Besides, ketosis (when the body turns to burning fat when insufficient carbohydrate is eaten) promotes water loss and curbs appetite. (Every gram of glycogen is stored with almost three grams of water, so as you deplete your glycogen stores, you lose a great deal of water.) Besides dehydration, ketosis also causes bad breath, light-headedness, dizziness, and fainting and can be dangerous in the long run.

Why do some athletes claim that they feel, and perform, better on a high-protein, low-carbohydrate diet? Obviously, we don't all have the same nutritional needs, and not everyone is an elite athlete who trains for hours every day. Some active people, especially those who have been on carbohydrate overload (eating, for example, fruit, salad, energy bars, bagels, pasta, and more bagels), may lose weight or perform better on high-protein diets simply because they're eating a more balanced diet. You'd be amazed at how getting enough high-quality protein, iron, zinc, calcium, and a little more fat can make you feel. Perhaps you've been "fat-phobic," that is, eliminating most protein-rich foods, such as meat and dairy products, because they also contain fat. Adding some protein and fat back to a very low-fat diet means that you may eat less because you feel more satisfied and can resist those urges to plow through a box of fat-free cookies in one sitting.

Keep in mind that deciphering complicated formulas and eating specific percentages of nutrients at every meal and snack most likely have little to do with your feeling healthier and performing better. The key lies in eating a balanced diet that tastes good; mixes carbohydrate, protein, and fat at every meal; and meets your energy needs. Eating plenty of carbohydrate, without going overboard, makes sense. Otherwise, someone should tell some of the world's fastest runners, the Kenyans, that they're doing it all wrong by eating a diet high in ugali, a starchy corn-based mash that's rich in carbohydrate.

The Body's Response to Training

Athletes of all ages and abilities often get caught up in manipulating their diets in hopes of performing better, rather than eating to support their training efforts. When you boil it down, the connection between your diet and your training program is simple. Food is fuel. To succeed you must train. To have enough energy to train, you must consume enough energy.

Sure, it's important to be knowledgeable about recommended nutrition guidelines, but those recommendations are just that—guidelines. We all know that simply eating properly doesn't guarantee a PR or put you on the winner's podium. You have to do the work. Take Lance Armstrong, winner of seven consecutive Tour de France races following successful treatment for testicular cancer. When asked what he was on that led to his success, he replied, "I'm on my bike!" Your diet plays a key role in your success by

Energy Nutrients Needed for Peak Performance

Relying on the food pyramid (refer back to chapter 1) and your common sense may be all you need to do to keep your eating habits on track most of the time. Sometimes, however, you might wonder if you're consuming the right mix of energy-supplying nutrients (carbohydrate, fat, and protein) to enable you to perform at your best. Use the following guidelines to help determine your caloric needs, and keep in mind that the food you eat serves three basic needs: it supplies energy (measured in calories); supports the growth, maintenance, and repair of tissues; and helps regulate the body's metabolism.

Carbohydrate (about 60 percent of total calories)

Training one hour per day—3 grams of carbohydrate per pound of body weight (6 to 7 grams per kilogram)

Training two hours per day—4 grams of carbohydrate per pound of body weight (8 to 9 grams per kilogram)

Training three hours per day—5 grams of carbohydrate per pound of body weight (10 to 11 grams per kilogram)

Protein (about 15 to 20 percent of total calories)

.55 to .75 grams of protein per pound of body weight (1.2 to 1.7 grams per kilogram)

Fat (at least 20 percent of total calories)

Approximately .5 grams of fat per pound of body weight (1 gram per kilogram)

Use the numbers you just calculated above to estimate your optimal daily caloric intake: (grams of carbohydrate × 4 calories/gram) + (grams of protein × 4 calories/gram) + (grams of fat × 9 calories/gram) = estimated total daily calories

enabling you to train consistently and recover quickly. Healthy eating habits also help you avoid losing days to injuries and upper-respiratory infections, such as colds.

Endurance training offers many benefits. Keep the following in mind when you're having a hard time riding one more mile, completing one more set of swimming intervals, or running along one more trail in the rain. Endurance training helps you in the following ways:

- Increases your cardiac output (the maximum amount of blood that the heart can pump every minute), which means that you supply your exercising muscles with more oxygen.

- Increases the capacity of your muscles to store more glycogen—the fuel that the body heavily relies on during prolonged exercise of moderate to high intensity (50 to 90 percent of $\dot{V}O_2max$).

- Increases the capacity of your muscles to store fat (triglycerides) and increases the rate at which it is released (as free fatty acids), thereby making free fatty acids more readily available for your muscles to use as fuel during exercise.

- Improves the aerobic energy system of your muscles by increasing the size and number of mitochondria (site of ATP production) in skeletal muscles, as well as the activity of oxidative enzymes needed to break down carbohydrate and fat to produce ATP. Consequently, a trained athlete has greater capacity to burn carbohydrate for fuel during intense endurance exercise and relies less on muscle glycogen and blood glucose as fuel during prolonged submaximal exercise.

- Raises your lactate threshold (the pace that you can maintain without causing lactic acid to accumulate significantly in the blood and contribute to fatigue) through certain types of training, such as fartlek, intervals, circuit training, and sustained tempo exercise, thereby helping to minimize anaerobic metabolism. A unit of glycogen burned aerobically (with oxygen) generates nearly 20 times the ATP that it could through anaerobic (without oxygen) metabolism. In practical terms, a higher lactate threshold means that your oxygen-dependent energy systems have improved and that your muscles are better able to clear lactic acid from the blood. You can exercise more intensely without accumulating lactic acid—an obvious benefit because the presence of lactic acid contributes to fatigue and inhibits the ability of the body to burn fat as fuel, which increases the rate at which glycogen is broken down.

All these adaptations help you become more efficient at using fat as a fuel source during exercise. Fats are mobilized and made available to working muscles more rapidly. Training also stimulates your muscles to store more carbohydrate in the form of muscle glycogen. The benefits are twofold: Muscles start out with larger glycogen reserves, and you use it at a slower rate. You can therefore exercise at a higher absolute level (for example, maintain your pace for longer) before experiencing the fatiguing effects of glycogen depletion.

Remember, making daily food choices that supply key nutrients and adequate calories sets you up to train consistently at a high level. Athletes who accomplish their training goals arrive at the starting line better prepared to handle the rigors associated with endurance sports. By coupling the benefits of endurance training with nutrition strategies that target the key time periods before, during, and after exercise (see chapter 4), you'll be able to succeed at whatever endurance endeavor you choose.

Boosting Your Strength-to-Weight Ratio

3

Are you training more than ever but just can't lose those last few pounds? Do you want to be stronger and faster next season? Athletes participating in endurance sports typically fall into two categories when it comes to body weight: those who wish they had less weight to carry around (especially less body fat) and those trying to boost their strength-to-weight ratio by adding muscle. In either case, you're wise to aim for a lean, healthy body through a combination of solid training and healthy eating habits. But if this quest becomes an obsession, you will perform poorly and may even do serious harm to your health (and happiness).

The Issue of Weight

If you're like most athletes I meet, whether you're a fitness nut, an elite competitor, or somewhere in between, you've probably tried to lose or gain weight at one time or another. You most likely set out to reshape your body in

"It's amazing how many strangers come up to me at races and tell me to lose weight. I've gotten to the point where I really like my body. It's strong and it works. I'm rarely injured. I sometimes wish I were thinner, but I don't want to be thin badly enough that I get hurt when I fall (running or skiing). Also, I want to still love running when I'm 60. Fearing food in order to run faster takes my love of the sport away."

—Nikki Kimball, ultraracer and U.S. Mountain Running Team Member (2001–2003), unbeaten in ultra trail races since 1999 hopes of performing better. Although most of us readily accept our height, we often spend a lot of time and energy trying to manipulate what we weigh. The important thing to remember is that your weight is influenced by more than what you eat and how much you exercise. Your sex, age, and height, as well as the thickness of your bones and your ratio of muscle to fat all affect how much you weigh. Obviously, most of these factors are genetically predetermined and out of your control, as is your inherited body type.

If you're using a typical bathroom or locker-room scale to monitor your weight, accept its limitations. The simple fact is that your bathroom scale cannot differentiate between fat weight and muscle weight. Besides, body weight is not static, remaining constant from day to day or even throughout a single day. Think of your body weight as a vital sign, like your blood pressure or body temperature, all of which vary throughout the day. To gain useful information from the scale, weigh yourself nude in the morning, once a week at most, after emptying your bladder and before you exercise or eat breakfast. Monitoring your weight over time (during a specific phase of your training, for example) can be valuable. An otherwise unexplained drop of weight over a few weeks or months, combined with less than satisfactory performances, for instance, can alert you to the dangers of becoming overtrained because of underfueling.

Daily weigh-ins, on the other hand, provide information only on shifts in body fluids. Many factors will affect your weight at a particular time. Sweating during exercise and vomiting or diarrhea because of an illness will temporarily decrease your weight, whereas you may appear to gain weight (literally overnight) because of water retention related to monthly hormonal changes or from eating a carbohydrate-packed meal the night before. If you still want to weigh yourself daily, put your time and energy to good use by weighing yourself before and after exercise to monitor your fluid losses. To rehydrate, drink at least 2.5 cups of fluid for every pound (1.3 liters for every kilogram) that you're down on the scale.

As a serious athlete, don't put too much stock into standard height–weight tables or even the more recent weight guidelines from the National Institutes of Health that are based on body mass index (BMI). Calculated with a formula that considers body weight relative to height, BMI does a better job of predicting a person's body-fat percentage than does body weight by itself. Health professionals developed BMI to help find people at risk for obesity-related diseases such as diabetes, coronary heart disease, and some cancers.

Many athletes and even regular exercisers, however, may show up on the charts as overweight (BMI of 25.0 to 29.9) or obese (BMI of 30.0 or above) even when they're not. You can blame your lean body mass, or muscles, which are denser than fat. If you're working out regularly and are really fit, don't worry about your BMI. Healthy bodies come in all shapes and sizes. What's important is your fitness level, not your weight.

Body Composition and Performance

Rather than relying solely on a scale to evaluate the effectiveness of your diet and training programs, look at your body composition. Simply put, the body is divided into two compartments, fat mass and fat-free lean body mass. You can distinguish the amount of body weight due to fat (expressed as percent body fat) from the nonfat tissue of the body, or lean mass (bones, muscles, organs, and connective tissue), using various techniques of body-composition analysis.

Generally, leaner athletes, or those with lower percentages of body fat, perform better on tests of speed, endurance, balance, agility, and jumping ability. For endurance athletes in particular, excessive body fat can be undesirable. It translates into extra weight that the athlete must transport for extended periods. The ideal body composition varies from sport to sport. In general, body-fat levels of elite endurance athletes, such as marathoners and triathletes, range from 5 to 9 percent in men and 8 to 15 percent in women. Keep in mind that these levels are simply what researchers have observed, not what all endurance athletes should strive for or necessarily attain.

Be careful not to confuse *correlation* with *causation*. The measured body-fat levels of elite athletes are observed to fall into (or correlate with) a particular body-fat range. These measurements, however, cannot prove (because observations simply don't have the scientific power to do so) that the low body-fat percentage is the reason (the cause) that these individuals are elite (effect). Doing whatever it takes to whittle your body fat down into these ranges doesn't guarantee that you'll enter the elite ranks. In fact, despite what athletes and those around them believe (or want to believe), rarely is an athlete's relative "fatness" the definitive limiting factor in his or her sport performance.

In fact, shaving your body fat level too low can be unhealthy and detrimental to your performance. Your body needs some essential fat to function. The American College of Sports Medicine estimates that men need a minimum level of 5 percent and women need at least 12 percent (females require higher body-fat levels to protect menstrual and child-bearing functions). If you choose to monitor your body-fat percentage, be realistic. The goal is to achieve an appropriate body-fat level that allows you to perform at your best without harming your overall health. As with weight, the top performers in any sport will vary in body-fat percentage. For example, I was involved in a comprehensive study of elite female distance runners. Most of the women were running well at body-fat percentages between 10 and 12 percent. But the most accomplished athletes at that time—the top collegiate 10K runner and the world's leading female marathoner—were both significantly above that range.

Methods of Assessing Body Composition

Several techniques are available for assessing body composition. The following section explains the advantages and drawbacks of the most common methods available to endurance athletes. Body fat can only be estimated in living humans, not measured directly. Analyzing a human cadaver is the only way to obtain a direct measure of body-fat percentage—obviously an impractical approach if you're reading this book! Keep in mind that even the best methods have an error of 2 to 3 percent. In other words, if your measurement is 12 percent, your predicted body-fat percentage is actually anywhere from 9 to 15 percent (assuming a 3 percent error).

Underwater (or Hydrostatic) Weighing

This method requires repeated tests in which you sit perfectly still for about 10 seconds while fully immersed underwater (in a special tank) after blowing all the air out of your lungs. The difference between your weight on land and your weight in water is used to estimate your body density. From that your body-fat percentage can be extrapolated. This test is a time when being found to be dense is OK, because denser bodies have less fat! If you're interested in underwater weighing, check with a local sports medicine center, a hospital with a wellness department, or a university with a physical education or exercise physiology program.

Underwater weighing has traditionally been the gold standard, the technique of choice by researchers when it comes to assessing body composition. All other methods are compared with it. Much of the success of this method, however, depends on the person's ability to tolerate being repeatedly underwater while expelling as much air as possible. Also, underwater weighing can be expensive (up to US$100 per test) and time consuming, and the formulas used may be less appropriate for some populations (such as older and non-Caucasian athletes).

Air Displacement (Bod Pod)

This technique relies on the same whole-body measurement principle as underwater weighing does; the overall density of the body is used to determine the percentage of fat and lean tissue. You sit in an enclosed egg-shaped capsule (the Bod Pod) for about one minute as computer sensors determine the amount of air displaced by your body. The Bod Pod quickly generates estimates of body-fat percentage, does not require the subject to get wet, and produces estimates that correlate closely with those produced by hydrostatic weighing for physically active people. Unfortunately, few facilities can afford the research-oriented version of the Bod Pod (which has the ability to measure actual lung volume), so this option can be expensive and may not be available in your area. Check university research laboratories and athletic facilities that serve professional and collegiate athletes. The Bod Pod version typically available in health clubs uses predicted lung volumes; thus athletes engaged in serious training may be led awry by skewed results. With either version, waiting at least two hours after exercising before being tested is advised.

Dual-Energy X-Ray Absorpiometry (DEXA)

DEXA is rapidly becoming the new gold standard because of its precision, accuracy, and reliability. DEXA looks at the body using a three-compartment model: lean muscle mass, fat, and bone. As you lie quietly for 10 to 20 minutes, a whole-body scanner that emits two types of low-dose x-rays (one for bone, one for soft tissue) passes across your body. Developed to measure bone density, DEXA assumes that the amount of photon energy being absorbed is directly proportional to the mineral content of the bones. Besides letting you know what shape your bones are in (compared with predetermined standards for people of the same sex and age group), DEXA provides relative measurements of fat and lean tissue. Furthermore, DEXA shows exactly where the fat (as well as the muscle) is distributed throughout your body.

Noninvasive and easy, DEXA does expose you to low amounts of radiation (as all x-rays do), and it can be relatively pricy because the equipment is expensive and trained professionals are required to operate it. Check universities, hospitals, and other research-based facilities.

Bioelectrical Impedance Analysis (BIA)

BIA involves having a low-voltage (undetectable) electric current passed through your body by electrodes attached to your hand and ankle. Your lean body tissue (primarily your muscles), containing most of your body's water and electrolytes, conducts the current faster and more easily than fat tissue does. The faster the current travels through your body, the less body fat you have.

Although quick and noninvasive, BIA has a higher error rate (3 to 5 percent) and can be particularly inaccurate when used with athletes. BIA tends to overestimate body-fat percentages in lean individuals, and fluid shifts in the body caused by dehydration from exercising or fluid retention due to a menstrual cycle can easily sway the results. To increase the probability of getting meaningful measurements, you must be well hydrated (although you should avoid eating and drinking for 4 hours before the test) and should avoid exercising for 12 hours before the test.

The same advice applies if you purchase a scalelike device based on BIA designed for home use (like the Tanita body-fat scale). You need to take readings at the same time of day, when you are in a hydrated state (with an empty bladder). Avoid getting on the scale when you are most likely to be dehydrated—early in the morning or late at night, following exercise, after a sauna, or within 24 hours of consuming large amounts of caffeine or alcohol.

Skinfold Caliper Test

A skinfold caliper test involves using hand-held calipers to pinch and measure the thickness of fat located right under the skin. Typically, three to seven sites are measured, for example, the abdomen, back of the arm, thigh, hip, and back of the shoulder. These measurements are plugged into a formula to estimate percent body fat. This simple, noninvasive, inexpensive technique can provide accurate and reliable readings, but only if the measurement taker is skilled and has lots of practice. Skinfold measurements are not the most valid predictor of body fat (3 to 5 percent error). Nevertheless, they can be very useful to athletes and coaches in monitoring changes in body composition over time.

Tape Measure

You can essentially accomplish what skinfold tests do by using a tape measure. This method requires no fancy scientific formulas, just precise measurements. Simply measure selected points on your upper arm, chest, waist, hips, thighs, and calves to the nearest eighth of an inch (three millimeters) with a tape measure and record those readings. You won't be calculating a specific body-fat percentage. Over time, though, as you repeat the measurements, you will be able to see your body respond as you adopt healthier eating habits or undertake a new training program.

If losing weight is your goal, for example, monitoring the amount that you lose (with your measurements getting smaller over time) can be gratifying and reassuring. If you lose fat and gain muscle at the same time, your weight as registered by a scale may not change at all. Female athletes who intensify their training or begin a strength-training program often struggle with this fact. A pound of muscle (think of a brick), however, takes up less space than a pound of fat (think of cotton balls), so a tape measure will more accurately reflect changes in body composition than a scale will.

Determining Healthy Body Composition

Many athletes I counsel want to know what they should weigh, especially those who are new to a sport or embarking on a challenging physical endeavor for the first time. I remind them that determining an exact weight or body-fat percentage isn't necessary or even desirable. Strive to keep your weight within an optimal *range*, within a few pounds for example, during a competitive season. Living on salad and rice cakes while training twice a day to reach or maintain a specific weight should be a red flag that your weight goal is unrealistic.

Remember that your weight and body-fat percentage will vary some throughout the year depending on the amount and type of exercise that you are engaged in. Measuring your body-fat percentage is better than knowing only your weight, but it's still just an estimated number. The most common mistake that I see athletes make is engaging in harmful behaviors, like crash dieting or overloading on caffeine or other stimulants to "burn fat," based on a single body-fat measurement. The second mistake that they make is comparing measurements compiled from different testing methods. Science tells us that if we want to track body composition, we must use the same method each time and follow the person over time. This approach allows us to monitor changes in body composition that truly occur in response to changes in training or eating habits. Because gaining muscle or losing body fat requires time and a lot of effort, most people won't benefit from having their body-fat percentage estimated more than twice a year. To make such measurements worthwhile, keep accurate notes on the type and volume of training that you were involved in at the time of each measurement.

Instead of focusing on your weight, which is merely an outcome of what you do, concentrate on what you need to be doing to reach the desired outcome.

Spend your energy on setting up and sticking to a sound training program and establishing smart eating habits. These two factors are what will carry you over the long haul. The weight that you end up at is your optimal healthy weight—one that you can realistically achieve and maintain, perform well at without compromising your health, and enjoy life with. You may not like what this healthy weight turns out to be, but that's another issue!

What's a healthy body-fat percentage to strive for? Check out the most current research-based standards, which take into account age and gender (see table 3.1).

Table 3.1   Body-Fat Basics

Health standards:
Body-fat levels considered healthy because they do not independently increase the risk for health problems, such as high blood pressure, diabetes, or heart disease.

Men < 55 yr: 8%–22%	Women < 55 yr: 20%–35%
Men > 55 yr: 10%–25%	Women > 55 yr: 25%–38%

Fitness and physical activity standards:
Body-fat levels that reflect greater physical training. No additional benefits to sport performance occur when body fat drops below 5% (< 55 yr) and 7% (> 55 yr) for men and below 16% (< 55 yr) and 20% (> 55 yr) for women, but health risks increase when body fat drops below those levels.

Men < 55 yr: 5%–15%	Women < 55 yr: 16%–28%
Men > 55 yr: 7%–18%	Women > 55 yr: 20%–33%

Athletes:

- No body-fat standards have been established for athletes in specific sports. Body-fat values for athletes vary widely depending on gender and the sport itself.

- All athletes need a certain amount of body fat, at least 5% for males and 16% for females, to insulate vital organs, regulate body temperature, and ensure adequate production of sex hormones.

- The optimal body-fat percentage for an individual athlete may be much higher than these minimums and should always be determined on an individual basis because of genetic differences in body type.

- In either gender, a too-low body-fat level (less than 5% for males, less than 12% for females) jeopardizes athletic performance and increases the risk for serious health problems.

- Athletes who strive to maintain inappropriate body weight or body-fat levels, or have body-fat percentages below the estimated minimal safe levels, may be at risk for an eating disorder or other health problems related to poor energy and nutrient intakes.

From V.H. Heyward and D.R. Wagner, 2004, *Applied body composition assessment*, 2nd ed. (Champaign, IL: Human Kinetics), and the American Dietetic Association, Dietitians of Canada, and the American College of Sports Medicine, "Nutrition and athletic performance—Position of the American Dietetic Association, Dietitians of Canada, and the American College of Sports Medicine," *Journal of the American Dietetic Association* 100: 1543–1556.

Changing Your Body Composition

I find that many athletes struggle when it comes to achieving a healthy weight. Some need to gain weight, whereas others want to lose weight (or body fat). Whether you maintain, lose, or gain is primarily a matter of energy balance. You'll maintain your weight if you consume roughly the same amount of energy, or calories, that you expend. To gain weight, you'll need to consume more calories than you burn off. To lose weight, you must expend more calories than you take in. In other words, you'll need to eat less and exercise more, or ideally, do both. The concept sounds simple, but in reality the process can be quite complex. After all, you're dealing with the human body, not a machine. And as you're probably aware, we eat for reasons other than being physically hungry.

Strategies for Losing Weight

Before embarking on a plan to lose weight, be sure that you really need to. Don't assume that your performance will automatically improve if you lose weight or that every time you weigh more on the scale you've gained fat. Determining your body-fat percentage or taking skinfold measurements can be particularly useful before you attempt to lose weight, especially if you're an athlete with a stocky, muscular build or a female who tends to look heavier because you carry weight on your hips and thighs. In any case, if your body fat is at a reasonable level, you won't gain anything from dieting or starving yourself to reach a new low on the scale.

You may instead need to concentrate on accepting your inherited body type or, if you're a coach or trainer, on accepting the body types of the athletes you work with. One of my collegiate teammates, the best female cross-country runner in her state as a high school senior, is a perfect example. Tall with a lean upper body, she carried all her weight on the lower half of her body. Despite completing a successful high school career at a certain weight, our coach decided that she would perform better in college if she lost 5 pounds (2.3 kilograms). Living on salad, air-popped popcorn, and a small dinner (accompanied by a scoop of ice cream as a reward for making it through the day), she did lose the weight. But she was constantly battling an upper-respiratory infection and even pulled some intercostal muscles (between the ribs) from coughing so hard! She never fully recuperated and ran poorly all year.

Second, I always remind active people, especially athletes who are serious about competing, that rapid weight loss isn't an option. If you lose more than one pound a week, or two pounds for males, you're not losing fat—you're losing water, muscle glycogen, and lean muscle mass. Your competitors are the only ones who benefit from this type of weight loss. Athletes who are chronically dehydrated and operating with low glycogen stores find it difficult to maintain their usual training pace, fatigue earlier in workouts and competitions, and suffer more injuries. Staying in peak mental shape is also difficult if you're depressed, anxious, weak, or preoccupied with food.

The long-term consequences of losing weight rapidly can be costly: loss of muscular strength and power, electrolyte disturbances due to dehydration, increased susceptibility to colds and other illnesses, iron deficiency anemia, amenorrhea (loss of menstrual periods), low bone density (due to hormonal imbalances and the lack of calcium), ketosis (an undesirable state that the body enters when it must use its fat to fuel the brain), and potential kidney problems. You may ultimately end up losing training time or even missing competitions, so don't try to lose weight during your competitive season or when you need to deliver a peak performance.

Repeated attempts to manipulate body weight or body fat below a level that is normal for you are counterproductive. Significant metabolic changes result from chronic dieting or loss of critical fat stores. For example, if you restrict your caloric intake too drastically, your body will resist your attempts to lose weight by immediately dropping its resting metabolic rate—that is, your body will use fewer calories to carry on essential vital functions and will store excess calories as fat. Because your body has no way of knowing how long this under-fueling will last, it will attempt to protect itself by adapting to the lower calorie intake.

Although this reduction in resting metabolic rate probably isn't permanent in most people, it may play a role if you lose and gain weight repeatedly. The body apparently receives messages through brain signals and hormones that help it become more efficient at extracting energy from food and storing it as body fat. Consequently, perpetual dieters often find it progressively harder to lose weight and must eat even fewer calories in the future to induce further weight loss. Muscles burn calories (fat doesn't), and you lose lean muscle tissue every time you diet, especially when you drop weight quickly. So, as your muscle mass decreases, your body requires fewer calories to remain at the same weight.

Set a realistic weight-loss goal. Work with a qualified expert, such as a sports dietitian, if you need help in this area. You can't lose body fat overnight. Focus on getting your weight into a realistic and healthy range that you can reach and maintain at this point in your life through healthy exercise and eating habits. Perhaps you've added children to your family or picked up additional hours at work that cut into your training time. If this is the case, don't assume that you can weigh what you did in college or even what you weighed last year!

Finally, keep in mind that how you eat is just as important as what you eat. Assuming that you have weight to lose, want to keep the weight off permanently, and want to have enough energy to exercise, calculate your calorie needs (see chapter 1) and put the following strategies into action.

You bite it, you write it: Keep a food diary

Keep a food journal, which serves the same purpose as a training log. A record of what you eat can help you or someone with a trained eye (like a sports dietitian) decipher your current eating patterns—what works for you and what doesn't. If you're serious about losing weight, this is your number-one tool. As in the exercise in chapter 1, simply write down everything that you eat or drink from the time you get up in the morning until you go to bed. Be sure to record the time of day or night too. Measure portion sizes at home so that you can more accurately estimate how much you're eating when you're away from home. Recording the reason that you are eating is also helpful. For example, are you eating because you are hungry? Bored? Nervous about an upcoming race? If you overindulge on weekends, a practice that can quickly erase the healthy choices that you've made all week, start by tracking those days.

Writing down everything that you eat can help you stay committed to your long-range goal of losing weight sensibly. One study followed 38 dieters who had been on a weight-loss program for a year through the danger zone, the two weeks before Thanksgiving (at the end of November) until two weeks after New Year's Day. The 25 percent of participants who consistently recorded all the foods that they ate during this period managed to lose 7 more pounds! The other 75 percent who weren't so vigilant gained back an average of 3 pounds.

The very act of writing down your daily choices, not the precise things that you record, is what counts. Self-monitoring forces us to be accountable for our daily actions. For example, you can't as easily forget the fact that you nibbled through a jar of peanuts while meeting a deadline at work if you write it down. You can also refer to your food journal to make certain that you're eating enough of the healthy foods that you need. For best results, leave your food journal in a visible place as a visual reminder (for example, on your desk or in your kitchen) or record what you eat in your day planner or training log.

Take the long road: Reduce what you eat by 200 to 300 calories a day

Losing one pound a week requires you to create a deficit of 3,500 calories, or the proverbial 500 calories a day, by eating less, moving more, or some combination of the two. If you're physically active, however, drastically reducing the amount that you eat isn't realistic and certainly isn't sustainable. For example, starving yourself while working out as hard as you can or swearing off all desserts or fun foods until you reach your ideal weight isn't likely to be a successful strategy. Unfortunately, the most common weight-loss strategy that athletes attempt is one that actually promotes weight gain. They diet all day by skimping on breakfast and lunch, become progressively hungrier as the day goes along, and then backload in the calories by beating a path to the refrigerator from dinner until bedtime.

Trimming the amount of calories that you currently consume by small increments shouldn't suppress your metabolism, and this approach helps protect against the loss of too much lean muscle tissue. You'll also still have plenty of energy to exercise consistently, which is essential if you want to keep the weight off permanently.

Keep in mind that athletes of all ages and abilities who want to lose weight should do so in stages. After you lose a few pounds, let your body become accustomed to your new weight and then decide whether you're feeling weaker or stronger before trying to lose more. Incorporating even small changes into new habits takes time and effort. Stop and assess how you are doing at maintaining the healthy changes that got you to a lower weight. Can you realistically continue them? Will you be able to do more? You may find that you would be better off directing your efforts elsewhere, into strengthening your mental skills or accepting your body type, rather than continuing to try to lose more weight.

Sit down: Eat real food

Don't throw your nutrition needs out the window because you're trying to lose weight. You still need to consume foods from all five food groups, just like everyone else. Many female athletes I know wouldn't dream of sitting down to eat a real lunch—a sandwich and a glass of milk, for example. Instead, they nibble their way though the day, racking up calories from small chocolate bars, energy drinks and bars, coffee beverages, and oversize bagels and muffins.

If you find yourself constantly eating out of a box, in your car, or while standing up, consider that these unfulfilling actions may be sabotaging your efforts to lose weight. You're more likely to feel full and experience less guilt or denial if you simply plan to eat meals (of at least three food groups) and snacks (aim for one to two food groups). You'll likely eat fewer calories too.

You may lack skills in the cooking and domestic department. I met one college athlete who lived off campus and was responsible for his own meals. He routinely boiled four hot dogs for lunch and followed that up with four more for dinner! If you're like me and can't afford to hire a personal chef, invest some time and energy into learning basic cooking and meal-planning skills. Alternatively, invest in cost-effective dinners offered by companies that provide preassembled meals that you cook at home. Because we eat what is available and convenient, your job is to keep a variety of nutritious and tasty foods on hand so that you can assemble meals quickly. This "skill power" is what keeps people from racking up excess calories from takeout and fast foods—not willpower.

Start out right: Eat breakfast

Eating breakfast is a habit—either you do it or you don't. If you're not a regular breakfast eater, start retraining yourself now. Why? One of the crucial habits of successful weight losers as tracked by the National Weight Control Registry (adults who have lost at least 30 pounds, or 14 kilograms, and kept it off it for more than six years) is eating breakfast every day. By eating breakfast, you jump-start your metabolism and set the stage for the rest of the day. If you allow yourself to become too hungry during the day (by skipping meals, for example), you'll likely always continue to struggle to reach and maintain a healthy weight. For that reason, eating breakfast is even more important for physically active people, because we tend to get hungry more often and more quickly. Remember, the less you eat in the morning, the more likely you are to overeat later in the day.

Be a portion master: Practice brings progress

Be aware of portion distortion, especially when you dine away from home. Because of the supersizing of food portions, an average bakery bagel now provides 320 calories—the equivalent of eating three to four slices of bread! Paying attention to serving sizes can be an easy way to reel in your calorie intake. Megasized cookies, muffins, sodas, and coffee drinks may appear to be a good buy, but can you afford the 500 to 800 calories that they provide? The bottom line: supersize portions lead to supersize people, including overweight athletes.

Even if you're training for an event such as your first marathon or century ride, you cannot afford to eat whatever foods you want in unlimited amounts. I constantly hear from fitness enthusiasts and recreational athletes who are disappointed because they assumed that they would inevitably lose weight while training for a new athletic challenge. If you snooze around food, however, you don't lose. If you don't also change the way that you eat (being mindful is required; being obsessed just backfires), you won't lose weight. Use a kitchen scale and measuring cups and spoons periodically at home so that you can estimate portion sizes when you dine out.

Look for easy ways to trim empty calories. If you eat out frequently, limit your intake of high-fat foods such as salad dressings, mayonnaise, cheese, fatty meats like hot dogs and sausage, and fried items. Inquire about how foods are prepared before ordering them to detect hidden fats, such as cream sauces, olive oil, and cheese. Watch out for carbohydrate overloading too. Ask yourself how many times you begin meals at home by eating a whole basket of bread! Divide your plate into thirds—and keep the starchy foods, like potatoes, rice, pasta, and bread, to one-third. Get a handle on how many calories you drink throughout the day too. Cutting back on soda, alcohol, health shakes, energy drinks, and even juice may be all you need to do.

Beef up: Include lean protein at every meal

It's no secret that many people lose weight on the popular carbohydrate-controlled (higher-protein, lower-carbohydrate) diets. It's also not a mystery why: They consume fewer total calories. People report feeling fuller longer when they eat ample amounts of protein, and that appears to translate into feeling less deprived and more motivated to stick with a lower calorie intake. Researchers are eagerly seeking the underlying mechanism to explain how protein works to increase the feeling of fullness. Include enough lean, quality protein such as fish (not fried), chicken (no skin), lean red meat, low-fat dairy and soy products, and beans of all kinds (pinto, black, kidney, and so on) at every meal. Stick to reasonable-size portions, such as 3 ounces (90 grams) of meat, at any one time. Unlike carbohydrate and fat, protein cannot be stored by your body. If you eat protein beyond your needs, your body breaks it down and converts the excess calories into body fat.

Key off the sun: Eat during the day and "diet" at night

Have you worked out today? Have you eaten today? Because most of us perform the bulk of our training, our work, and our family obligations between nine o'clock and six o'clock (even earlier if you train first thing in the morning), why do most of us insist on eating most of our calories after six o'clock? Concentrate on eating your calories when you need them most, which is during the day. Our muscles and our brain cells thrive on having a steady, constant supply of fuel available. To avoid becoming too hungry and devouring everything in sight, stagger your calories throughout the day. Plan to eat a meal or healthy snack every three to four hours so that your blood sugar doesn't dip too low. Otherwise, you'll be racing for the nearest vending machine or fast-food outlet.

Be creative with your eating schedule. Even if you're trying to lose weight, you still need to be well fueled before you head out the door, and you still need to replenish your glycogen stores following exercise. For instance, if you train after work, eat less at lunchtime and save some calories for an afternoon snack closer to your workout time. A sports drink or energy bar after you finish takes the place of that second helping or extra dessert at dinner. You can "diet" by eating reasonable size portions (a good reality check is the serving size listed on the label), by selecting lower-fat items, and by eating fewer calories at night when you don't really need them.

Make friends with fat: Good fats aren't bad

The fat that you eat in foods doesn't inevitably reappear as body fat. You can still obtain a desirable level of body fat if you snack on half a bagel spread with peanut butter or a salad with dressing drizzled over it. Be sure to keep enough fat in your diet. Besides supplying energy and essential fatty acids, fat allows your body to absorb and use fat-soluble vitamins.

Fat also heightens the flavors of food, curbs cravings, and helps you feel full. Without enough fat in your diet, you will feel unsatisfied and will be more likely to overeat, especially in the carbohydrate department. How many times have you passed on eating a burger or a piece of pizza because you tell yourself that it's too fattening only to end up an hour later reaching for another sugary, caffeinated drink (or two) or answering an out-of-control chocolate craving? The fact remains that we do not gain weight simply from eating foods or meals that contain fat. Excess calories, whether they come from fat, carbohydrate, or protein, are the culprit.

Eating a diet that contains an appropriate amount of fat, at least 20 percent of total calories or one-half gram per pound (one gram per kilogram) of body weight, is not overdoing it. The key is to concentrate on eating the right kind of fat. Nuts and nut butters, seeds, avocados, and oils such as olive, canola, and flaxseed are rich in heart-healthy monounsaturated fat. Of course, even these heart-healthy fats supply concentrated calories (nine calories per gram), so use small amounts spaced throughout the day.

Fats that we all need to limit in our daily diet are saturated fats and partially hydrogenated fats, or trans fats. To reduce the saturated fat in your diet, choose low-fat dairy products and lean cuts of meat. Limiting traditional fatty foods such as fried food, fast food, and processed foods containing partially hydrogenated vegetable oils such as stick margarine, snack foods, and bakery goods will help keep the amount of trans fat that you consume under control.

Pick it up: Complement aerobic training with anaerobic training

Don't fall into the trap of believing that you must train at a slow pace to burn fat and lose weight. Although exercising at lower intensities (aerobic exercise) uses a higher percentage of fat than exercising at high intensity (anaerobic exercise, such as interval or speed work), the picture is not that simple. Exercise does more than just help you burn fat. It helps create a calorie deficit in the body; in other words, it helps you expend more calories than you consume. Remember that to lose one pound, you need to create a deficit of 3,500 calories, either by eating less, exercising more, or some combination of the two. No matter what fuel you burn during exercise, the body can pull from its fat stores later to make up for the calories expended during exercise.

The amount of calories that you burn during exercise depends on many factors—your body weight, the type of exercise that you do, the intensity and duration of exercise, and whether you are a novice or a trained athlete. As an endurance athlete, you're most likely focusing on putting in the distance. But strength or resistance training and higher-intensity exercise, such as intervals, tempo workouts, and fartlek training (breaking your normal pace up with fast bursts), can help you lose weight as well as boost your performance. Don't forget that during exercise you burn both fat and carbohydrate for energy. Given the same time period, lower-intensity exercise uses a greater percentage of fat, but it also burns fewer total calories than higher-intensity exercise does. During faster paced activities, a greater percentage of calories come from carbohydrate than from fat, but the overall amount of calories that you use is higher. What matters most is the total number of calories used, not the percentage of fat to carbohydrate. Higher-intensity exercise helps you lose weight because it uses more calories per minute.

Think about it this way: A large percentage of a small number can be smaller than a small percentage of a large number. For example, a 150-pound (68-kilogram) cyclist averaging a leisurely 12 miles (19 kilometers) per hour may burn 380 calories an hour, and about 70 percent of the energy is derived from fat. The same cyclist may burn approximately 780 calories per hour riding at 18 miles (29 kilometers) per hour, and fat provides about 50 percent of the necessary fuel. But 70 percent of 380 is 266, and 50 percent of 780 is 390, so the more intense ride burns over 100 more fat calories. More important, because few people have unlimited time to exercise, riding more intensely burns 400 more calories in the same period (780 versus 380).

Trained athletes burn more fat for two reasons. They use fat sooner during exercise (training helps you store more fat within muscles for easy access), and they have the ability to work at higher intensities (thanks in part to an elevated lactate threshold) than recreational athletes do, thus burning more calories and proportionally higher amounts of fat. Of course, you can't just go flying out the door and start training frantically every day in an attempt to lose weight. You won't burn many calories from the couch if you come down with an injury.

Working at lower intensities until you can handle workouts that are more intense helps you avoid injuries and prepares your body for future stress. As you work up to handling higher-intensity workouts, duration becomes a greater factor in losing weight, not to burn more fat but to burn more calories. In other words, you need to exercise longer to make up for the lower number of calories used per minute. Consider increasing your training volume by adding more distance to your weekly training program. Or simply become more active during the day, such as by taking the stairs instead of the elevator or by walking instead of driving to complete errands.

Visiting the weight room while trying to lose weight is especially beneficial. Strength training builds muscle mass, which boosts your resting metabolic rate. This means that you'll be burning more calories throughout the day, even when you're not exercising. Weight training also helps ensure that the weight you lose is primarily from body fat, not muscle.

Keeping It Off During the Off-Season

If you're like most athletes, you're ready for the off-season when it arrives. This recovery period provides your body—and your mind—with a well-deserved and, for many athletes, a much-needed break, from training. Whether you totally kick back, engage in active rest (a perfect time to try new activities), or enter a period of lighter training, decreases in exercise volume and intensity also mean decreases in caloric intake. Otherwise, unwanted extra weight is the result. The off-season is also the best time to reexamine your nutrition goals, establish new eating habits, lose weight if you need to, or work on increasing your muscle mass.

1. Skip the sports foods. Save energy drinks, bars, and gels for their intended purposes—before, during, and after exercise. If you're not exercising continuously at a moderate pace for at least an hour or longer, however, you don't need them. Coordinate any exercise or training that you do so that you can refuel by sitting down to your next meal within 30 to 60 minutes.

2. Keep moving. Besides workouts and races, many athletes are quite sedentary, especially those tied to a desk all day. With fewer planned exercise sessions, you may need to remind yourself to get up and get moving. To hold yourself accountable, buy a simple step counter. Aim to walk at least 10,000 steps a day, approximately five miles, by taking the stairs, running errands on foot, and pacing back and forth while on the phone. To keep your weight within a healthy range (3 to 5 pounds), establish your baseline (average steps walked weekly) and then increase your weekly step goal as needed.

3. Weigh yourself weekly—on the same scale, at the same time of day, and under the same conditions. Modest weight gains are acceptable and expected. Be alert to rapid or large gains in unnecessary weight (for example, those not associated with a strength-training program or the restoration of healthy weight lost during the competitive season). Take responsibility for your body and take action before small gains lead to an unreasonable amount of extra pounds.

(continued)

(continued)

4. Eat a fruit or vegetable at every meal and snack. Fill up without filling out. A good habit any time becomes an essential habit during the off-season. Commit to filling half your plate at lunch and dinner with fruits and vegetables. And french fries don't count! For snacks, start with a fruit or vegetable (carrot cake, strawberry Pop Tarts, corn chips, and the like do not qualify) and then decide whether you're still hungry.

5. Eat your calories; don't drink them. It's easy to overload on calories by guzzling down coffee drinks and other caffeinated beverages, like soda and energy drinks, especially if you're doing so to "not eat." Bursts of caffeine and sugar will temporarily dull cravings, but hunger always comes roaring back. Don't go longer than five hours (when awake) without eating. Commit to eating three balanced meals (each containing at least three food groups) every day, with snacks as needed.

Strategies for Gaining Weight

Gaining weight can be an advantage if speed, power, leverage, or mass come into play in your sport or activity. Of course, you most likely want to gain lean muscle tissue, not fat. Adding muscle mass can increase your strength-to-weight ratio, which ultimately increases your strength and power, enabling you to perform at a higher level. Depositing extra body fat does little to enhance power or strength. On the other hand, some endurance athletes find that carrying a little extra padding may help them fend off illness and better weather the rigors of hard training.

Like athletes who are trying to lose weight, you need to be realistic about the amount of weight or lean body mass that you can gain. Adding a few pounds before you head off to an ultrarun or adventure race is one thing, but expecting to transform your physique is a completely different ball game. Your genes, gender, diet, training program (including the amount of strength training that you're willing to do), and motivation all count. Look at the other members of your family, especially your parents, to get a clear picture of your potential. If you're a well-trained athlete or simply a "hard gainer," you may find it difficult, if not impossible, to gain weight without substantially increasing the amount of calories that you eat or cutting back on your exercise.

The bottom line, of course, is that to gain weight you must consume more calories than you expend. In general, you'll need to eat an extra 400 to 500 calories a day to gain about one pound of lean muscle in a week. Don't look to supplements as a substitute for hard work and good nutrition. No magic nutrients exist that promote substantial gains in strength and muscle mass. (See chapter 5 for a complete review of creatine and other supplements that are touted for their potential to enhance lean muscle mass in athletes.) Keep the following guidelines in mind as you attempt to gain lean muscle mass.

Boost what counts: Increase calorie intake and strength training

Contrary to popular opinion, your calorie intake, not the amount of protein that you consume, is the determining factor when it comes to gaining muscle. Bulking up, or building muscle, requires you to have enough calories on board to meet your energy demands as well as support the growth of new tissue. If you don't take in enough calories, the protein that you consume will be used to satisfy your energy needs rather than build new muscle tissue. You must also commit to a well-designed strength-training or weight-training program. Eating extra calories or protein, or ingesting vitamins, amino acids, or other supplements, won't magically do the trick. Strength training helps muscle cells become more efficient at using available protein to synthesize new cells.

If you're training and eating appropriately, most of the weight that you put on will be muscle. Of course, if you simply overeat (literally consume more calories than you burn off), then the extra calories from any source—carbohydrate, protein, or fat—will help you gain weight by increasing your body fat.

Make eating a priority: Start early and eat often

Many athletes need to make eating a higher priority to ensure that they get enough calories. Aim to eat frequently throughout the day (starting within an hour or two of when you arise) and eat well at meals, even if you don't feel hungry. Don't let mealtimes slip away on weekends, business trips, or during busy times, like the holidays. Also consciously plan to eat minimeals (snacks) two to three times a day. Be smart and plan by buying and keeping healthy snacks on hand at home, at the office, and in your car. (See chapter 8: Performance-Enhancing Snacks, page 175.) Refuel promptly after all training bouts—don't wait until your hunger returns.

Take the hearty route: Choose higher-calorie but still-healthy foods

You can easily boost your calories by choosing heartier versions of various foods, such as granola over cornflakes, cranberry juice over orange juice, and split-pea soup instead of chicken noodle soup. Eating larger than normal portions of healthy foods, such as another helping of baked beans or an extra sandwich, will also add calories. If you're crunched for time or planning to exercise soon, drink your calories. Liquid meal products, homemade milk shakes and fruit smoothies, and even 100 percent fruit juice can be easy ways to down additional calories.

Double up: Eat both carbohydrate and protein with each meal or snack

Special protein powders or weight-gainer supplements aren't essential when you're trying to put on muscle or gain weight. Eating more protein, such as meat or eggs, won't necessarily translate into more muscle either. Most athletes have trouble gaining weight not because they lack protein but because they fail to consume enough calories or enough carbohydrate in their day-to-day diet. Although protein requirements do increase when gaining muscle is the goal, most athletes naturally consume enough extra protein from the additional food that they eat to boost their calorie intake. Carbohydrate-rich foods should still supply most of your calories. Your body relies on carbohydrate to fuel your weight-training sessions as well as the endurance activities that you participate in. Consuming adequate carbohydrate also replenishes your muscle glycogen stores so that you can continue to train effectively day after day.

To meet your protein and carbohydrate needs simultaneously, eat a variety of foods. Meat, poultry, fish, eggs, cheese, and tofu all supply quality protein (as well as fat, obviously), but virtually no carbohydrate. Few foods, though, are composed of one nutrient. Milk (regular and soy), yogurt, cottage cheese, dried beans, and lentils are good sources of both protein and carbohydrate. Vegetables and other carbohydrate-rich foods like pasta, rice, bread, and cereal contain relatively small amounts of protein, but it really adds up if you eat large portions.

To remind yourself of the importance of eating enough carbohydrate and protein, include a protein-rich food (from the milk group or the meat and beans group) with your carbohydrate-rich meals and snacks. For example, melt cheese on a bagel; add tuna, chicken, or a hard-boiled egg to a salad; top pasta with a meat sauce; or eat baked beans over rice or on top of a baked potato. Adding a strength-training program to an already ambitious training schedule will substantially increase your body's need for protein initially, so pay particular attention to your food choices when you first hit the weight room.

If you're still concerned that you're not eating enough protein, consider sports shakes or complete meal replacement powders. These products offer a more complete nutritional package than straight protein powders or supplements. They're relatively expensive, so you might consider saving them for travel or for days when a busy schedule would otherwise result in missed meals. If you don't have a milk sensitivity, you can add nonfat dried milk powder to just about anything, such as homemade shakes or smoothies, or stir it into oatmeal, soup, or cooked rice. Nonfat dried milk is a high-quality, inexpensive protein supplement (a quarter cup provides about 11 grams of protein) without the unproven additives that many other supplements provide.

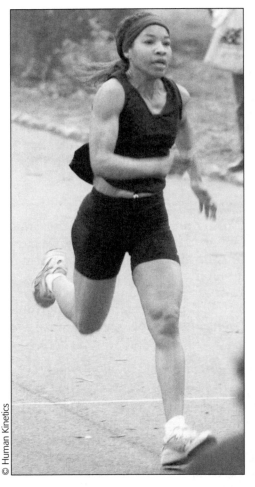

© Human Kinetics

Endurance athletes come in all body types, but most share a common trait—lean muscle mass.

Time it right: Fuel your muscles before and after workouts

Feed your muscles when they need it most—before and after exercise. During exercise, muscle fibers are ripped apart and broken down. Repair of damaged muscle fibers and formation of new muscle tissue happen only postexercise, when you allow your body to recover. To optimize gains of lean muscle and strength, eat a small amount of protein (along with carbohydrate, of course) just before and after you strength train. Your muscles are primed at these times, so give them what they need. Scientists at the University of Texas, for example, found that drinking a protein-fortified sports drink (containing only 6 grams of protein—slightly less than the amount of protein contained in an ounce of meat or a cup of yogurt) before a weight-training workout resulted in greater gains in lean body mass than drinking it afterward. Researchers theorize that a ready supply of essential amino acids in the bloodstream combined with the increased blood flow to muscles during exercise translated into the amino acids being ready and waiting in the muscle for postexercise repair.

We also know that consuming a carbohydrate-rich sports drink or meal immediately after training (during the carbohydrate window) enhances the replenishment of muscle glycogen. By adding some protein during that time, you can jump-start muscle repair and growth too. The carbohydrate (which is broken down into glucose) stimulates the release of insulin, a powerful hormone that directs glucose out of your bloodstream and into your cells. Insulin also decreases the rate at which body proteins are broken down and simultaneously the rate at which they are rebuilt—a perfect scenario for an athlete seeking to gain lean muscle mass. Researchers aren't certain of the ideal ratio of carbohydrate to protein (3:1 to 7:1 have been used in studies), although it appears that a small amount (about 10 grams) can have a significant effect. Opt for lean animal-based protein sources because they provide ample amounts of the essential amino acids that our bodies cannot make.

Three Dangerous Ds: Body Dissatisfaction, Dieting, and Disordered Eating

A chapter about athletes and weight would not be complete without a discussion about disordered eating. That's right—*disordered eating*, not *eating disorders*. (For more on eating disorders, such as anorexia and bulimia nervosa, see chapter 6). The National Eating Disorders Association defines disordered eating as "attitudes about weight, food and body size and shape that cause a person to have very strict or rigid eating and exercise habits that jeopardize their health, happiness and safety." Sports-minded people who are constantly at war with food, dissatisfied with their body size and shape, and obsessed with controlling their weight (which usually means wanting to lose weight) are often trapped in disordered eating.

Disordered eating involves trying to consciously control what, when, and how much you eat, not by tuning into your body's signals of hunger or fullness (as normal, healthy eaters do) but by tuning them out. Adhering to external rules and guidelines (like diets, prepackaged drinks and meals, and self-imposed rules about good and bad foods) takes precedence over listening to what your body needs. As a result, disordered eaters become overly preoccupied with eating a certain way, such as avoiding all sugar and white flour or eating as little fat as possible. They may obsessively count calories or fat grams, or eat in irregular and chaotic ways, such as skipping meals, fasting, or bingeing. Dieting or restrained eating—eating less than the body needs at a given time or actively resisting the intake of specific foods or entire food groups—also fits the definition of disordered eating. In fact, many experts who specialize in food, body image, and weight issues believe that dieting itself is the chief cause of most disordered eating.

According to nutrition and body image experts, two main styles of disordered eaters exist: deprivation eaters and emotional eaters. I routinely see both in the clients with whom I work. Deprivation eaters have a history of dieting (usually with accompanying "fat" and "thin" weights), of disliking their bodies and trying to change them with exercise or restricting the foods that they eat. They divide foods into good and bad categories and then attempt to eat only the good or legal foods. They spend a great deal of time worrying about whether the foods that they eat are going to make or keep them fat or berating themselves from not being able to stay away from their forbidden foods.

Of course, you can't stay on a diet or avoid all your favorite foods forever, especially when you expect your body to perform physically, nor can you drastically alter your inherited body type. The natural response to deprivation or restrained eating is bingeing or overcompensating, particularly on all the foods that you've deprived yourself of. Deprivation eaters, however, use this as further evidence that they are controlled by food or out of control when it comes to food. They thus believe that they need a diet or meal plan to follow. Their own body signals of hunger and fullness certainly can't be trusted when it comes to figuring out what, when, and how much to eat. Deprivation eaters can also engage in emotional eating. For example, feeling guilty about eating a food that they "shouldn't" eat drives them to eat even more. As long as they hold on to the diet mentality, deprivation eaters tend to be miserable around food and on a constant quest to change their bodies.

Emotional eaters eat either less or more than their bodies need in response to intense or uncomfortable emotions. Emotional overeaters attempt to numb distressing thoughts and feelings by distracting or comforting themselves with food. Because food is a temporary solution at best and doesn't resolve the true issues (the feelings come back or the problems remain), eating continues. If you overeat to cope with emotional needs, you easily can eat past feeling full and will struggle to lose weight and keep it off.

Emotional undereaters also numb themselves. They are trying to stay away from feelings altogether—which includes feeling hungry. Emotional undereaters do this by finding ways to ignore their hunger, such as staying busy and "forgetting to eat," using caffeine, and going places where food isn't allowed or available, like the gym. Although emotional undereaters may lose weight, they don't do it in a healthy, sustainable manner.

Why do some fitness enthusiasts and competitive athletes become trapped for years in the world of disordered eating? As an athlete or person interested in fitness, you can easily hide or rationalize disordered eating behaviors under the guise of improving health or as a means of improving your performance or fitness level. Furthermore, the culture surrounding many endurance sports emphasizes, even worships and rewards, lean physiques and low body weights, helping to fuel disordered eating. Sadly, so many sports- and fitness-minded people are currently engaged in disordered eating that you may believe that these disordered beliefs, attitudes, and behaviors are normal or essential to performing at your best. The oft-promoted tagline that the thinner you are, the faster you'll run (bike, swim, climb, or whatever) is difficult to ignore, especially for adolescent girls and anyone else for whom weight and self-esteem are closely linked.

Although disordered eaters do not meet the strict diagnostic criteria of a full-blown eating disorder, disordered eating has serious consequences, including the increased risk of spiraling out of control into an eating disorder. According to the NCAA's *Sports Medicine Handbook*, disordered eating can lead to semistarvation and dehydration, resulting in loss of muscle strength and endurance, decreased aerobic and anaerobic power, loss of coordination, impaired judgment, and other complications (like iron-deficiency anemia, menstrual irregularities, and stress fractures) that decrease performance and impair health. Obviously, this is a poor approach for anyone whose happiness or job performance (such as a student–athlete) depends on his or her body.

Compulsive exercise is another complicating factor typically intertwined with disordered eating habits. Are you dedicated and training hard, or are you training beyond your coach's knowledge or more intensely than athletes of similar fitness levels? People who are struggling with compulsive exercise and underfueling include those who pass out during workouts or races, those with a history of stress fractures, active females with exercise-induced amenorrhea (loss of three or more consecutive menstrual cycles or failure to start menstruating by age 16), and people drawn to endurance activities primarily as a way to burn calories and control their body weight.

I've counseled numerous pregnant women, for example, who even before they deliver, commit to endurance-type races that will take place just two to three months after their expected due date. With a history of not trusting themselves around food and feeling anxious about their weight, they view enforced exercise and an eating plan from a sports nutritionist as the only way to get their bodies (and life) back under control. Many experts in the field of preventing and treating eating disorders believe that one way to uncover disordered eating is to determine whether the person is exercising compulsively. Although not all compulsive exercisers are disordered eaters (some middle-age men, for example), experts think that most (particularly girls and women) are.

As a sports dietitian, I look for other disordered eating patterns besides compulsive exercise among endurance athletes. These include unbalanced vegetarian eating styles; multiple self-diagnosed food allergies; numerous or chronic stomach problems that interfere with preexercise fueling; undertaking prolonged training efforts and races (like marathons and century rides) on water alone because of being unable to tolerate sports drinks; avoiding food-related social situations such as family gatherings, team outings, or eating at restaurants; being excessively critical about one's body (characterized by lots of negative body talk); and weighing oneself more than once or twice a week.

Disordered eaters are not simply misinformed eaters—that is, eaters who are concerned about nutrition and eating habits yet operate with a great deal of misinformation. Misinformed eaters, when sufficiently self-motivated, are generally capable of improving their daily eating habits by using basic nutrition information and following appropriate guidance. For those struggling with disordered eating, however, more rules, plans, diets, and nutrition information isn't helpful and may do more harm than good. Guidance from a credible health professional, such as a sports dietitian or therapist, is needed for learning how to invest time and energy into something other than attempted weight control (see "Selected Resources").

Do You or Does Someone You Know Struggle With Disordered Eating?

You don't have to suffer from a full-blown eating disorder, such as anorexia or bulimia nervosa, to do yourself harm. Abnormal eating habits alone can impair your health, performance, and quality of life. To get a handle on your attitudes about food and your body, answer the following questions honestly.

Do you eat when you're not hungry or wait until you're extremely hungry to eat?

Do you frequently diet or avoid certain foods or food groups?

Are you aware of the calorie content of the foods that you eat?

Do you eat until you are physically uncomfortable?

Do you find yourself excessively preoccupied with food, dieting, your body image, or your weight?

Are you terrified about being overweight or gaining fat?

Do you feel guilty, disgusted with yourself, or out of control when you eat?

Do you avoid social situations because you fear food or your eating behaviors?

Are you uncomfortable eating in front of others?

Do you think about burning up calories when you exercise?

Do you feel that food controls your life?

The more yes answers that you gave to the preceding questions, the more you need to consider seeking help from a qualified professional, such as a mental health expert or a sports dietitian, to deal with your restrictive eating attitudes and behaviors.

Timing Fuel and Fluids for Optimal Results

4

You've logged many miles and set your sights on completing some personal challenge. It may be scaling a 14,000-foot (4,200-meter) peak, finishing your first century ride, or surviving an open-water swim. Or, if the competitive bug has bitten you, the possibilities are endless. Choose your weapon—racing flats, a bike helmet, swim goggles, oars, snowshoes, skis, or trekking poles.

Of course, before you pack all that gear, you want to make certain that you don't leave home without your most important piece of equipment—a well-hydrated and well-fueled body. And you must have a fluid and fuel plan in place for what lies ahead. Otherwise, you won't be going anywhere very far or very fast. Dehydration and glycogen depletion are two foes that all endurance athletes constantly battle as they push their bodies to perform. Just remember, fancy and expensive equipment may get you to the starting line, but adequate fluid and fuel is what it takes to get to the finish line.

"I was doing fine on the early climbs. I was fine even halfway up Mount Cole de Marie Blanque. Then I got the chills . . . and that's a sure sign you don't have enough fuel."

—American Levi Leipheimer, winner of the Deutschland Tour (Tour of Germany) and three-time top-10 finisher of the Tour de France

The Importance of Timing

To illustrate the critical role that nutrition plays, especially on race day, read the following account about a world-class athlete who was at the top of her game.

Colleen De Reuck, a three-time Olympian for South Africa, has been one of America's top female marathoners since becoming a U.S. citizen in December 2000. At the 2004 U.S. Olympic Marathon Trials, just 10 days shy of her 40th birthday, she was the surprise champion ahead of overwhelming race favorite Deena Kastor (the American record holder with a PR of nearly seven minutes faster than anyone in the field). Blowing past Kastor at mile 24, De Reuck ran to a stellar Olympic trials course record of 2:28:25. A lot can change in a year. On the same course the year before, De Reuck herself had been the prerace favorite to win the U.S. Women's Marathon Championship. Instead, she was passed at mile 25 and struggled to hold on to finish second in 2:37:41.

What did she learn from her bad experience? What did she plan to do differently at the 2004 trials race? It was simple. She answered, "I'm going to make sure I get all my fluids, and I'm going to start taking my Clif Shots earlier in the race. I'm going to try some glucose tabs also."

This real-life account illustrates several important points about hydrating and refueling for peak performance. First, not even the best athletes always get it right. De Reuck was able to rely on her superb fitness level, her considerable experience as a marathoner, and her honed mental skills to pull her through the U.S. Championships. If you're less gifted genetically, less fit, or less experienced as an endurance athlete, you have even more need to go by the book when it comes to nutrition. You simply don't have the knowledge or the experience to fall back on.

Second, there's usually more than one way to get the job done. Your job is to start with the science and apply it to yourself. No one else can do the work for you. At least once a week I meet an endurance athlete who is in denial—who is convinced that the basic laws of physiology and nutrition science simply do not apply to him or her. Obviously, this isn't true. Paying attention to your need for fluid and fuel is always important. After all, success on the big (in this case long) day hinges on your ability to work out or train consistently day after day. During these workouts and training sessions throughout the week, you must practice and hone your nutrition strategies. This chapter provides a general nutrition foundation for three particularly critical periods—before, during, and after exercise. The second half of the book (chapters 9 through 16) provides more detailed nutrition tips, as well as tried-and true strategies from well-known and successful athletes and coaches, on successfully navigating the various distances and conditions that you will undoubtedly find yourself in as an endurance athlete.

Timing is everything, especially for endurance athletes who often need to squeeze eating in among work and family responsibilities, social commitments, and workouts that can last for hours (perhaps even more than once a day) and involve more than one sport or activity. The fueling cycle (see figure 4.1) depicts an easy way for you to remember when it is most critical for you to be

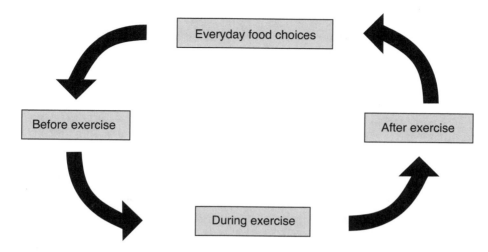

Figure 4.1 The fueling cycle illustrates the key times for active people and competitive athletes to pay attention to their body's need for fluid and fuel.

nutritionally prepared—before, during, and immediately following exercise. Although most people I counsel during sports nutrition checkups can readily tell me what they will be doing on a certain day (their work or school schedule, for example) and what they have planned for a workout (for example, masters swim workout at noon or hilly ride with the group or a rest day), few can state what their nutritional game plan is for the day. Most nutritionally challenged athletes fall into one of two camps. Some say, "I eat whenever I find the time." The others say, "When I get hungry, I grab whatever I can find." No wonder people often view food as the enemy, responsible for everything undesirable and disastrous—from indigestion to dropping out of a race.

Glycemic Index

Some people are extremely sensitive to the initial lowering of blood sugar produced by eating within a half hour to even a few hours before exercise. They complain of sugar lows (hypoglycemic reactions) such as sweating and feeling light-headed, dizzy, or shaky. Besides the timing of preexercise meals, the type of carbohydrate eaten at preexercise meals may play a role, too. The glycemic index (GI), a system that ranks carbohydrate-rich foods on how they affect our blood glucose levels, may help athletes enhance their endurance without suffering any negative consequences.

Carbohydrate-rich foods and beverages that are quickly broken down or digested in the intestine cause blood glucose to rise rapidly and thus earn a high glycemic index rating. In contrast, foods that are broken down more slowly and therefore enter the bloodstream more slowly have a low glycemic index. Don't be fooled into thinking that this system neatly divides carbohydrate-containing foods into simple and complex categories, or that less healthy simple carbohydrates (sugar in a candy bar) rapidly raise glucose and consequently insulin (which causes the rebound lowering of blood sugar that some people are sensitive to), or that wholesome complex carbohydrates (starch in potatoes) produce the desired slow release of glucose (and insulin). On the contrary, potatoes produce a rapid blood-glucose response (high GI) and chocolate induces a slow rise in blood glucose (low GI).

The glycemic index, however, is no longer the only important factor to keep on top of when it comes to carbohydrate-containing foods. The GI system tells you only part of the story, that is, how rapidly a particular carbohydrate turns into sugar (a quality issue). The GI doesn't tell you how much of that carbohydrate is in a serving of a particular food (a quantity issue). Scientists have felt for some time that calculating the glycemic load, which takes the quantity of available carbohydrate into account, is just as important as the GI because you really need to know both things to understand the effect of a food on blood sugar.

The glycemic load (GL) measures the effect of the GI of a food multiplied by the available carbohydrate content (in grams) in a standard serving. GL rankings are as follows: high (20 or more), medium (11 to 19), and low (10 or less). Foods that have a low GL almost always have a low GI too. Foods with medium or high glycemic load, however, can range from a very low GI to a very high GI. The glycemic index, for example, of one-half cup of carrots and an 8-ounce Coca-Cola are similar (47 and 58), but the GL of the soda (15) is five times that of the carrots (3). For a sample list of foods with their corresponding GIs and GLs, see table 4.1. (The GL of more than 1,600 foods for which GI numbers have been previously calculated has now been completed. If you want to pursue this topic further, visit www.mendosa.com/gilists.htm.)

If you're sugar sensitive, try experimenting with preexercise meals based on low-GI foods. *Think low before you go.* Choosing low-GI foods before exercise, particularly before prolonged efforts, may benefit your performance because of the sustained release of glucose that these foods promote. Conversely, carbohydrate-rich drinks or foods with a moderate to high GI that makes glucose readily available work best during exercise. Eating high-GI foods after exercise may also help you more quickly replenish the glycogen that you used during exercise.

As easy as this method sounds, it may not work for all athletes in all cases, so the glycemic index should not be your only criterion when selecting what to eat. Combining foods at meals, including the presence of other nutrients such as fat, protein, and fiber, and even the way that carbohydrate-rich foods are prepared, can affect the GI. Practical concerns, such as taste, how easily the food can be prepared and toted around, and how well you tolerate the food, are also important considerations in choosing what to eat before (as well as during and after) exercise.

Experimenting in training is the best way to find out what works and what doesn't. Besides, you really need to pay attention only to the major carbohydrate players in your daily diet, that is, foods that provide the most carbohydrate. If you're like most active people I meet, that means breakfast cereals, breads, potatoes, pasta, rice, energy bars, and soft drinks, not high-GI foods like watermelon, carrots, honey, or overripe bananas.

Table 4.1   Glycemic Index by Glycemic Load of Common Foods

Low GI	Medium GI	High GI
Grains		
Spaghetti, whole wheat 15/37 Barley 11/25 Rice, brown 18/55 All-Bran 9/38	Rice, instant 28/69 Pancakes 39/67 Bran muffin 14/60 Spaghetti, white 27/61 Rice, white 23/64 Couscous 22/65 Life 17/66 Oatmeal, instant 17/66	Waffle 10/76 Bagel 25/72 White or wheat bread 10/70 Whole-wheat bread 9/71 Rice Krispies 21/82 Cheerios 15/74 Grape Nuts Flakes 17/80 Shredded Wheat 15/75 Cornflakes 21/81 Grape Nuts 15/71
Fruits		
Pear 4/38 Apple 6/38 Orange 5/42 Banana 12/52 Grapes 8/46	Pineapple 7/59 Raisins 28/64	Watermelon 4/72
Vegetables		
Carrots, cooked 3/47 Green peas 3/48 Sweet corn 9/54 **Beans** Baked beans 7/48 Butter beans 3/31 Kidney beans 7/28 Chickpeas 8/28 Lentils 5/29 Soybeans 1/18	Sweet potatoes 17/61	Potatoes, baked 26/85 Potatoes, mashed 14/74 Potatoes, instant 17/85 French fries 22/75
Dairy		
Milk, skim 4/32 Milk, chocolate 12/43 Milk, full fat 3/27	Yogurt, sweetened 3/66 Ice cream, regular 8/61	

(continued)

Table 4.1 *(continued)*

Low GI	Medium GI	High GI
Other		
Chocolate 12/43	Angel food cake 19/67	Rice cakes 17/78
Banana cake 18/47	Wheat crackers 9/67	Graham crackers 14/74
Peanuts 1/14	Corn chips 17/63	Microwave popcorn 8/72
Potato chips 11/54	PowerBar 23/56	Pretzels 16/83
Oatmeal cookies 10/55	Table sugar (sucrose) 7/68	Pop Tarts 25/70
Peanut M&M's 5/33	Cola soft drinks 15/58	Jelly beans 22/78
Honey 10/55		Gatorade 12/78
Orange juice 13/50		
Apple juice 12/40		
Ensure 16/48		

Notes: The first number listed is glycemic load (GL); the second number is glycemic index (GI).

GL: low = 1–10; medium = 11–19; high = 20 or more

GI: low = 1–55; medium = 56–69; high = 70–100

Foods with higher glycemic values produce a faster rise in blood sugar (glucose) than do foods with lower values. Nothing produces a faster rise in blood glucose than pure glucose, which has a glycemic index of 100. A slow, steady rise in blood glucose is generally better than a sudden rise in blood glucose. Therefore, foods with a glycemic index below 70 are preferable for usual consumption.

Adapted, by permission, from J.W. Rankin, 1997, "Glycemic index and exercise metabolism," *Sports Science Exchange* 10(1).

Strategies Before Workouts

Many athletes I meet would rather not eat than risk being stuck in the bathroom before workouts. Obviously, no one wants to start out with a stomachache, cramps, or diarrhea from eating the wrong thing or eating too much of the right thing too close to heading out the door. On the other hand, studies repeatedly show that athletes who consume carbohydrate up to one hour before exercise improve their performance in endurance events. Why does this work? It's simple. This extra dose of carbohydrate helps maintain blood sugar levels and tops off glycogen stores.

As expected, eating a carbohydrate-rich food before you exercise, such as cereal, yogurt, an energy bar, or a glass of juice, raises your blood sugar (glucose) level. In response, your body releases insulin (a hormone produced by the pancreas). The job of insulin is to move glucose rapidly out of the bloodstream and into cells, where it's typically used right away for energy. In the case of the liver and muscle cells, excess glucose can be stowed away as glycogen for later use. In the old days (the 1970s) people thought that athletes should avoid eating before exercise because a high insulin level would be responsible for lowering the blood glucose level (perhaps too low), as well as suppressing the ability of the body to access its fat stores. This was bad news for endurance athletes, who need to use fatty acids for fuel to spare limited glycogen stores. Numerous studies since then have revealed that this isn't the case. Although blood glucose levels may be lowered and insulin levels may be high following a preexercise meal, the condition is only temporary. Within 15 minutes after the start of exercise, insulin levels fall and glucose levels rise to normal. In most cases, the person exercising doesn't feel a thing, nor is performance negatively affected.

Keep in mind these general guidelines for eating before exercise: The longer you have, the more you can eat; the closer you are to the start of your workout, the more important it is to choose carbohydrate. Eating at least an hour before exercise should allow your glucose and insulin levels to normalize before you head out the door. If you don't have that much time, say before an early morning training ride, run, or swim workout, try to eat or drink something containing readily digestible carbohydrate, such as a glass of juice or sports drink, an energy gel, or even a piece of toast with jam, as close to the start of exercise as you can.

This preexercise carbohydrate may be just the fuel you need to finish strongly, because—depending on when you last ate—your liver glycogen stores can be cut in half by the time the morning rolls around. Remember, your body breaks down liver glycogen to keep your blood sugar level constant—during the day, while you're sleeping, and during exercise. Liver glycogen also provides extra fuel to working muscles. Being well fed during exercise keeps your brain happy. The pool won't feel quite as cold; the wind won't feel quite as strong.

Eating before exercise: the longer you have, the more you can eat; the closer you are, reach for some carbohydrate.

If you have:	Choose:	Containing:
3 hr–4 hr	Meal	Carbohydrate, protein, fat
2 hr	Minimeal or snack	Carbohydrate, protein
1 hr	Fluids	Carbohydrate
5 min–10 min	Fluids or energy gel	Carbohydrate

You'll also benefit from staying adequately hydrated. Many athletes walk around in a chronically dehydrated condition, especially if they train in the heat more than once a day or complete long exercise bouts on successive days. (Being in an air-conditioned environment all day doesn't let you off the hook, because that comfortable environment may make acclimatizing to the heat more difficult.) Weighing yourself before and after exercise (especially during warm weather) is an easy way to monitor how well you are matching your fluid losses. Any weight loss following exercise represents fluid lost as sweat or urine. If you progressively lose weight over the course of a few days, you're most likely dehydrated. Replace every pound lost during daily exercise with at least 2.5 cups (replace every kilogram lost with at least 1.3 liters) of fluid as soon as possible, or better yet, try to consume that amount of fluid while you exercise. Incidentally, you should be able to urinate before and after you exercise. If you're unable to do so or your urine is dark yellow, work on drinking more throughout the day and while you exercise.

Strategies During Workouts

You don't need to worry about the effect of consuming carbohydrate *during* exercise. Other hormones released during exercise suppress insulin production and single out muscles as the main recipient of glucose. This way, the sports drinks and any carbohydrate-rich foods that you consume during exercise help stabilize your blood sugar and provide additional fuel to working muscles, extending the limited glycogen stores of the body. You definitely need to plan to consume carbohydrate if you will be engaged in continuous exercise lasting 60 to 90 minutes or longer, especially if you'll be pushing the pace or really exerting yourself.

Hitting the Wall and Bonking

Remember, if you eat a normal athlete's diet with about 60 percent of your calories from carbohydrate, you can store 1,400 to 1,800 calories worth of glycogen in your muscles on any given day. An athlete can burn through that in one to three hours of moderate- to high-intensity continuous exercise. When muscle glycogen stores become depleted during exercise, a situation typically referred to as hitting the wall, muscle fibers lack the fuel needed for contraction and fatigue takes over. Depleted muscle glycogen stores force you to reduce your pace drastically and may even prevent you from finishing what you set out to do. Sure, your body continues to burn fat, but it can't turn it into energy quickly enough. If you've ever watched or run a marathon, you may have witnessed even top athletes shutting down and basically shuffling to the finish, running on almost-empty muscle glycogen reserves.

Your blood sugar level during exercise depends on a balance between the release of glucose by the liver and the uptake of glucose by the muscles. Keep in mind that glucose is the sole source of energy for the brain and nervous system. If exercise continues to the point that the liver can no longer release glucose fast enough to fuel the brain and working muscles, you're in real trouble. Your body needs some carbohydrate to burn as a pilot light while burning fat as the main fuel. What happens if no carbohydrate exists to prime the engine? Your nervous system shuts down, making exercise difficult, if not impossible. Now you know what it means to bonk.

Because your brain isn't receiving enough energy to function properly, you feel irritable, lose focus, and find it difficult to concentrate. You may become dizzy, disoriented, and even hallucinate. Your vision begins to close in, and maintaining your balance becomes difficult. When you bonk, molehills turn into insurmountable mountains. Feeling miserable, you can easily make a costly error, such as taking a wrong turn or riding your bike right off the road, or find yourself forced to stop altogether.

The length and intensity of your chosen activity will dictate what foods and fluids you need to consume during exercise. Stopping to eat a sports bar during a 45-minute run doesn't make much sense, but having a bunch on hand for a daylong ski fest does. Dehydration, hitting the wall, and bonking don't happen only during prolonged races and adventures. Every time you head out the door you need to be prepared to battle two major foes: dehydration and glycogen depletion.

Meeting Your Fluid Needs During Workouts

The loss of body fluids, typically referred to as dehydration, can stop you in your tracks long before your fuel reserves run low. If you exercise, you'll sweat, especially on a warm day, which can mean a loss of as much as 2 to 4 pounds (.9 to 1.8 kilograms) of water per hour. As the water content of the body drops, blood volume drops, which means that the heart pumps less blood with every beat and less blood is delivered to exercising muscles and the skin. Muscles receive less oxygen, and waste products, such as lactic acid, build up. The core temperature of the body rises because less heat is being carried (in the blood) to the skin where it can evaporate as sweat. Your body attempts to compensate by working harder. Your heart rate increases as much as seven extra beats per minute for each 1 percent loss in body weight due to dehydration.

Athletes of all abilities battle the fatigue associated with dehydration as an elevated body temperature and increased heart rate take their toll. Studies have shown that athletes slow down by about 2 percent for each 1 percent loss in body weight. For example, a 150-pound (68-kilogram) runner would slow down by 4 percent after sweating off only 3 pounds (1.4 kilograms) of water (2 percent loss in body weight). At a pace of eight minutes per mile (five minutes per kilometer), slowing down by 4 percent means an additional 20 seconds per mile (12.4 seconds per kilometer). Greater losses, in the range of 6 to 10 percent of body weight, can lead to life-threatening conditions such as heat exhaustion and heat stroke (see chapter 14).

Even being mildly dehydrated can affect your ability to make decisions and perform complex skills. Keep that in mind the next time you head out on your bike to bomb down a route with hairpin curves at 45 miles (72 kilometers) per hour, or negotiate a trail in the dark, or need to get yourself to safety under whiteout conditions. Dehydration also increases your risk for stomach problems, even vomiting, because it slows the rate at which fluids empty the stomach and move to the intestinal tract for absorption.

Although your risk for dehydration increases the longer you push your body to perform, you need to stay on top of your fluid needs every time you exercise. The closer your fluid intake comes to matching your sweat losses, the better you will feel and perform. Unfortunately, left to their own devices, most athletes don't do a very good job, ingesting only half to two-thirds of the fluid that they need. The following guidelines on drinking during workouts apply to all endurance athletes. Be prepared, however, to do some experimenting to find a program that suits the specific needs of your activity or sport. For additional condition-specific recommendations, see chapters 9 through 16.

What You Should Drink

Water is acceptable for workouts lasting 30 to 60 minutes. Ingesting a flavored beverage, such as a sports drink, shouldn't do any harm and can be a plus if it leads you to consume more fluid. If you plan to be on the move at a moderate to fast pace for longer than 60 to 90 minutes, use a sports drink. Sports drinks designed for use during exercise provide modest amounts of carbohydrate (6 to 8 percent) and electrolytes (for example, sodium). The carbohydrate extends your limited glycogen stores and may be just what you need to finish workouts strongly. Sodium helps you absorb and retain water and stimulates you to drink more.

Although dehydration is still the most common foe, hyponatremia (low blood sodium) is a real possibility if you exercise continuously for three to four hours or longer, especially in hot, humid weather. This condition, which causes you to become confused and disoriented, and possibly faint, arises if you rely only on water or other low-sodium drinks to replace your fluid losses during prolonged exercise bouts. Because the body can lose substantial amounts of both sodium and fluid through sweating, drinking plain water dilutes the remaining sodium in the blood to a dangerously low level.

The sodium supplied by sports drinks (and foods eaten before or during exercise) is usually enough to protect most athletes from hyponatremia during endurance exercise. If you sweat excessively, have had problems in the heat, or will have access only to plain water, you may need to experiment with salt or electrolyte tablets. (For more information on preventing hyponatremia and taking salt tablets, see chapters 5 and 14.)

When You Should Drink

As a rule, you should drink at least every 15 to 20 minutes from the start of your workout. Follow a predetermined drinking schedule instead of relying solely on thirst. If you wait until you feel thirsty, you've waited too long. The goal is to minimize the effects of dehydration instead of trying to reverse it later. Athletes often falsely blame their sports drink for causing stomach upset or diarrhea when dehydration may be the real culprit. Dehydration slows the movement of fluids out of the stomach and their subsequent absorption from the intestinal tract. You can get caught in a self-perpetuating cycle in which you become increasingly dehydrated because you avoid drinking something that you believe is causing the discomfort. If need be, set an alarm on your watch as a reminder to drink frequently.

Be especially diligent when exercising in warm weather and during activities that jostle the stomach, such as running. Cold-weather events and sports during which you maintain a relatively stable or horizontal position, such as swimming or cycling, tend to present less risk for developing abdominal pain and diarrhea.

How Much You Should Drink

As a rule, drink 2 to 8 ounces (60 to 250 milliliters) at a time. Think in terms of gulps instead of ounces. For most adults, one gulp equals roughly 1 ounce (30 milliliters). For younger athletes, two gulps equal roughly 1 ounce. Most standard water bottles hold 20 ounces (600 milliliters). The amount that you will need to drink during exercise is highly individual. We all sweat at different rates, and the rate at which fluids (and food) empty the stomach also varies widely among individuals. Your fluid requirements will also depend on the weather and how fit you are to deal with it.

Try to begin exercise with the largest volume that you can comfortably tolerate and continually refill your stomach as a portion of this empties. Larger volumes of fluid (for example, 8 ounces) tend to empty from the stomach faster, as do colder fluids.

How to Tell Whether You're Drinking the Right Amount

Weigh yourself before and after exercise. Fluid losses should be modest, a few pounds (a kilogram) at most. If you lose more than that, you need to do a better job of rehydrating while you are exercising. To determine whether you're drinking enough during exercise bouts lasting several hours, monitor your ability to urinate and the color of your urine. It should be pale yellow, not as clear as water or dark yellow like straw. Weighing more after you exercise or feeling increasingly bloated during exercise (with rings and watches getting tighter) indicates that you are drinking too much and increasing your risk of developing hyponatremia. If you're struggling or simply want to improve in this area, make the time now to determine your individual sweat rate (see page 80).

How to Drink While on the Move

Because going without fluid isn't an option for endurance athletes, you need to become proficient at meeting your fluid needs without expending a lot of energy. Practice simple techniques, such as drinking on the run. Grab a paper cup and pinch it slightly on the sides to create a funnel from which to drink or add handles to your water bottles. On a bike, grip the handlebar next to the stem when reaching for your water bottle to avoid veering or swerving as you ride one-handed. Endurance swimmers must master drinking while doing a resting backstroke.

Adventure racers can conserve energy by sharing water bottles when traveling in single file while walking or running. Reach forward to grab the water bottle from the carrier worn by the person in front of you, instead of struggling to reach around your back. (Obviously, the first person in line must drink from his or her own bottle, but you should be swapping the lead anyway!)

Situations in which you need to carry your own fluids (such as long rides and runs and backcountry travel) present an extra challenge. Experiment with hip-mounted water-bottle carriers, fluid belts, sport vests, or fluid-toting bladders worn backpack style (for example, a Camelbak) to determine what works and what doesn't.

How to Estimate Average Hourly Sweat Rate
to Minimize Fluid Loss During Exercise Without Overdrinking

Preexercise weight − postexercise weight (in pounds or kilograms) + fluid intake during the activity (in ounces or liters) = individual hourly sweat rate

Notes

1. Body weight pre- and post-exercise is taken in the nude.
2. Every pound lost equals 16 ounces of fluid; every kilogram lost equates to approximately one liter of fluid.
3. This formula assumes no urine output during this period.

Example One

Preexercise weight: 60 kilograms

Postexercise weight: 58.5 kilograms

Volume of fluid consumed during exercise: 1 liter (1 kilogram)

Exercise duration: two hours

1. Fluid deficit in the body: 60 kilograms − 58.5 kilograms = 1.5 kilograms or 1.5 liters
2. Total sweat loss: 1.5 liters + 1 liter (consumed during exercise) = 2.5 liters
3. Sweat rate (liters/hour) = 2.5 liters/2 hours = 1.25 liters/hour
4. Drink to match sweat losses = .31 liters (310 milliliters) every 15 minutes

Example Two

Preexercise weight: 140 pounds

Postexercise weight: 139.5 pounds

Volume of fluid consumed during exercise: 24 ounces

Exercise duration: one hour

1. Fluid deficit in the body: 140 pounds − 139.5 pounds = .5 pounds or ~ 8 ounces
2. Total sweat loss: 8 ounces + 24 ounces (consumed during exercise) = 32 ounces
3. Sweat rate (ounces/hour) = 32 ounces/1 hour
4. Drink to match sweat losses = ~8 ounces every 15 minutes

Why a Smart Athlete Chooses to Put in the Effort

First, keeping your body hydrated proves that you really do respect it and want to treat it well. Second, you drink because you want to enjoy your workout and get the most out of it. Third, you accept the need to drink because this is the time to practice any fluid-replacement strategies that you intend to rely on during important events or race situations.

Some Other Tips to Keep in Mind

Pouring water over your head or body or using sponges can help you feel cooler and provide a psychological boost, but it doesn't help you stay hydrated. Given the option of drinking or pouring fluid over your head—drink it.

Drinking carbohydrate-containing beverages during intense exercise or competitions (as well as before and after) appears to lessen the effect of stress hormones on your immune system, which may help protect you against colds and other upper-respiratory infections.

Your sensation of thirst always lags behind the body's need for fluid. Cold weather further depresses thirst, so adhere to a predetermined drinking schedule when exercising in cold weather. You lose a substantial amount of fluid on cold, dry days through rapid breathing (expired air contains water) and sweating, especially if you're working intensely and wearing the proper amount of clothing for the cold. Other confounding factors include exercising at altitude and on windy days when sweat evaporates so quickly that you may not realize how much fluid you are losing.

Drinking fruit juice and defizzed soft drinks during exercise may increase your risk for nausea, cramps, or diarrhea because of their high sugar content (10 to 12 percent carbohydrate). Some athletes dilute them to half strength with water or ice. If you can tolerate it, however, fruit juice or a defizzed soft drink could provide a welcome change from sports drinks during long workouts and races. Be aware that these beverages contain minimal sodium and that cola drinks may contain more caffeine than you may want.

If you will be traveling into the backcountry (ski trips, hikes, trail runs, adventure race practices), check beforehand on the quality and availability of water along the way. No matter how clean the water looks, you need to protect yourself from microorganisms, which can cause significant gastrointestinal problems. Educate yourself on how to use a water filtration device and iodine and neutralizing tablets (in case your filter breaks) to purify backcountry water sources. Water filters and iodine treatment kits are available at stores that sell camping or outdoor adventure gear. Water bottles that contain small filters are also available, but they weigh considerably more than a standard water bottle. Be prepared to lug at least two to three quarts of water per person per day if no water is available.

Meeting Your Fuel Needs During Workouts

If you're eating every three to four hours and timing your meals and snacks around your workouts (for example, eating within a reasonable time frame before and after you exercise), you should have plenty of glycogen stored in your muscles and liver to handle workouts lasting an hour or less. People used to think that sports drinks wouldn't improve an athlete's performance in exercise bouts as short as an hour because we have enough glycogen to last about one and a half to two hours of hard exercise. Researchers have found, however, that taking in carbohydrate and water may be more beneficial than ingesting water alone. One study looked at cyclists who pedaled intensely (80 percent of maximal effort) for 50 minutes and then tried to kick the last several minutes. Cyclists who consumed 6 ounces (175 milliliters) of a sports beverage were 6 percent faster than cyclists who consumed 6 ounces of water. Cyclists who consumed 32 ounces (1 liter) of the sports beverage were an additional 6 percent faster, or 12 percent faster than those who only drank water. Drinking a sports beverage is worth testing in prerace situations, such as interval workouts or other short, intense efforts, to see whether it works for you. If your performance improves, consider whether the improvement is enough to offset the time that it takes to drink and the extra weight if you must carry the beverage.

As the time that you plan to be on the move exceeds 60 to 90 continuous minutes at a moderate or faster pace, you will have to monitor the need of your body for extra fuel in addition to staying on top of your fluid needs. Drinking or eating carbohydrate-rich foods during prolonged exercise is crucial on two accounts: to maintain an adequate blood sugar level and to provide an extra source of fuel for working muscles. Establishing and practicing an effective refueling routine in training is the key to being successful in endurance races.

A properly formulated sports drink (6 to 8 percent carbohydrate plus sodium) should definitely be part of your refueling plan for longer events and competitions, so you need to practice with one now. Sports drinks are the most practical way to get the carbohydrate and fluid that you need during exercise that exceeds 60 minutes. High-carbohydrate beverages, such as Ultra Fuel, and liquid food supplements, such as Ultramet and Metabolol Endurance, are generally best used before and after, but not during, exercise.

The high carbohydrate concentration of these beverages (along with the fat and protein) means that they empty from the stomach more slowly, which increases your risk of dehydration, nausea, cramps, and diarrhea. Ultra-endurance athletes often include them during long-duration events, though, when the need for calories is almost as high as the need for fluid. Although research is building that including a small amount of protein in sports drinks used before or after exercise is helpful, the evidence is far less compelling for including protein during exercise. If your favorite sports drink includes protein and you tolerate it well during exercise, go with it. If not, don't worry that you're missing out.

Other carbohydrate-rich foods, such as energy gels and bars, fruit, candy, cookies, bagels, and other solid foods, can be equally effective at supplying carbohydrate (as well as various amounts of sodium) during extended bouts of exercise, and they can help you feel more satisfied than drinking just fluids.

Foods with low water content such as cookies and energy bars are compact and easy to carry, but they can be difficult to chew when you're working hard. On top of that, solids take longer to empty the stomach, which could lead to more intestinal problems, especially if you're running. Remember, the most important nutrient that you need during exercise is water. Solid foods (including semiliquid energy gels) don't help in that regard, so you will have to drink plenty of fluid along with these foods.

The following guidelines for refueling during workouts apply to all endurance athletes. Every athlete, however, should be prepared to develop (and practice) his or her own unique refueling plan for undertaking endurance events and competing in endurance races. Read Chapters 9 through 16 for additional condition-specific recommendations.

When You Should Refuel

To delay fatigue, you need to replace carbohydrate throughout exercise before your muscle glycogen reserves become depleted. Don't wait until you begin feeling poorly or can't maintain your pace. Begin supplementing with carbohydrate immediately (within the first 30 minutes) if you know that you will be moving (at a moderate to fast pace) for 60 to 90 minutes or longer. Do what you can to protect what is usually an endurance athlete's weak link at some point—the stomach. Try to drink and eat (if applicable) small amounts continually.

How Much You Should Take In

The general rule is to consume 30 to 60 grams of carbohydrate every hour that you exercise. Sports drinks supply fluids and carbohydrate simultaneously. Most supply 14 to 20 grams of carbohydrate (50 to 80 calories) per 1-cup serving or 35 to 50 grams per one standard 20-ounce water bottle (140 to 200 calories). The longer you're on the move, the more your body will need a readily available supply of fuel of at least 200 to 300 calories per hour. Aim for 60 grams or more of carbohydrate per hour in the latter stages of long (over four hours) workouts.

Options for Refueling While on the Move

Sports drinks and sports foods like energy gels (25 grams of carbohydrate per packet) and bars (20 to 50 grams) are the easiest and most convenient ways to refuel while on the move. Many exercisers and athletes find that sports drinks made with maltodextrins (small glucose chains) are more palatable because they taste less sweet. Depending on your activity, however, any familiar and well-tolerated solid or liquid carbohydrate-rich food can help you meet the need, such as a banana (30 grams of carbohydrate), one-quarter cup of raisins (30 grams), or a meal replacement beverage (20 to 50 grams per 8 ounces). Other options for temporarily boosting a falling blood sugar level include hard candy, glucose tablets, sport jelly bellies, fruit juice, and nondiet soda.

As you go longer, listen to your body and eat what you crave or can keep down. Many athletes perform perfectly well eating foods and drinking fluids that fall outside the established guidelines. Getting down some type of nourishment is better than consuming nothing during endurance exercise.

How to Avoid Gastrointestinal Problems

To get a handle on how to meet your carbohydrate and calorie needs while avoiding intestinal problems, you simply have to experiment in training, ideally under conditions similar to any upcoming race or event. This is a trial-and-error endeavor. How much and how frequently you need to eat to maintain a readily available supply of blood glucose for fuel varies widely among individuals. If you participate in several sports (for example, a triathlon) you'll need to develop and practice strategies for each activity.

Again, pay particular attention to your fluid needs early on. Dehydration wreaks havoc with your gastrointestinal tract and isn't an immediately reversible situation. Practice drinking ample amounts of a sports drink and then supplementing with solid foods (if applicable) as the duration of your workout increases. If you've got a really sensitive stomach, beware of caffeine and fructose, a form of sugar found in fruit, honey, and products made with high-fructose corn syrup (including some energy bars). Even small amounts can cause some athletes abdominal distress and diarrhea.

What You Need to Know About Energy Gels

Energy gels need to be taken with water; otherwise, they end up as a thick syrup sitting in your stomach. Ideally, to produce an absorbable sports drink that falls into the optimal 6 to 8 percent carbohydrate range, try to drink at least 6 to 8 ounces of *water* with every packet of energy gel that you consume. You can carry the contents of three to five gel packets in a small, plastic closeable container that you can clip onto your shorts or store in a bike jersey pocket until you need it. For backcountry adventures, get a refillable tube (like a toothpaste tube) from a camping supply store that you can fill yourself.

Another energy food option for long outings is Shot Bloks® offered by Clif Bar®. These simple-to-handle, easy-to-chew jellylike blocks provide similar nutrition to a gel (three blocks provide 24 grams of carbohydrate and 100 calories) and can make tracking your caloric intake easy and fun.

How to Replace Electrolytes

Sodium appears to be the most important electrolyte that endurance athletes need to monitor. Sodium supplied by the foods that we eat daily, as well as sports drinks and sports foods consumed during exercise, will satisfy the needs of most exercisers. If you're a heavy sweater, have had problems dealing with heat in the past, or engage in outings that last four hours or longer, you may need to experiment with consuming extra sodium, as in actual table salt; salty foods like soup, tomato juice, pickles, and pretzels; or electrolyte tablets. (See chapter 5 for more information on electrolyte tablets.)

Why A Smart Athlete Chooses to Put in the Effort

You work diligently to refuel because you want to complete and enjoy as much as possible what you set out to do.

You also want to decrease your risk of getting injured or coming down with an upper-respiratory infection afterward by avoiding prolonged periods of low blood sugar during exercise. If competing is in your plans, accept that you must first practice in training what you're going to do during the race. You need to train your stomach just as you train your muscles and your brain. This is the time to develop a cache of tried-and-true foods that are familiar (that is, they passed the test in training) and enjoyable to eat during exercise.

For workouts that include teammates or partners, you realize that others are depending on you and you want to send a strong message that you're committed to doing your part. Last but not least, getting yourself (and others) home or back to the car safely can literally be a matter of life and death. A well-fueled brain and the ability to think clearly and solve problems while on the move could be the definitive factor during endurance outings.

Other Tips to Keep in Mind

Exercising under extreme conditions, such as heat and humidity, cold, and at altitude, also boosts the body's need for carbohydrate and calories. You'll need extra calories to counter an increased metabolic rate at altitude (especially for extended stays), with an emphasis on carbohydrate as your skeletal muscles shift to relying more on carbohydrate for fuel than they do fat. In cold weather, muscle glycogen, supplemented with carbohydrate-rich foods and fluids, remains the most important fuel. Exercising in the heat (especially if you're not acclimated) increases the rate at which you burn muscle glycogen. (For specific strategies for exercising in extreme conditions, see chapters 14 through 16).

Consuming carbohydrate during exercise is particularly important in certain situations. Relatively speaking, supplemental carbohydrate appear to be more critical during prolonged cycling (two hours or longer) than during prolonged running or walking. You may have a harder time maintaining your blood glucose level when cycling because a smaller active muscle mass uses glucose at a faster rate. Eat often instead of loading up every few hours. Eat by your watch when fatigue or sleep deprivation dampens your appetite. For example, snack every 20 to 30 minutes, aiming for 125 to 200 calories each time (for example, one or two bananas, or three or four fig bars).

Learn to recognize the signs and symptoms of bonking, or hypoglycemia (low blood sugar). If you or a teammate (or an athlete whom you coach) is acting exceptionally irritable, combative, disoriented, indecisive, or lethargic, suspect hypoglycemia. For the quickest relief, stop and immediately ingest rapidly absorbable carbohydrate, such as a sports drink, soft drink or juice, a packet of energy gel, glucose tablets, sugar cubes, or candy (gumdrops, jelly beans, and so on). If you have only energy bars or other solid food on hand, eat those. Pay extra attention to your food and fluid intake from that point on and keep an eye on susceptible individuals in your group. During exercise in the cold, hypoglycemia impairs shivering, thereby increasing the risk of hypothermia (low body temperature).

After you have a defined eating and drinking program in place, be flexible and keep an open mind. Your tastes may change after hours of exercise, during warm weather, or at altitude. You may need to abandon your intention to eat wholesome fruits and sports bars and instead try M&Ms and potato chips. Forcing the same routine or giving up on eating altogether usually spells disaster.

Develop a taste for a liquid meal replacement product if you're training for a single-day ultraendurance event, such as a 100-mile running race, or a multiday or multistage event, such as a hut-to-hut ski trip or the Race Across America (RAAM) individual and team cycling race. When you feel exhausted or have no appetite, liquid meals are easier to consume than solid food is. They make good prerace meals and reduce the need to defecate. You first need to become accustomed to drinking liquid meals during long training efforts. Foods containing moderate amounts of fat and protein can also help satisfy cravings and provide a much needed psychological boost during ultraendurance outings.

Have a long chat with yourself if you have any doubt about the value of drinking and eating during endurance events and races. Be prepared for the little voice in your head that squawks, "You're wasting time," when you think about slowing down or stopping to drink and eat, especially in the early stages when everything is going well. Switch over to a new mental tape, the one that says, "I'm increasing my chances of going faster or farther or both."

Does Coke Make the Grade as a Sports Drink?

You've seen it happen. An athlete at the top of his or her game drinks Coke during a long race. Is it a smart idea or just something the good guys (and gals) can get away with? One year, to see just how many athletes rely on Coke as a sports drink, researchers at the Australian Institute of Sport surveyed 11 of the 19 men's cycling teams in the U.S. Professional Championships. How widespread was the use of Coke? Every athlete on 6 of the 11 teams and almost two-thirds of the riders on 4 other teams drank Coke. Only one team went for the gold without the beverage in the red and white can. Most of the athletes drank the Coke defizzed in the last half of the two- to six-hour-long competitions. Fast forward 10 years and not much has changed. Despite the bevy of sports drinks on the market, endurance athletes are still reaching for cola drinks.

When it comes to being a winning sports drink, Coke appears barely qualified to enter the contest. It contains excessive carbohydrate (11 percent), limited electrolytes, carbonation, acidity, and artificial colors. Why then does the stuff continue to be the drink of choice for many endurance athletes? Does the science back up the athletes who say that it works? Obviously, Coke supplies performance-enhancing carbohydrate, but the real appeal is most likely the caffeine (30 to 45 milligrams in a 12-ounce can). Ditto for Mountain Dew (55 milligrams) and drinks like Red Bull (80 milligrams). Caffeine has been shown to reduce fatigue and enhance muscle strength at the end of exhaustive exercise by working on the nervous system or perhaps by stimulating muscles. And that's not the only good news for athletes who drink Coke during exercise. Research has shown that carbonation doesn't substantially interfere with the rate at which fluids empty the stomach to be absorbed, nor does caffeine taken during exercise act as a diuretic and increase the need to urinate (as it can before or after exercise).

Scientific studies have shown caffeine to enhance performance in a variety of sport situations. Since being dropped from the International Olympic Committee's banned drug list, caffeine vies with creatine as the hottest legal ergogenic aid available to competitive athletes. Caffeine was once thought to help endurance athletes perform better by promoting the release of free fatty acids from muscle and fat stores (thereby conserving muscle glycogen), although scientists no longer believe this to be true. Caffeine most likely works by helping the body maintain better blood glucose levels (energy for muscles and the brain) and by stimulating the release of two powerful hormones, epinephrine and norepinephrine, which helps increase blood sugar levels and enhance the strength of muscular contractions.

Coke certainly isn't the ideal sports beverage for everyone (and it's not a great everyday choice), but keep the following points in mind if you like the taste of it and want to try it during prolonged exercise. Diluting Coke with a sports drink (which many athletes do) or water will lower the carbohydrate concentration into the desired range. Drinking it defizzed is the safest and most comfortable way to go, especially if you're running. When it comes to the amount of Coke that you need to consume, researchers have shown that a far smaller dose (1.5 milligrams per kilogram, or .7 milligrams per pound) than originally thought, when taken in the latter stages of endurance exercise, can produce a worthwhile performance boost. Regular caffeine users, however, may not get the same jolt that caffeine neophytes do from the modest amount of caffeine in Coke. Keep in mind that Coke is also low in the sodium department (only 50 milligrams per 12-ounce can). On the other hand, if you strongly believe that swigging the stuff helps you perform better, you may get the lift that you've been looking for.

Adapted from O. Anderson, 1998, "Athletes use Coca-Cola as sports drink, but does running really go better with Coke®?," *Running Research News* 14(6), and D.T. Martin, 1997, "Coca-Cola preferred by top endurance cyclists," *Sportscience News*.

Recovering Your Fuel Needs After Workouts

Unfortunately, your job isn't done as you flop down on the sofa or stagger back to your car. You need to make some small efforts now to rehydrate and refuel to reap large dividends later, such as a faster recovery from your workout. Keep in mind that the effects of dehydration and muscle glycogen depletion are cumulative. If you plan to head back out in several hours, hit the road or trail again the next day, or just want to rejoin the land of the living quickly, you need to pay attention to your fluid and fuel needs even when you least feel like it. Exercising on dehydrated and depleted muscles increases your risk for soft-tissue injuries, and you can make poor decisions when you try to function in a depleted state.

Replacing both fluids and glycogen are the immediate priorities as you set about trying to recover and prepare for tomorrow. (Yes, there is a tomorrow.) Your muscles are most receptive to reloading glycogen in a 15- to 30-minute window immediately following exercise. The blood flow to muscles is enhanced immediately following exercise. Muscle cells can pick up more glucose and are more sensitive to the effects of insulin, a hormone that promotes the synthesis of glycogen (by moving glucose out of the bloodstream and into cells).

You may be able to boost the rate at which your muscles store glycogen, as well as speed up the recovery and repair of muscle fibers, by ingesting protein in combination with carbohydrate at this time. This carbohydrate–protein combo appears to produce a greater secretion of insulin than eating either carbohydrate or protein alone. Along with glucose, insulin also stimulates greater uptake of protein into muscle cells. Eating the exact right balance of protein and carbohydrate isn't necessary or even required (scientists haven't even definitively figured it out). A good rule of thumb is to consume one gram of protein per four grams of carbohydrate. By the way, chocolate milk fills the bill perfectly!

Because you will need at least 20 hours of refueling with carbohydrate-rich foods to replenish your muscle stores fully, you need to start as soon as possible. Don't neglect your fluid needs either (even when you do a good job during exercise, you can only hope to match 80 percent of what you lose by sweating) because you can suffer with headaches and nausea for hours after you finish simply because you're still dehydrated.

The following strategies will help all endurance athletes meet their fluid and refueling needs following exercise.

How Much You Should Drink to Rehydrate

Drink at least 2.5 cups of fluid for every pound you lost during exercise. Weighing yourself periodically in training (before and after exercise) can help you estimate how much fluid you typically sweat off. If you haven't urinated within a few hours after an endurance activity or you feel headachy or nauseous, you most likely need to concentrate on taking in more fluid.

Be careful not to consume copious amounts of plain water, however, because you also need to replenish electrolytes, especially sodium. Again, fluid replacement drinks containing sodium are a convenient option. Alcoholic beverages are a poor choice, particularly if you're dehydrated, so if you consume them do so only after you've filled up with adequate amounts of nonalcoholic beverages.

When You Should Refuel After Endurance Outings

After vigorous or prolonged bouts of exercise, whether you eat or drink your carbohydrate doesn't matter as long as you do it quickly. Aim to consume .5 to .75 grams of carbohydrate per pound (1.1 to 1.65 grams per kilogram) of body weight (at least 50 to 100 grams for most athletes) within the carbohydrate window, particularly the first 15 to 30 minutes (of the first 2 hours) immediately after you finish.

Just as you can't rely solely on thirst to tell you when you need to drink, don't wait until you feel hungry or your appetite returns to start the refueling process. The longer you wait to eat, the less glycogen you store and the longer it takes to recover. Intense or exhaustive exercise, especially in warm weather, depresses your appetite. You need to anticipate and prepare for a reduced appetite by having on hand foods that you like and can tolerate. A good rule to follow is to drink or eat at least 50 grams of carbohydrate as soon as possible after exercise and then follow up with a well-balanced meal within two hours or less.

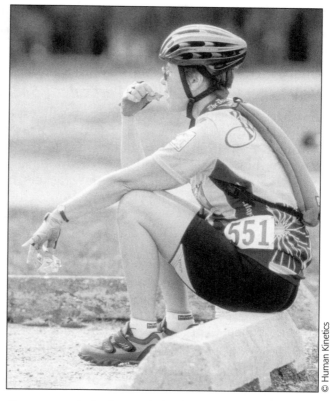

© Human Kinetics

Consume carbohydrate-rich foods and drinks immediately after the event to replenish glycogen stores.

What Options Exist for Refueling

Sports drinks are probably the most efficient and convenient way to meet your needs because they also provide both fluid and carbohydrate. Because most sports drinks intended for use during exercise (Gatorade, PowerBar Endurance, Cytomax, and so on) contain only 14 to 20 grams per cup, make sure that you drink enough of them or choose a high-carbohydrate sports drink (50 grams per cup), fruit juice (25 to 40 grams per cup), or, in a pinch, a nondiet soft drink (40 or more grams in a typical 12-ounce can). Low-fat milk shakes and smoothies will also do the trick.

The best recovery plan also includes eating carbohydrate-rich foods as soon as you can tolerate them. For example, ease in some postrecovery favorites, such as yogurt, pudding, fresh fruit, a milk shake, an energy or breakfast bar, or a bagel. Aim to consume an additional 50 to 100 grams of carbohydrate every two hours until your next full meal. Some healthy examples include a bagel with jam (about 50 grams), a banana with four fig bars (about 70 grams), a cup of yogurt with cereal stirred in (about 60 grams), or a baked potato (about 50 grams).

Carbohydrate-rich foods with moderate or high glycemic index ratings should, at least in theory, enhance glycogen storage after exercise. Examples of moderate and high glycemic index foods include ripe bananas, mangoes, orange juice, sports drinks, cornflakes and muesli cereals, white rice, oatmeal, baked and instant mashed potatoes, cooked carrots, white or wheat bread, jelly beans, and ice cream. (Refer to table 4.1 for more options.)

How to Replace Electrolytes, Particularly Sodium

Go ahead and satisfy your cravings for salt, especially if you've lost substantial weight during exercise or if you're a heavy sweater. The salt will help you hold onto fluid and stimulate you to drink more. Use salt on foods at meals and include salty foods, such as soup, vegetable or tomato juice, salted pretzels and popcorn, pickles, low-fat crackers, baked goods, spaghetti sauce, and pizza. (If you have high blood pressure, check with your physician about consuming some salt following prolonged bouts of exercise or during periods of hot weather.)

How to Add Protein During the Recovery Period

Plenty of recovery drinks with protein are now available for use following exercise, but you can get the job done just as easily by drinking a glass of milk or eating a cup of yogurt. Including small portions of meat, poultry, or fish at your next meal (3 ounces, or 85 grams, the size of a deck of cards, provides 20 to 25 grams of protein) can also do the trick. For example, a postrace meal of rice with a small portion of chicken, a bowl of cereal with milk, a bagel with a thick slice of cheese and a piece of fruit, or a tuna sandwich with a piece of fruit provides the optimal combination of carbohydrate and protein.

Complete meal replacement products such as Ensure and Boost and other liquid food supplements such as Metabolol II and GatorPro are another convenient option. These products provide a balance of energy nutrients with approximately 40 to 70 percent carbohydrate, 15 to 30 percent protein, and 5 to 25 percent fat. Choose one whose taste you enjoy.

Why A Smart Athlete Chooses to Make the Effort

Replenishing your fuel stores after workouts signifies that you respect your body and want to treat it well. You understand the value of training consistently, especially if you're serious about preparing for a particular endurance race or event. By refueling promptly, you acknowledge that smart day-to-day nutritional recovery habits lessen your risk of becoming injured or catching a cold. You also want to feel good afterwards and have enough energy to do something other than lie around on the couch for the rest of the day (or significant others want this for you). Basically, you refuel after a workout because you're committed to doing whatever it takes to be ready to get out there again tomorrow.

Keep Written Notes on Your Refueling Plan

Even if you want to forget the whole experience of the outing or workout, quickly jotting down some notes immediately following it will help you prepare for and succeed in future endurance endeavors. As soon as you can, record fluid and refueling strategies that worked well (for example, one bottle of sports drink and one energy gel per hour) and those that didn't (cookies were too dry or the cold made the candy bars too hard to eat). Note how your tastes and cravings changed as the time that you exercised progressed. Write down any intestinal problems that you incurred, note your ability to handle the elements, and list the drinks or foods that you want to have available next time.

Strategies Before Long Events and Races

Congratulations! After months of deliberation, you finally registered for that killer century ride, mountain run, or your first triathlon. Now that the check is in the mail, it's time to start eating smart. Here is a preevent or prerace nutritional countdown that will get you to the starting line a step ahead of the competition.

In Advance (Weeks to Months)

The best way to prepare for a long event or race is to do some backward planning. You can't get the job done by stuffing in some pasta the night before or waiting until the race to experiment with a new food or sports drink. Make the most of your daily food choices and workouts. Just as you experiment with and develop new mental and motor skills in training, you need to experiment with sports foods, including drinks, bars, and gels, to establish the types and amounts that you will tolerate in competition or under stressful conditions. Do you really want to lug around your favorite sports bars only to find that they're hard as rocks and inedible because of the cold or that after being on the road for three hours you can no longer tolerate your favorite candy?

Learn what you can about your event before you arrive at the starting line. Talk to other participants and read race applications closely. Find out what will be provided at aid stations and what you will be expected or allowed to provide for yourself. Adventure races, for example, provide no outside assistance, whereas standard road-running races and cycling events supply fluids and foods along the way. If you don't currently use the sports drink that the organizers will provide, get used to it during your training. Familiarize yourself with the ever-expanding options for toting fluid and food, such as bladder systems, multiple-bottle waist belts, flask belts, and fluid reservoirs that affix directly to a bike. Rehearse drinking out of a bottle or grabbing cups and swallowing liquid on the move without choking. Your main job is to test in training what you plan to do during the race.

Travel, particularly to another time zone or country, can interfere with your preparations and routines. Gather information about restaurants, food stores, and other resources near your lodging and talk to athletes and coaches who have previously been to the area. If you're traveling into the backcountry, be sure that your water filtration device is in working order or have a supply of iodine and neutralizing tablets on hand. Scan outdoor and adventure travel magazines and cookbooks or visit your favorite camping store to research the latest options for lightweight, portable meals.

In some cases, you may find it advantageous to gain a few pounds of padding before you participate in an endurance activity. An extended stay at high altitude or a prolonged backcountry trekking or skiing trip can lead to extensive weight loss when you burn extreme amounts of calories with limited or inadequate options for proper refueling. An experienced mountaineering friend often reminisces about eating a stick of butter every couple of days during his final preparations for expeditions to Everest and other Himalayan adventures.

To put on weight before you depart, you need to increase the amount of calories that you consume or reduce the amount that you burn through physical activity. If you desire to gain lean weight (muscle mass), you will need to increase the amount of calories that you consume and engage in a substantial strength-training or weight-training program. Otherwise, most people can expect to gain a few pounds by eating larger portions of foods than they currently consume, adding more snacks or minimeals throughout the day and before bedtime, and supplementing with high-calorie foods such as commercial or homemade liquid meals or shakes. Tapering your training will also help you create and store excess calories.

Week Before the Event

The goal the week before endurance adventures and races lasting longer than 90 to 120 continuous minutes is to carbohydrate-load—a process of loading muscles with the glycogen that will be needed to fuel the activity. The greater your preexercise muscle glycogen stores, the greater your potential to perform well. What you may not know about smart carbohydrate loading is that it involves more than just eating some extra pasta and bread. Traditionally, endurance athletes prepared for long races by doing a long, hard effort seven days before their event. The scientific rationale behind this exhaustive bout of exercise was to reduce muscle glycogen stores intentionally because endurance training itself is known to provide a powerful stimulus for the resynthesis and storage of muscle glycogen.

After following a high-protein, high-fat, low-carbohydrate diet for the next few days (the depletion phase) while continuing to exercise (or at least trying to), endurance athletes then fed their by-now totally starved muscles a high-carbohydrate diet for the remaining three days before the race (loading phase). The muscles would rebound by stocking up on every gram of carbohydrate that they could get. Although this approach worked well for some athletes, timing it just right was challenging. Feeling poorly so close to an important event or race (which occurs during the low-carbohydrate depletion phase) is mentally taxing, and some athletes couldn't tolerate the growing stiffness and muscular discomfort associated with superpacked glycogen stores.

Today, a modified carbohydrate-loading regimen appears to be the way to go. This method has proved just as effective at maximizing muscle glycogen stores, and you're more likely to get it right. Skip the last strenuous exercise bout (unless it's part of your typical training program) and the depletion phase. With a week to go, gradually taper your training while eating your normal diet. For the last few days of the week, further reduce your training, perhaps even resting completely for one to three days, while consuming a high-carbohydrate diet, defined as up to 5 grams of carbohydrate per pound of body weight (10 grams per kilogram). Keep in mind that if you don't simultaneously cut back on your training, you run the risk of using the dietary carbohydrate that you hope to stockpile for the long event as fuel for your last few exercise sessions. This approach will help superload your muscles with glycogen, and it can increase endurance by about 20 percent. If your competitive season involves several races longer than 90 to 120 minutes and you cannot reduce your training each time for the full week, try to back off for at least the three days before the event and eat more carbohydrate than usual. You need about three days of eating a high-carbohydrate diet to achieve maximum glycogen stores.

Many athletes I meet hesitate to cut back their training or eat more carbohydrate-rich foods because they fear gaining weight or feeling heavy the week before a competitive event. You need to realize that gaining weight means that you are carbohydrate loading properly. Every gram of glycogen is stored with almost three grams of water, which can result in a gain of up to 5 pounds (2.5 kilograms). Remind yourself of the benefits of carbohydrate loading. You'll arrive at the starting line well fueled, and the extra fluid will help delay dehydration during the event. The stiffness and heavy legs that you may feel with glycogen loading will dissipate as you exercise. If the stiffness or heavy feeling is worrisome to you, take a rest day two days before the event (rather than the day before) and exercise lightly the day before the event.

You don't need to sit around and eat boxes of bonbons for three days either. Use your common sense. You don't even need to consume that much extra food because by cutting back on your exercise bouts, you will be expending fewer calories than normal. What does need to increase, however, is the proportion of your caloric consumption from carbohydrate. Although bonbons and other chocolate-covered treats provide carbohydrate in the form of sugar, they also contain a lot of fat and little else in the way of useful nutrition. You don't have to stop eating these familiar foods but save the extra helpings of high-fat candies, cookies, muffins, pastries, doughnuts, chips, and ice cream for after your event or race.

For example, if you typically consume 3,000 calories a day, with 60 percent of your calories coming from carbohydrate, you eat about 450 grams of carbohydrate a day. (Here's the math: .6 × 3,000 = 1,800 carbohydrate calories. 1,800 carbohydrate calories / 4 calories per gram = 450 grams of carbohydrate.) To boost your carbohydrate intake to 70 percent of your total calories, you would need to eat about 525 grams of carbohydrate. What should you eat to boost your carbohydrate intake? Concentrate on consuming ample servings of complex carbohydrates. Starchy foods, such as bread, cereal, rice, pasta, beans, and potatoes, and all types of fruit deliver plenty of carbohydrate (15 grams or more) in a relatively small amount of food—one additional slice of bread or one-half cup of fruit, for example. (See chapter 1 for more information about serving sizes.) Milk and yogurt weigh in next at 12 grams of carbohydrate per cup. If you're having trouble consuming enough carbohydrate from food group sources, add an energy bar or supplement what you eat with liquid carbohydrate, such as fruit juice, sports drinks, high-carbohydrate recovery drinks, or a meal replacement beverage.

The key is to load up on carbohydrate, not fat (see table 4.2, High-Carbohydrate, Low-Fat Meals). For instance, opt for low-fat frozen yogurt over premium high-fat ice cream, pasta with marinara sauce rather than Alfredo sauce, and thick-crust pizza topped with vegetables instead of meat. Check the nutrition facts label of your favorite snack foods too. As a rule, snacks that supply at least four grams of carbohydrate for every gram of fat can be considered low-fat, high-carbohydrate foods. A chocolate-covered doughnut, for example, doesn't fill the bill. It supplies only 21 grams of carbohydrate (40 percent carbohydrate) for 13 grams of fat (59 percent fat). A cup of instant pudding made with low-fat milk is a better choice, offering 56 grams of carbohydrate (75 percent carbohydrate) and five grams of fat (15 percent fat).

Carbohydrate loading will not help you run faster, but it can help you maintain your pace longer before tiring. If your race or event will last less than 90 continuous minutes, a 10K road race or one leg of a relay race, for example, you won't gain any advantage from carbohydrate loading. Eating normally, along with a substantial prerace meal, will ensure that you have enough glycogen on board to complete short-duration events and races.

If you will be on the move or engaged in low- to moderate-intensity endurance exercise for several hours, your fat stores can provide most of the energy that you need to perform, but only if you have enough carbohydrate on board to oxidize the fat. Fat loading with a week to go will not enable you to burn more fat, instead of glycogen, during endurance activities. In fact, eating too much fat makes it more difficult to load up on the carbohydrate that you definitely need. Aerobic training, of course, teaches your body to prefer fat and spare your limited glycogen reserves, but you can't influence that factor with only a week to go.

Be alert to situations or factors that can put you at additional risk for dehydration during the week leading into your long event or race. Running a low-grade fever, being nauseous and vomiting, menstruating, or having a sunburn can promote fluid loss. Other situations that increase your risk for dehydration include traveling by airplane, acclimating to altitude, and working out in hot and humid weather, especially if that isn't your normal training environment. Carry bottled water or a personal water bottle with you throughout the day to remind yourself to drink.

Keep an eye out for the early warning signs of dehydration: flushed skin, trouble tolerating the heat, feeling light-headed or unusually fatigued, loss of appetite, or being able to produce only small amounts of dark yellow urine. You want to be well hydrated without being overhydrated. Drink healthy beverages with your meals and snacks because the fluid will stay in your body longer rather than run right through you. Be sure to drink before you head out

Table 4.2 High-Carbohydrate, Low-Fat Meals

Waffles with fruit and syrup	Chili with beans
Bagel	Rice
Low-fat milk	Lemonade
	Sherbet

Cereal with banana and granola	Grilled chicken sandwich
Whole-wheat toast with jam	Baked potato
Orange juice	Iced tea
	Frozen fruit bar

Roast beef sandwich on whole-grain roll with tomato and lettuce	Pizza with mushrooms
Applesauce	Salad with veggies
Fruit juice	Breadsticks
Low-fat vanilla milk shake	Soft drink

Spaghetti with tomato sauce	Chicken on romaine salad with sliced apples
Garlic bread	Oatmeal raisin cookie
Garden veggie salad	Low-fat yogurt
Low-fat frozen yogurt	Soft drink
Low-fat milk	

Bean burrito	Turkey sub
Low-fat chips and salsa	Low-fat chips
Lemonade	Apple
	Sports drink

Pasta with vegetables	Rice with vegetables and black beans
Italian roll	Garden veggie salad
Strawberries	Fruit cup
Iced tea	Low-fat milk

Reprinted, by permission, from S. Nelson Steen, 1998, "Eating on the road: Where are the carbohydrates?," *Sports Science Exchange*, #71, 11(4): 1-5.

Carbohydrate Loading—Out With the Old and In With the New

It's a good idea to get advice from an endurance athlete who really knows what he's doing. Pete Pfitzinger fills the bill. During a career marked by consistency, the wily veteran was the top American finisher in two Olympic Marathons (2:13:53, 11th place in Los Angeles and 2:14:44, 14th place in Seoul, South Korea). Today, Pfitzinger is a sought-after exercise physiologist and coach. He serves as the director of the UniSports Centre for Sport Performance in Auckland, New Zealand.

The Old Days: "I did the full carbohydrate depletion and loading diet (three to four days of depletion, three to four days of loading) for 12 of my 18 marathons. The pattern for a Sunday morning marathon would be as follows: following a long depleting run (17 to 20 miles) the previous Sunday, I would start the depletion phase. For example, a big omelet for breakfast, tuna salad with mayonnaise for lunch, cashews and diet soda (a relative luxury) for a snack, most of a chicken and a salad with diet dressing for dinner. The carbohydrates were low, the calories pretty low, the protein content was high, and the fat content was fairly high also. I would taper my training back during the week and do most of my runs in the morning as I would be too tired to run in the afternoon or evening.

Wednesday I would run eight to nine miles, with the last three miles at close to race pace to burn off the last bits of glycogen, and I would start to load at either Wednesday dinner or following Thursday morning's run. Loading would consist of a lot of bread, pasta, rice, sweet potatoes, crackers, and cookies. It took a while to realize what was carbohydrate and what was fat. I gradually learned that lasagna was not a good option. I never experienced any particularly negative effects commonly associated with depleting and loading—maybe I was just lucky. The benefit of the depletion phase had a strong psychological component. I thought it worked and, perhaps more importantly, it made me think that if I adhered to it religiously that I deserved to run well in the marathon."

Now: "What I recommend today is a one-day depletion phase. The last week of training before a Sunday marathon looks like this: 13- to 14-mile run on Sunday, 6 miles on Monday and Tuesday, a minidepletion run on Wednesday of 8 miles with 3 miles close to marathon pace, followed by a 5-mile run before breakfast on Thursday morning. Then you start to carbohydrate load. [Lightly jog or rest completely on Friday and Saturday.] There is evidence this one-day depletion provides most of the stimulus of the longer depletion with little or no side effects such as the danger of becoming overtired during depletion or compromising your immune function from the extreme swing in nutrient composition. It also provides the mental reinforcement that the runner has done everything in preparation."

to exercise (1 to 2 cups, or 250 to 500 milliliters, of fluid 15 to 30 minutes before-hand), during exercise if need be (a couple gulps every 15 to 20 minutes), and enough afterwards to replace 150 percent of body weight lost during exercise (this translates into at least 2.5 cups for every "lost" pound, or about 1.5 liters for every kilogram). You should be able to urinate before and after exercise, and your urine should run pale yellow if you're properly hydrated. Alcoholic drinks, as well as caffeinated beverages for those who don't typically imbibe, promote loss of body fluids, setting the stage for dehydration and early fatigue. Alcohol negatively affects how the liver metabolizes carbohydrate as well.

Remember to consider how travel will affect your nutritional game plan. Most airlines can accommodate special requests if you notify them at least 48 hours in advance (even better, reserve a special meal when you make your airline reservation). Of course, your flight may not include a meal. Make your visits to airport concession stands worthwhile by choosing healthy low-fat, high-carbohydrate snacks such as frozen yogurt, unbuttered popcorn, bean burritos, baked potatoes, soft pretzels, bagels, fruit juices, low-fat milk and smoothies, and fresh or dried fruit. Another smart move is to pack your own supply of nonperishable foods. Depending on the destination and length of your trip, include such items as cold cereals, instant oatmeal, instant breakfast powders, low-fat cookies and crackers, pretzels, dried fruit, prepackaged puddings, granola, breakfast and energy bars, canned fruit or fruit juices, instant soups, a peanut butter and jelly (or honey) sandwich, bottled water, and sports drink powders, including high-carbohydrate and meal replacement options. If you need it to perform well, bring it with you.

International travel, in particular, can cause unwanted problems. Don't test your immune system after you arrive by experimenting with local "bugs." Drink only bottled water (even for brushing teeth), avoid swallowing shower or pool water, turn down ice cubes made from the local water supply when ordering beverages, and stick to familiar foods if possible. Your best bets are foods that have been well cooked, fruits that can be peeled (bananas, grape-fruit, oranges, kiwi, and mangoes), and prepackaged ready-to-eat items. Avoid salads and other uncooked foods that kitchen staff workers handle directly and abstain from milk and milk products if pasteurization and refrigeration practices are questionable.

Day Before the Event

The main goal when it comes to eating the day before your endurance adventure or race is to eat in a way that leaves you physically ready and mentally prepared. Top off your glycogen reserves and avoid any last-minute pitfalls. No experimenting! Trying new foods the day before an important race or event is risky. Jen, an avid runner I met while receiving physical therapy, learned this lesson the hard way. After diligently training for months for the Boston Marathon, including experimenting for the first time with using a sports drink, Jen was on pace to set a new PR when I left her office a few days before the marathon. When I paid her a visit the following week, I was shocked to hear that she didn't finish the race. Her enthusiastic friends and husband had taken her to a new ethnic restaurant the night before, and she awoke with stomach pains and diarrhea. She started the race but ended up dropping out at the eight-mile mark.

Keep it simple. Eat foods that you like and that you eat all the time. Eat them in normal-size amounts. Graze or eat frequently throughout the day, so that you don't feel as if you have to stuff yourself at the evening meal. Your last meal should be high in carbohydrate and contain modest amounts of fat and protein. A pasta dinner is a proverbial favorite, but it's not a magical meal. Choose foods that you feel comfortable with or that you believe enhance your performance. I routinely eat pizza before my races, dating back to my first year in college when my coach, Jack Bacheler, the ninth-place finisher in the 1972 Olympic Marathon, recommended it. Other elite athletes dine on baked potatoes, or fish or poultry with vegetables and rice. Choose what works best for you. You have enough on your mind at this point, so your last meal shouldn't be something that causes added anxiety.

Here are some other tips to keep in mind the day before the event:

- Drink a healthy beverage with every meal and snack. Don't overload with plain water. (See chapter 14 for a discussion on how overloading with water increases your risk of hyponatremia.)
- Avoid beans, broccoli, cabbage, radishes, and other gas-causing foods if you suffer from bowel problems.
- Avoid high-fiber foods such as raw fruits and vegetables with thick skins, bran cereals, nuts, and seeds.
- Avoid sugar substitutes like sorbitol and mannitol (in gums, candies, and other foods), which may cause diarrhea.
- Limit alcohol or avoid it altogether.
- Set out, prepare, and pack everything that you need. Don't wait until the morning of the race!
- Eat or drink a bedtime snack to squeeze in a few more calories and help you sleep better.

Morning of the Event

You don't want to be stuck in the bathroom when the gun goes off or hold back the group because you're running on empty after only the first hour. The most important step that you can take is eating a light to moderate prerace meal. If you've satisfied your carbohydrate and fluids needs throughout the week, you should be well hydrated and your muscle glycogen stores should be at their peak. Your liver glycogen stores, however, may be substantially depleted, especially if you were tossing and turning all night. Liver glycogen is converted back to glucose to maintain normal blood sugar (the fuel used by the brain) and provide fuel for exercising muscles, especially during prolonged endurance exercise. In other words, eating a meal before you compete helps you make wise decisions while you're on the move, like staying on course or remembering to change shoes between events.

Eating a single carbohydrate-rich meal can quickly restore your liver glycogen reserves to normal. Your job will be to find a happy medium in terms of the foods and the amounts that you can tolerate; you don't want to suffer from stomach problems or diarrhea, nor do you want to arrive at the starting line feeling hungry and light-headed. Choose familiar foods that you enjoy. I'll never forget my first international race, an all-women's 10K road race that took place in the United States. The Russian women downed a full breakfast of eggs, toast, and bacon, and they didn't seem to suffer one bit during the race. Obviously, they knew what they were doing. (Remember, you have plenty of opportunities to practice what you'll eat before an endurance endeavor or race. They're called training days.)

Plan to eat one to four hours before start time (you can always go back to bed after you eat), and aim for 50 grams of carbohydrate for each hour before the start. For example, down 150 grams of carbohydrate three hours before the race by eating a large bagel (50 to 60 grams) with jam (13 grams per tablespoon), 8 ounces of fruit yogurt (34 grams), and 16 ounces of fruit juice (50 to 60 grams). Some athletes feel satisfied longer if their prerace meal also contains higher-fat foods, such as peanut butter or cheese. Eat early enough, especially if you'll be exercising or competing intensely, because these meals take more time to empty the stomach. If you do well by eating closer to the starting time, make it a carbohydrate-rich snack (50 grams of carbohydrate), such as an energy bar (30 to 45 grams) or instant oatmeal (12 grams) with a medium banana (27 grams) and 8 ounces of low-fat milk (12 grams). Be sure to drink ample fluids with your meal. Aim for at least 2 cups of fluid two hours before exercise and another cup as close to the time of the race as practical.

If your stomach is tied in knots on race morning, or you have an ultra-sensitive stomach and simply cannot eat before prolonged exercise, make an effort to eat extra food the day before, including a substantial bedtime snack. Liquid meals, such as breakfast shakes, high-carbohydrate sports drinks, or meal replacement beverages (for example, Ensure or Boost) empty from the stomach faster than solid foods do and contain less fiber, which may cause discomfort during exercise. Liquid meals are usually well tolerated up to one to two hours before exercise and are handy if you are in transit or have an early start time.

If you shy away from eating before races because you seem sensitive to swings in blood sugar, try experimenting with a prerace meal based on low-glycemic, carbohydrate-rich foods, such as milk, flavored yogurt, whole-wheat bread, bran cereal, pasta, baked beans, apples, and oranges. High-glycemic, carbohydrate-rich foods eaten before exercise, such as honey, white bread, corn flakes, and sports drinks, may cause undesirable reactions in sensitive individuals (refer back to table 4.1).

What Is Available to Eat Out on the Trail?

Stacy Allison, the first American woman to reach the summit of Mount Everest, offers the following advice to day hikers and expedition-bound trekkers alike who set out to enjoy the great outdoors.

- Bring foods that you really like. Allison, for example, never leaves home without fancy dark chocolate.

- Bring enough of your favorites to share with others. Sharing food builds trust and cements the bonds that form (we hope) between group members during a trip.

- Bring fun foods, like popcorn. There is no better way to make friends or alleviate boredom on days when bad weather keeps you in your tent than sharing a pot of freshly popped popcorn.

- Bring a variety of foods so that no one ever goes hungry. Food takes on a whole different meaning on the trail. The quality and types of food on hand can boost morale or cause a whole trip to fall apart.

- Adding spices to your pack adds barely any weight, but they can give new life to the same old foods that you normally bring.

- Take seriously the job of staying properly fueled and hydrated. Keep foods and water accessible (not buried in the bottom of your pack), force yourself to eat when necessary (plan at least three mealtimes a day), and try drinking your calories (sports drinks and shakes) when the going gets really tough.

- On extended trips, get everyone to sign off beforehand on the types and quantities of food that the group is taking. The time to find out about likes, dislikes, and possible food allergies is before you leave home.

- Add butter to foods to boost the calorie intake and help foods go down when eating gets really tough, for example, at high altitudes. Allison maintains that this is her secret to never losing weight on an expedition.

Using Supplements Effectively

5

"I am practicing taking water. I have been using more drinks than I needed in all of the half marathons I have done just to train myself in picking them up."

—Paula Ratcliff, world-record holder in the marathon (2:15:25, a time that would have won every men's Olympics marathon until 1960), before her debut at the distance

Taking supplements is nothing new. For centuries, athletes have attempted to improve their performance by eating just the right foods or taking dietary supplements or other ergogenic (performance-enhancing) aids. Endurance athletes are no exception. Unfortunately, more often than not, supplements don't deliver on their promises. The response that I hear most often from athletes is, "Big deal, what's the harm in trying?" First, investing time, energy, and money on supplements that don't work is, well, not a good use of your time, energy, and money. On top of that, taking supplements could prove harmful to your health, hurt your performance, or result in your disqualification from competition.

Of course, if you're like the athletes I meet, you don't intend to harm yourself or your performance when you jump on the latest nutrition bandwagon. Rather, you rationalize that taking supplements compensates for a less-than-ideal diet or lifestyle, or you believe that you have special nutrient needs resulting from strenuous exercise. If you're highly competitive, you may think that supplements will help you avoid colds and injuries, as well as give you that little extra competitive edge. Let's face it: You're not out there to lose.

The first part of this chapter presents the most current information on the supplements that endurance athletes most commonly use—some with proved benefits and others with potential benefits for improving your performance. In the second part of this chapter, you will learn how to determine whether a supplement is safe, effective, and legal to take, and how to evaluate claims made by supplement manufacturers.

Understanding the Supplement Hype

Unfortunately, the extraordinary drive that endurance athletes possess to improve and excel (you know, the drive that keeps you going hour after hour) can leave you particularly vulnerable to the lure of dietary supplements. The supplement industry capitalizes on this weakness by spending vast sums of money to market the latest promise of the day, including vitamins, minerals, herbals, botanicals, amino acids, and other substances such as phytochemicals, extracts, and glandular concentrates and metabolites. On top of that, the opinions of those who perform better than we do can easily sway us, so advertisers target us by using successful athletes and coaches to represent products. To make matters worse, you probably have at least one friend or teammate who swears by how well a particular supplement is working. This influence, coupled with the fact that you may not have had a nutrition course since ninth grade, makes it easy to see how myths regarding nutrition supplements are perpetuated.

My friend Peter, an avid and dedicated trail runner, performed a ritual every morning and evening. He religiously swallowed a tablespoon (15 milliliters) of a smelly, vile-tasting concoction that he affectionately called bark juice. He didn't miss a day for over seven years. He took this awful-tasting stuff because he was convinced that it helped him recover from his weekly training volume of 60 or more miles (100 kilometers) of running and 150 miles (240 kilometers) of cycling.

Whether it worked or not may be hard to prove. As with many supplements, the scientific evidence doesn't yet exist to rule definitively on what effect, if any, taking a particular substance may have on an athlete's health or performance. What can you do? What should you do? If you rely on your body to perform, I recommend learning as much as possible about the substances that you wish to take. With knowledge comes power. On top of that, you'll also need a healthy dose of skepticism and a bit of common sense to sidestep potential minefields when evaluating supplements. After all, vitamin T (where *T* stands for *Training*) is the most important vitamin of them all. (See figure 5.1.)

Popular Supplements for Endurance Athletes

The following section contains information on specific supplements that may help you stay healthy and perform better during endurance activities. Before looking to supplements for a boost, however, make sure that you have in place a smart sports diet and a sound training program—and even then don't expect miracles. (See figure 5.1.) My advice is based on the guidelines developed by

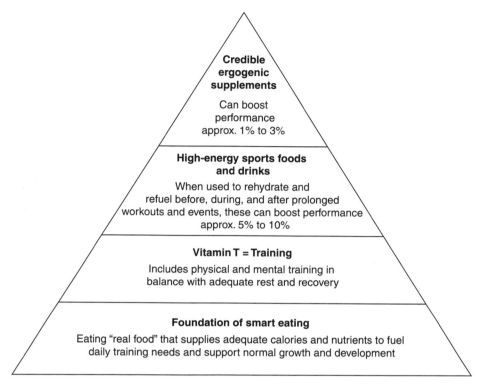

Figure 5.1 Supplements and sports foods are like the icing on a cake. You first need to build a strong base (from the bottom up) because the most important nutritional benefits come from eating in a way that leaves you physically ready and mentally prepared to train.

Adapted with permission from the Australian Sports Commission.

the Department of Sports Nutrition at the Australian Institute of Sport (AIS), the world leader in the sports nutrition field. AIS has an active research program that includes scientific evaluation of dietary supplements and nutritional ergogenic aids to find practical nutrition strategies that athletes and coaches can use to achieve optimum performance. Keep in mind, however, that you may fail to respond positively or to gain any performance-enhancing effect from a supplement, despite using it as recommended.

Supplements With Scientifically Proven Benefits

I consider the following supplements to be safe healthwise when used as directed. They are backed by enough science to be proved reasonably effective and are legal to experiment with in terms of boosting your athletic performance. One caveat, however, is that any seemingly harmless dietary supplement can be contaminated with a banned substance. The presence of prohormones, compounds that can be converted in the body into an active hormone such as testosterone, continues to be a particular problem. (See "Banned Substances in Nutritional Supplements: Athletes Pay the Price" on page 123.)

Fluid Replacement Drinks, Energy Bars, and Energy Gels

The most powerful supplements that you have at your disposal may be fluid replacement drinks, energy bars, and energy gels. During exercise, you can't last long without fluid, and you won't get far without adequate fuel for your muscles. Water is adequate for exercise bouts lasting an hour or less, but a properly formulated sports drink does triple duty by providing fluid, electrolytes, and carbohydrate. As your athletic adventures and races stretch past an hour, your success (from setting a personal record to just plain finishing) can hinge on consuming a fluid replacement drink.

The closer you come to replacing your fluid losses during exercise, the better you'll perform, especially in hot weather. An adequate fluid intake helps your heart beat efficiently, attenuates the rise in body temperature that results from exercise, and delays the onset of dehydration. Study after study has shown that athletes offered either water or a sports drink during exercise will drink a greater amount of the sports drink.

Bars, gels, and sports drinks also provide carbohydrate that helps stabilize your blood sugar and acts as fuel for your muscles during exercise. To perform at their best during events lasting longer than 90 to 120 minutes, endurance athletes need to consume at least 30 to 60 grams of carbohydrate per hour of exercise. Most sports drinks provide 14 grams of carbohydrate per 8 ounces (250 milliliters), gels offer 25 grams per packet, and bars (if you can tolerate solid food during your event) range from 20 to 50 grams per bar. Thanks to powders and convenient packaging, you can now refuel easily during most endurance endeavors.

Fluid replacement drinks and sports bars can also be used as part of a carbohydrate-loading regime before exercise and to help replenish muscle glycogen stores following exercise. Recent research also suggests that drinking carbohydrate-containing beverages in events and races lasting longer than 90 to 120 minutes can bolster the immune system to the physiologic stress initiated by prolonged exercise.

Possible side effects   Fluid replacement drinks, energy gels and sports bars may cause gastrointestinal distress, such as nausea and diarrhea, during exercise. Energy bars may compromise overall nutrient intake if they routinely replace meals and snacks based on real foods from the five food groups.

Advice   The best fluid replacement drink is the one that you will drink the most of. Experiment during training sessions with different flavors and brands to find products that taste good and sit well with your stomach. Fluid replacement drinks formulated for use during exercise (6 to 8 percent carbohydrate concentration), such as Gatorade, Cytomax, and Powerbar Endurance, are generally tolerated best (see table 5.1 for a comparison of some of the fluid replacement drinks on the market).

During exercise lasting 90 minutes or longer, consuming a sports drink (or water and an energy gel) to prevent precipitous dips in blood sugar is particularly important. A low blood sugar level causes the body to release large quantities of stress hormones, particularly cortisol. Elevated cortisol levels

Table 5.1 Comparison Chart of Fluid Replacement Drinks (per 8 oz, or 250 ml, serving)

Beverage	Carbohydrate type	Calories	Carbohydrate (g)	Carbohydrate concentration	Sodium (mg)
Accelerade	Sucrose, trehalose	80	16	6.6%	110
Cytomax	Maltodextrin, polylactate, fructose	80	15	6%	70
Endura	Glucose polymers, fructose	60	15	6%	48
Enervit G Sport	Fructose, maltodextrin, glucose, sucrose	60	14.6	6%	112
1st Endurance EFS	Maltodextrin, glucose, sucrose	64	16	6.6%	166
Extran Thirst Quencher	Fructose, maltodextrin	60	14.6	6%	81
Gatorade	Sucrose, glucose	50	14	6%	110
Gatorade Endurance	Sucrose, dextrose	60	15	6%	200
Hydralyte (Gookinaid)	Glucose, fructose	39	10	4%	69
GU20	Maltodextrin, fructose	50	13	5%	120
Hammer Heed	Maltodextrin	50	13	5.5%	31
PowerBar Endurance	Maltodextrin, dextrose, fructose	70	17	7%	160
Shaklee Performance	Maltodextrin, fructose, glucose	100	25	10%	115
Red Bull	Sucrose, glucose	113	28	12%	215
Revenge Sport	Maltodextrin, amylopectin starch, fructose	45	11.5	5%	50
Succeed! Ultra	Maltodextrins, sucrose	64	14	6%	Trace
Ultima	Maltodextrins	20	5	1.7%	25
XLR8	Glucose, fructose, glucose polymers	50	12	5%	40
Compared with					
Coca-Cola	High-fructose corn syrup or sucrose	100	27	11%	35
Orange juice	Fructose, sucrose	120	29	12%	trace
Water	N/A	N/A	N/A	N/A	N/A

profoundly suppress the immune system, leaving you vulnerable to colds and other upper-respiratory infections in the days following the exercise bout.

Experiment with energy bars and gels, too. Reduce your risk of having stomach problems during exercise by taking energy gels with plenty of water, ideally 6 to 8 ounces (175 to 250 milliliters), rather than a sports drink. To avoid "flavor fatigue" during daylong or multiday events, develop a taste for more than one flavor of your favorite brand of energy bar or gel. In terms of your training diet, energy bars make handy snacks, but use them to supplement, not replace, wholesome foods in your diet.

Liquid Food Supplements

High-carbohydrate beverages, such as UltraFuel and Extran, supply a concentrated dose of carbohydrate (40 to 50 grams per 8 ounces) to help build muscle glycogen stores before exercise and to replenish those stores following exercise. Other products, such as Ensure, Metabolol Endurance, and EnduroxR4, provide a variety of nutrients—carbohydrate, protein, and fat, as well as various vitamins and minerals. Consume them two to five hours before exercise as a low-fiber preevent meal, immediately afterward to enhance recovery, or to provide a concentrated dose of energy, carbohydrate, and nutrients during periods of heavy training or when you need to gain weight. These products can also be easily ingested sources of calories and nutrients during ultraendurance events (see table 5.2 for a comparison of some of the liquid food supplements on the market). Powdered varieties provide portable, convenient nutrition while traveling.

Possible side effects Liquid food supplements may cause gastrointestinal problems and dehydration when consumed during exercise, nutrient deficiencies or excesses if routinely used to replace foods in meals, and weight gain from consuming excess calories.

Advice To recover more quickly from daily training bouts and reduce your risk of injury, get in the habit of replenishing your muscle glycogen stores as soon as possible. Drink either a high-carbohydrate beverage or a meal replacement product within 15 to 30 minutes following exercise, especially if you don't plan to eat a meal within an hour or two. Aim to consume .5 grams of carbohydrate per pound (~1.0 gram per kilogram) of body weight. High-carbohydrate beverages and meal replacement products also come in handy as prerace meals and as part of a carbohydrate-loading regimen before endurance races lasting longer than 90 to 120 minutes.

Liquid food supplements are also the easiest and most convenient way to meet your energy needs during ultraendurance events, such as a 100-mile ultrarun or a century bike ride. Experiment in training with any product that you intend to consume during an event or race so that you know what it will taste like and how it will settle in your stomach. Ingesting both carbohydrate and protein in the latter stages of ultraendurance events may help lessen the breakdown of muscle tissue associated with those endeavors.

Round out a healthy sports diet with these products, especially if you need extra calories or are trying to gain weight. Homemade milk and yogurt smoothies, beverages fortified with nonfat dried milk powder, or instant

Table 5.2   Liquid Food Supplements

Beverage	Serving size	Calories	Carbohydrate (g)	Protein (g)	Fat (g)
Boost	8 oz (250 ml) bottle	240	41 (68%)	10 (17%)	4 (15%)
Carbo Pro	2 oz per 20 oz–24 oz (600 ml–720 ml)	224	56 (100%)	0	0
Clif Shot Recovery	2 servings per 16 oz (500 ml)	290	62 (86%)	10 (14%)	0
Cytomax Pre-Formance	2 scoops	260	25 (54%)	26 (40%)	2 (6%)
EAS Catapult Pre-Race	1 serving	90	21 (100%)	0	0
Endura Optimizer	2 scoops per 12 oz (350 ml)	306	61 (80%)	10.5 (14%)	2 (6%)
EnduroxR4	2 scoops per 12 oz (350 ml)	270	53 (78%)	14 (20%)	1 (3%)
Enervitene	3 scoops per 16 oz (500 ml)	180	44 (100%)	0	0
Ensure	8 oz (250 ml) bottle	250	40 (64%)	9 (14%)	6 (22%)
Extran Carbohydrate	1 box	320	80 (100%)	0	0
Hammer Recoverite	2 scoops	166	32.5 (77%)	10 (23%)	0
Hammer Perpeteum	2 scoops	260	54 (83%)	6 (9%)	2 (7%)
infinIT Ironman	2 scoops	305	72 (95%)	4 (5%)	0
Interphase	2 scoops	161	13 (32%)	25 (62%)	1 (6%)
Metabolol (Met) Endurance	2 scoops per 12 oz (350 ml)	200	24 (48%)	15 (30%)	5 (22%)
OS Endurance	1 pouch per 24 oz (720 ml)	355	100 (100%)	0	0
OS Re-Load	1 pouch per 24 oz (720 ml)	370	65 (65%)	31 (33%)	2 (4%)
PowerBar Endurance Recovery	1 scoop	90	20 (88%)	3 (12%)	0

(continued)

Table 5.2 *(continued)*

Beverage	Serving size	Calories	Carbohydrate (g)	Protein (g)	Fat (g)
Succeed! Amino	2 scoops per 20 oz (600 ml)	150	36 (97%)	1.2 (3%)	0
Sustained Energy	3 scoops per 8 oz–12 oz (250 ml–350 ml)	334	73 (88%)	10.5 (12%)	0
Spiz	4 scoops per 20 oz (600 ml)	517	94 (75%)	20 (16%)	5 (9%)
Ultramet	1 packet per 12 oz (350 ml)	280	24 (34%)	42 (60%)	2 (6%)
Ultra Fuel	4 scoops per 16 oz (500 ml)	400	100 (100%)	0	0
1st Endurance Ultragen	2 scoops per 12 oz (350 ml)	320	60 (75%)	20 (25%)	0

Note: 1 cup = 250 ml

breakfast drinks can serve the same purpose. Keep in mind that you need adequate protein, carbohydrate, and calories (along with a weightlifting program, of course) to build lean muscle mass. Consuming protein beyond your needs (as supplied by high-protein drinks) will be stored as fat instead of contributing to muscle growth, and it will increase your need for fluid. If you're trying to lose weight, watch out for the calories packed into these products.

Finally, keep a supply of meal replacement products on hand to use as backup meals while recovering from exhausting efforts or races, when traveling, or on busy days when you would otherwise skip meals or eat poorly.

Multivitamin/Multimineral Supplement

Take a multivitamin/multimineral supplement to bolster a diet that is sometimes less than adequate, especially if you are dieting, are lactose intolerant (possible riboflavin, calcium, and vitamin D deficiencies), or if you avoid foods because of food allergies. Multivitamins are also appropriate for vegetarian athletes (who run the risk of being low in iron, zinc, and other nutrients) and women who are trying to become pregnant (you need at least 400 milligrams of folic acid daily to help prevent birth defects).

Possible side effects Some athletes may rely too heavily on a multivitamin to compensate for a poor diet. Multivitamins may supply too little or too much of key nutrients.

Advice Along with taking a multivitamin/multi-mineral supplement, work on making better food choices. Vitamin and mineral supplements don't give you energy (calories), fiber, phytochemicals, or yet-to-be-discovered magic bullets that occur naturally in foods. Eating right is still key. Choose a brand with 100 percent of the daily value for most nutrients and be sure that it carries the United States Pharmacopeia (USP) stamp of approval to guarantee that it will dissolve properly (but not necessarily be absorbed effectively) in the body. Take your daily multivitamin/multi-mineral supplement with a meal to enhance absorption.

Men and nonmenstruating women may need to consider a supplement with little or no iron (10 milligrams or less) to avoid iron overload. Most multivitamins contain negligible amounts of calcium (the pill would be too big to swallow), so you may need a calcium supplement too.

Calcium

Besides building strong bones and teeth, calcium helps muscles contract, helps nerves send messages, and helps blood clot properly. Consuming an adequate amount throughout life, especially during adolescence and the early adult years, reduces the risk of osteoporosis (a condition characterized by brittle bones that break easily). Calcium may also play a role in alleviating symptoms of premenstrual syndrome and hypertension (high blood pressure).

Possible side effects   Calcium supplements may contribute to kidney stones in some people. Some athletes may rely too heavily on a calcium supplement to compensate for poor eating habits.

Advice   Calcium can be found in foods from all the food groups, so work on including alternative sources if you don't drink milk or eat dairy products (see "Best Bets: Calcium" in chapter 1). Aim for 1,000 milligrams a day (1,300 milligrams per day for younger athletes ages 9 to 18, 1,200 milligrams for adults over age 50). People gain peak bone mass between the ages of 16 and 25. The more calcium that you deposit into your bones, the more withdrawals you can withstand (as you get older) before you get into trouble.

If you can't get all the calcium that you need from your diet, you should take a supplement. To get the best absorption, take your calcium supplements at mealtimes and divide your dose throughout the day, taking no more than 500 milligrams at a time. (Pay attention to the amount of *elemental* calcium listed per tablet.) Don't take more than you need and be careful not to think of your supplement (like Tums or Viactiv soft calcium chews) as candy.

Choose a calcium supplement that contains vitamin D (needed by the body to absorb calcium efficiently) or, if you take a multivitamin, check to make sure that it contains 200 to 400 IU of vitamin D. Calcium carbonate is generally well absorbed, but choose calcium citrate if you plan to take your supplements between meals. If you take a multivitamin containing iron as well as a calcium supplement, don't take both at the same time if you have problems with low blood iron (anemia). High doses of calcium from the supplement can impair your ability to absorb iron. If you want to experiment with alleviating mild to moderate premenstrual symptoms, take 1,200 milligrams of calcium a day for at least two to three months.

Iron

Iron is an essential component of the oxygen carriers hemoglobin (found in red blood cells) and myoglobin (found in muscle cells), as well as some of the oxidative enzymes needed to convert food into fuel for working muscles. Inadequate hemoglobin or body iron stores (ferritin) affect how the body transports and uses oxygen and impairs performance in endurance activities.

Possible side effects Iron supplements may cause constipation or diarrhea, or contribute to hemochromatosis (iron overload) in susceptible individuals.

Advice Work at obtaining adequate iron by eating foods rich in heme iron (meat, fish, and poultry) and nonheme iron (plant sources such as dark green leafy vegetables, tofu, dried beans, dried fruit, and fortified foods). Keep in mind that heme iron is absorbed better than the iron from plant foods or supplements is. To increase the absorption of the nonheme iron in plant foods, consume these foods with heme-rich foods, such as three-bean chili with a small amount of meat added, or eat foods high in vitamin C along with foods that provide nonheme iron. Drink a glass of orange juice, for example, with a bowl of iron-fortified cereal.

Monitor your iron status through blood tests that measure hemoglobin, hematocrit, and ferritin (iron stores). Female endurance athletes and athletes training at altitude, in particular, often need to supplement with at least the recommended daily dose of iron to prevent iron depletion during training. The recommended daily amount is 18 milligrams for teenage and adult females, 11 milligrams for teenage males, and 8 milligrams for adult males.

If your hemoglobin and ferritin levels are normal, taking large doses of extra iron through supplements will not boost your performance, and it could be harmful. Hemochromatosis, or iron overload, is a genetic disorder that affects as many as 1 in every 200 people. Hemochromatosis disrupts iron metabolism in such a way that the body absorbs too much iron. The excess iron deposits in the liver, heart, joints, and other tissues, damaging those tissues and potentially increasing the risk for heart disease and cancer. Because this disorder is not routinely screened for, take large doses of supplemental iron only if your physician has diagnosed you as iron depleted or anemic, and then only until your iron status normalizes.

Antioxidants

Antioxidants, such as vitamins C and E, protect cells and tissues by working to neutralize the damaging effects of free radicals (by-products of strenuous aerobic exercise, pollution, cigarette smoke, and so on). Consuming supplemental doses of antioxidants at key times might translate into less muscle tissue damage, speedier recoveries, and a bolstered immune system. Antioxidants have not been found, however, to improve athletic performance directly.

Possible side effects Excessive vitamin C (such as 1,000 to 3,000 milligrams) can cause diarrhea and kidney stones in some people. Because vitamin C enhances iron absorption, high doses may also lead to harmful or excessive iron levels in the body (especially for those at risk for hemochromatosis). Excessive vitamin E (over 1,000 milligrams) can lead to fatigue, headaches, and diarrhea, as well as impaired immunity and excessive bleeding. Vitamin E supplements also interfere with anticlotting medications, including daily low-dose aspirin.

Advice   Antioxidants found in food cannot always be replicated in a pill. For example, not only did vitamin E supplements fail to reduce the risk of chronic diseases in studies of reducing heart disease and cancer, they may actually increase the risk by working as pro-oxidants. Because nutrients tend to work in concert, consuming too much of a single nutrient through a supplement might do more harm than good by creating an imbalance in the body. Your best bet to obtain vitamin C is to eat a daily diet rich in nutrient-dense fruits and vegetables. Develop a taste for brightly colored fruits and vegetables such as papaya, cantaloupe, berries, apricots, oranges, kiwis, mangoes, sweet potatoes, carrots, spinach, collard greens, red peppers, and kale.

Meeting your recommended daily intake for vitamin E (15 milligrams or 22 IU from natural source E or 33 IU of the synthetic form) can be difficult, however, for even the most nutrition-conscious athlete. Vitamin E is found primarily in vegetable oils, margarine, and nuts and seeds. Consider supplementing your diet with a small daily dose of vitamin E (if you don't take anti-clotting medications or daily low-dose aspirin), especially if you eat a very low-fat diet or exercise in heavily polluted areas. To get the most from your vitamin E supplement, choose one that contains natural vitamin E (also called d-alpha tocopherol or RRR-alpha) rather than synthetic vitamin E (dl-alpha-tocopherol or all-rac alpha).

Antioxidants work quietly behind the scenes. Don't take megadoses to try to see an effect. The AIS suggests an initial two-week booster dose (500 milligrams of vitamin C and 400 IU of vitamin E) may be helpful to combat stress, which may temporarily overwhelm the antioxidant defense system of the body. For example, antioxidants may be helpful when you substantially increase your training volume or intensity or shift your training to a stressful environment (altitude training or hot environments). Taking a vitamin C supplement (about 600 milligrams) for at least one week before participating in an ultraendurance event may help protect important immune cells and reduce your risk of an upper-respiratory infection.

Supplements That Might Be Helpful

The following section profiles several popular supplements that may boost your health or improve your performance in endurance activities, but research results are either mixed or athletes may find it difficult to obtain positive results. I consider these supplements reasonably safe (within limits as noted), backed by enough science to warrant another look, and legal for endurance athletes to experiment with (with limits as noted). Keep in mind that I'm not suggesting nor advocating the use of any particular supplement. The decision to take a supplement always lies with you.

Caffeine

Sound evidence shows that caffeine can reduce times in marathon and cycling time trials, as well as increase the duration over which trained elite and recreational athletes are able to exercise vigorously—at least in the laboratory. Small but credible performance boosts have been shown across a wide spectrum of exercise protocols of interest to endurance athletes: prolonged high-intensity events (20 to 60 minutes), endurance events (90 or more minutes of continuous exercise), and ultraendurance events (4 or more hours).

Until recently, the enhancing effects on endurance performance were primarily attributed to the ability of caffeine to promote an increase in the use of fat as fuel during exercise, thereby conserving muscle glycogen, which would allow exercising muscles to keep working at a high level for longer periods. Athletes were always warned, however, that caffeine-containing drinks acted as diuretics and would lead to dehydration. Scientists now discount both of these effects of caffeine. Not all athletes respond to caffeine during submaximal exercise by demonstrating a glycogen-sparing effect; thus, other mechanisms must be at work. Most likely it is the ability of caffeine to stimulate the brain and alter our perception of fatigue or how hard we are working, thereby making exercise seem easier, as well as the direct effects of caffeine on the muscles themselves. Furthermore, an extensive review of the scientific literature to date confirmed what many people commonly report—caffeine-containing beverages (coffee, tea, and cola drinks) routinely provide a substantial source of fluid on a daily basis with minor, if any, effect on urine losses. This effect is particularly true for die-hard habitual caffeine users.

Possible side effects   Caffeinated beverages or supplements used before or during exercise may cause nausea and abdominal cramps, as well as increased urination in some people. Excessive caffeine may cause you to feel dizzy, jittery, or nauseous; experience heart palpitations; and interfere with your sleep patterns. Habitual users can experience headaches and insomnia when they consume less caffeine than they normally do. Consistently consuming excessive amounts of caffeinated beverages can lead to poor nutrient intake (if other more nutritious beverages or foods are routinely passed over), calcium loss from bones, impaired iron absorption, and problems trying to conceive. For collegiate athletes, high caffeine consumption can result in a failed drug test.

Advice   Studies investigating the effect of caffeine on performance during real-life sports and athletic events are scarce, so solid caffeine supplementation protocols do not currently exist. You'll really need to experiment with caffeine as a potential performance aid. Some people feel no lift at all, and the physical side effects outweigh the benefits for others. Try it in training first under various conditions. Don't wait until the morning of your big event. The caffeine content of tea and coffee, as well as herbal products and sports foods, varies widely depending on the brand, the way that beverages are prepared, and the size of the cup or mug (hence laboratory studies don't use caffeine in any of these forms). In general, studies use a caffeine dose based on body weight (about 3 milligrams per pound, or ~6 milligrams per kilogram, which is 300 to 500 milligrams for the typical athlete) one hour before exercise.

To decrease your tolerance to caffeine and receive the maximal boost, some researchers believe that habitual caffeine users may need to reduce or abstain from caffeine for three to four days before competition. Avoiding the headaches and general malaise associated with caffeine withdrawal can be tricky though. During exercise, don't underestimate the potential side effects of caffeine (from drinking caffeinated sodas, for instance), such as nausea and abdominal cramps, because those issues already occur with high frequency during endurance events and races. Recent studies reported that athletes involved in prolonged exercise (lasting 60 minutes or longer) experienced benefits when they ingested small to moderate amounts of caffeine (70 to 150 milligrams of caffeine) at numerous times before and/or throughout exercise, or toward the end of exercise when they became fatigued.

For elite athletes subject to drug testing following competitions, the World Anti-Doping Association removed caffeine from its prohibited list in January 2004. The National Collegiate Athletic Association (NCAA), however, still restricts caffeine (and guarana). A caffeine concentration in the urine that exceeds 15 micrograms per milliliter is considered positive (performance enhancing) and would result in a failed drug test. Athletes metabolize caffeine at very different rates, and some medications (such as Vivarin, No Doz, and Tylenol, or acetaminophen), supplements, and energy drinks contain appreciable amounts of caffeine, so caffeine intake can add up.

No evidence exists that if a little caffeine boosts performance, then more caffeine will produce even more performance benefits. Your goal should be to find the lowest effective dose. All exercisers need to be careful not to combine caffeine with other stimulants that are like or similar to ephedrine, which can lead to an irregular heartbeat as well as increase your risk of heat illness.

Don't abuse caffeine on a daily basis. No credible health experts support consuming large amounts of caffeine (more than 500 milligrams per day) long term. Low-fat milk, 100 percent fruit juice, and sports drinks make far healthier choices than tea, coffee, soda, and chocolate-covered espresso beans. (The average caffeine content in 8 ounces, or a 250 milliliter cup of brewed coffee is 80 milligrams; in 8 ounces of instant coffee, 60 milligrams; and in 8 ounces of tea, 27 milligrams). Caffeine can leach calcium from your bones, so boost your calcium intake with at least two extra tablespoons of milk or yogurt for every cup of coffee that you drink. If you have problems with iron-deficiency anemia, drink your caffeinated beverages between meals so that the caffeine doesn't interfere with your absorption of iron. Women trying to conceive should consume as little caffeine as possible and continue to restrict themselves while pregnant (two cups or less per day) to reduce the risk of miscarriage or giving birth to an underweight baby.

Glucosamine and Chondroitin Sulfate

Synthesized by the body, glucosamine plays a major role in building and repairing joint cartilage, as well as inhibiting the breakdown of existing cartilage. Chondroitin reportedly helps joints remain fluid and inhibits enzymes that break down cartilage. Short-term (four- to eight-week) controlled trials have found glucosamine sulfate as effective as ibuprofen in relieving pain and increasing range of motion in people with osteoarthritis, a degenerative joint disease.

Possible side effects Glucosamine and chondroitin sulfate may cause gastrointestinal discomfort and diarrhea in some people. Some athletes may gain a false sense of security that a supplement will heal or cure an exercise-induced injury.

Advice Glucosamine appears to be safe, but no long-term studies have been done on either supplement or the combination together. Don't be fooled by claims that glucosamine or chondroitin sulfate can cure osteoarthritis. The evidence doesn't exist, especially because glucosamine apparently can't influence the repair of cartilage when little or no cartilage remains. If you decide to try these substances for relief of everyday aches and pain or a more serious injury, the commonly recommended dose is 500 milligrams three times a day. Just don't neglect or abandon well-established treatments for athletic or overuse injuries, such as stretching, massage, physical therapy, strengthening exercises, orthotics, and so forth.

Glycerol

This substance may help reduce dehydration and fatigue during exercise by prompting the body to store more water than possible by ingesting plain water alone (glycerol attracts and holds water like a sponge). Some studies have shown these benefits: greater fluid retention, lower core temperatures during exercise, and improved performance during prolonged exercise. Other studies have shown no physiological benefits or positive effects on performance. Research is lacking on the effects of ingesting large doses over a prolonged period.

Possible side effects Glycerol may cause headaches, nausea, vomiting, bloating, dizziness, and muscle stiffness.

Advice Experiment with a commercially prepared sports drink that contains glycerol or mix a premeasured amount (obtained from a pharmacist) with water or a sports drink as directed. Don't exceed the recommended amount—the dosages are based on body weight (see the package label for exact amounts). If you're pregnant or have diabetes, high blood pressure, or kidney problems, check with your physician first. The potential benefits of glycerol are greater during events of longer distances and in hot and humid weather. You are unlikely to see any benefit in races lasting less than one hour.

To hyperhydrate, consume the glycerol–fluid mixture one and a half to three hours before an endurance event. Experiment in training before using it in competition. Keep notes on how long it takes you to drink the mixture comfortably, how long you feel that it takes the mixture to clear your stomach, and how long any feeling of bloating lasts. Be aware that you will still need to replace your fluid losses by drinking water and fluid replacement drinks throughout the race.

Branched Chain Amino Acids (BCAAs)

BCAAs (leucine, isoleucine, and valine) are located primarily in muscle, and they can be broken down and burned for energy during prolonged exercise (e.g., over two hours) as muscle glycogen levels fall. Supplementing with BCAAs may improve performance by preventing muscle protein breakdown and damage or by delaying the mental fatigue that arises in the latter stages of prolonged exercise when blood levels of BCAAs fall. Findings of research studies are promising but inconclusive on the effect of BCAAs on performance.

Possible side effects   Large doses may cause gastrointestinal distress. Routine consumption might interfere with the absorption of other amino acids into the body.

Advice   Supplementing with BCAAs to alleviate mental fatigue during exercise is promising for endurance athletes. Studies to date, however, have found that carbohydrate-containing beverages are just as effective in improving performance as are drinks containing both carbohydrate and BCAAs. To capitalize on potential benefits, experiment with supplements, powders, or sports drinks that contain added BCAAs during prolonged exercise, when blood levels of BCAAs decrease and you're most likely to be in a glycogen-depleted state. BCAA supplementation appears to be safe, but the effects of long-term use, if any, are unknown. Don't overdo it because large doses can contribute to stomach upset.

You can maintain your muscle mass most effectively by consuming enough calories and adequate protein each day. Protein-rich food sources, which provide 10 to 15 grams of protein per serving (meat and milk in particular), provide ample amounts of BCAAs as well. A sound training program and a carbohydrate-rich diet will also help spare your protein stores from being converted to fuel during exercise. Ingesting large doses of individual amino acids on a daily basis could influence the absorption and metabolic balance of other amino acids, so choose supplements or powders that provide a full complement of amino acids. Don't be duped by the large numbers on labels. For example, 10,000 milligrams of amino acids may sound like a lot, but this is only 10 grams of protein, an amount that you can get more easily (and for a lot less money) by drinking a glass of milk.

Electrolyte (Salt) Replacement Supplements

Traditionally given to athletes who are exercising in the heat to prevent muscle cramps, salt tablets can help endurance athletes maintain an adequate sodium level in the body during prolonged activities, such as marathons, ultraruns, and triathlons. Sweating causes you to lose electrolytes, primarily sodium. You can lose as much as 1,000 milligrams of sodium for every 2-pound sweat loss.

Electrolyte deficits, particularly of sodium, can result from repeated training bouts in extreme heat and humidity, when you're initially acclimating to a hot climate, and during endurance and ultraendurance events, especially if you consume only plain water. Hyponatremia (a low blood sodium concentration of 135 milliequivalents per liter or less), a potentially dangerous condition that can arise during prolonged exercise, can result from excessive loss of sodium (through sweating), excessive intake of plain water, or both.

Possible side effects   Salt tablets may cause nausea, vomiting, and dehydration.

Advice   Moderately salting your food (a half teaspoon of table salt provides 1,200 milligrams of sodium), choosing salty foods in the few days before competition, and consuming a sports drink that contains sodium during exercise will be more than adequate most of the time. Use caution if you decide to experiment with salt tablets or other electrolyte replacement supplements or powders during exercise. Save them for intensive exercise (bouts lasting three hours or longer) or for when you exercise in extreme conditions (temperature above 80 degrees Fahrenheit, or 27 degrees Celsius, and 70 percent humidity or higher). If you plan to take them during races, be sure to try them in similar training situations first.

No definitive guidelines exist, but start with the recommended dose (typically one salt tablet 30 to 60 minutes before prolonged exercise and then one tablet per hour depending on the weather and how heavily you sweat) and be sure to consume plenty of fluid at the same time. Otherwise, your body draws water away from your muscles and into your stomach to dilute the tablets, negating the effect of taking them. Choose a buffered variety to reduce the risk of nausea and vomiting. Salt tablets don't increase your thirst as salty foods do, so don't overdo it. Most salt tablets supply 200 to 350 milligrams of sodium per tablet. Other electrolyte replacement supplements (tablets and powders) provide varying amounts of sodium (check the label) to allow you to customize the amount that you take.

MCT Oil

Consuming high-fat foods during exercise provides inefficient fuel for working muscles because of the extended time required to digest and absorb regular fats. Medium chain triglycerides (MCTs), on the other hand, a unique form of fat characterized by shorter-than-normal fatty acids, are digested and burned for fuel at a much faster rate, similar to carbohydrate. Consuming MCTs during endurance events and races may enhance performance by sparing the limited glycogen stores of the body. Other purported benefits of consuming MCTs, such as an increase in metabolism, less weight gain, and a lower level of body fat have been demonstrated only in animals, using relative doses of MCTs that humans could not reasonably consume.

Possible side effects   Large doses (more than 30 grams) can cause intestinal discomfort, such as cramping and diarrhea, and MCT is unsafe for athletes with diabetes or liver function problems. Essential fatty acid deficiencies can arise if MCTs are the sole source of fat in the diet.

Advice   MCT oil is expensive (US$25 to US$30 per quart) and may be diluted with water or other ingredients. Try to find a product that contains only MCT oil. Start by stirring small doses into a carbohydrate-containing sports drink or experiment with a commercially prepared sports drink containing MCTs, such as Succeed! Increase your intake gradually, because large doses can cause gastrointestinal problems, including cramping and diarrhea. Don't wait until race day to experiment with MCT oil. If you need extra calories while training, supplementing with MCT oil is a possibility. Just don't rely on it as the sole source of fat in your diet, because MCT oil lacks essential fatty acids.

Glutamine

As the most abundant amino acid in the body, glutamine plays a key role in maintaining a healthy gastrointestinal tract and immune system. Glutamine reserves (particularly in skeletal muscles) are depleted in times of stress, such as infection, surgery, trauma, and possibly even exercise. Prolonged strenuous exercise, running a marathon, for example, depresses blood levels of glutamine, with several hours of recovery needed to restore proper levels.

Typically synthesized by the body, glutamine may become conditionally essential during illness and acute stress when the body can't make enough to keep up with its needs. Low glutamine levels have been measured in athletes suffering from overtraining syndrome. Glutamine supplementation may improve athletic performance by helping the body build and maintain muscle mass, by decreasing muscle damage and shortening recovery time, by strengthening the immune system, and by stimulating the accumulation of muscle glycogen.

Possible side effects   Glutamine may give athletes a false sense of security or lead them to abandon lifestyle factors that prevent poor health or overtraining syndrome. Free-form L-glutamine is unsafe for athletes with kidney or liver dysfunction.

Advice   No standard dose exists, but research suggests potential benefits with 5 to 20 grams a day. Experiment with meal replacement powders or nutrition bars containing glutamine mixed with other amino acids to aid absorption. To obtain an adequate dose, glutamine should be among the first five protein ingredients listed, because many companies do not indicate the exact amount that the product contains.

Don't let the emerging role of glutamine as an indicator of exercise stress and overtraining lead you to abandon other healthy practices. Low blood levels of glutamine appear to be linked with the overtraining syndrome but do not necessarily cause it. Supplementing with glutamine isn't a substitute for time off from training, a healthy diet, adequate sleep, or learning how to manage stress appropriately.

Creatine Monohydrate

Creatine supplementation helps the body increase and rapidly replenish its stores of readily available energy (phosphocreatine and ATP)—the primary fuels needed for short, high-intensity efforts such as sprinting and lifting weights. For endurance athletes, the ability of creatine to increase muscle strength and help buffer lactic acid buildup in the blood and muscles could improve the quality of interval workouts and other training efforts, which could ultimately translate into improved race performances.

Possible side effects   Weight gain (from tissues holding onto extra water), dehydration, and an increased risk of muscle cramps, tears, and pulls.

Advice   Humans need approximately two grams of creatine a day. Animal foods, such as meat, poultry, and fish, are rich sources of creatine. Our bodies also synthesize creatine from nonessential amino acids at the rate of approximately one gram a day. As far as endurance athletes are concerned, creatine supplementation has been shown to have no effect on maximal aerobic capacity (VO_2max), nor has it been shown to improve endurance. Some researchers believe, however, that creatine supplementation might indirectly improve an athlete's ability to perform in endurance events. Creatine supplementation may lift an athlete's lactate threshold (the speed or intensity above which lactic acid accumulates in the blood), thereby allowing more intensive interval-type training. By facilitating strength and cardiovascular improvements in this manner, creatine supplementation could improve overall performances in endurance events.

Short-term creatine supplementation (up to eight weeks) appears safe, but the American College of Sports Medicine recommends that all athletes check first with a physician. Be aware that although studies fail to support an increase in muscle cramps and pulls with creatine supplementation, anecdotal information from athletes abounds! Dehydration may be the culprit, so athletes who are taking creatine need to consume more fluids than usual during training and competition. The safety of prolonged creatine supplementation has not been completely established.

Two loading techniques that purportedly induce less water retention (and thus less weight gain) than the traditional 20-gram-per-day strategy include 6 grams per day over 5 to 6 days (.5- or 1.0-gram doses) with a maintenance dose of about 2 grams a day or 3 grams a day over 30 days. Supplementing with creatine will not build muscles or improve performance on its own. Coordinate creatine supplementation with your training schedule by starting just before you begin a period of high-intensity training. Keep in mind that 20 to 30 percent of people fail to respond even when creatine is taken correctly and training is appropriate.

Probiotics

Probiotics are live bacteria from certain foods or supplements that when ingested can enhance the growth of good bacteria in our intestines. The two most common species of probiotic bacteria are lactobacillus acidophilis and bifidobacterim bifidum, two species that already live in our intestines. Consuming extra probiotics should boost their numbers and may enhance the digestion and absorption of nutrients, reduce lactose intolerance, decrease allergies in susceptible individuals, and bolster the immune system.

Possible side effects   Consuming probiotics presents few, if any, risks for healthy adults. An upset stomach or bowel problems are possible.

Advice   As a preventive measure, eat more fermented milk products such as yogurt (with live cultures), acidophilus milk, and kefir on a daily basis. Probiotics are measured in colony forming units (CFUs). For health effects, no official recommended dosages currently exist, nor are there established limits for safe consumption. According to the research to date, 1 billion CFUs is the minimum per day thought to benefit health. A recent *Consumer Reports* feature on probiotics found that yogurt products provided 15 billion to 155 billion CFUs per 6- or 8-ounce (175- or 250-gram) serving and probiotic supplements supplied about 20 million to 70 billion CFUs per daily dose. Keep in mind that besides providing probiotic bacteria, yogurt products also dish up calcium, protein, and other nutrients.

Add probiotics gradually to your daily diet, taking two to three weeks to build up to the recommended dose. Because probiotics pass through the intestine, a daily dose is needed. The shelf life of most supplements is a year, although probiotic levels probably drop significantly during this time. The American Academy of Pediatrics has no guidelines for probiotics use with children or teens. Women who are pregnant or lactating should check with their health care provider first. Athletes can benefit from taking probiotic supplements when traveling to help ward off traveler's diarrhea, when under extra stress (after surgery, for example), or when taking antibiotics because they kill both bad and good intestinal bacteria.

HMB (ß-hydroxy ß-methylbutyrate)

Chemically related to the essential amino acid leucine, HMB also appears to play a role in muscle protein metabolism. HMB supplementation has been shown to decrease protein breakdown after strenuous exercise (studies have looked at strength training), contributing to gains in muscle size and strength. Most of the original studies focused on previously untrained people, although recent studies also reported gains in experienced athletes engaged in strength-training programs. A proposed benefit for endurance athletes is quicker recoveries because less exercise-induced muscle damage would mean less muscle tissue to repair and rebuild.

Possible side effects Supplementation with HMB has minimal side effects at the recommended dose.

Advice Extrapolation of the scientific studies is tricky because naturally induced adaptations to training, particularly regular resistance training, produce similar results—less breakdown or damage of muscle tissue and increases in strength. The typical suggested dosage of HMB is three grams per day in three divided doses of one gram each (upon waking, with lunch, and at bedtime). Don't fall for overpromises of major strength gains, losses of body fat, and greatly enhanced athletic performance, particularly if you're not engaged in a sound strength-training program. HMB supplementation is most effective during fairly strenuous exercise. You also must be consuming adequate dietary protein, or you're wasting your money on what is typically an expensive supplement.

Theoretically, well-trained endurance athletes could benefit from HMB supplementation when significantly increasing the intensity or volume of their training—if it helps to preserve muscle mass, if accelerated recovery leads to an increase in quality training, or if it improves strength that effectively translates into more power during athletic performance. Nevertheless, the AIS cautions athletes and coaches to expect minor effects at best on strength, body composition, and exercise performance.

Just the Facts Please

Supplements fall into a special category that lies somewhere between foods and drugs. Although supplements are required to carry a supplements facts label and an ingredient list similar to the nutrition facts label found on food packages, dietary supplements do not have to meet the same tough standards regarding health claims, manufacturing processes, and product safety that apply to all food additives and drugs.

Keep these facts about supplements in mind, as written in the Dietary Supplement Health and Education Act (DSHEA), as you reach for the latest magic potion.

> **Fact number one:** Proof that a supplement works is not required. In other words, the stringent guidelines set by the Food and Drug Administration (FDA) for drugs and food additives do not apply to supplements.

> **Fact number two:** Supplement manufacturers do not have to prove that their products are safe. Don't be fooled just because supplements look like drugs that the FDA has thoroughly tested and approved.

> **Fact number three:** Supplement manufacturers can put health claims on their labels. Health claims on supplement packages must be "truthful and not misleading." Unfortunately, the definition of this phrase continues to evolve. In other words, as long as a claim does not promise that the supplement will prevent or cure a disease, almost anything goes. For example, claims that do not relate to disease, such as "helps you relax," "for muscle enhancement," or "maintains a healthy circulatory system," are allowed without FDA approval. Remind yourself to read the small print on product labels and ads that states, "This statement has not been evaluated by the Food and Drug Administration. This product is not intended to diagnose, treat, cure, or prevent any disease."

> **Fact number four:** Supplements do not have to conform to any manufacturing standards. In other words, each company can decide for itself how to prepare and package its supplements, leaving the potency and quality of dietary supplements up in the air. In other words, just because the label says that the product contains certain ingredients doesn't guarantee that it does. Nor does it guarantee that undisclosed substances couldn't have been deliberately added (or introduced by cross-contamination during manufacturing) and not appear on the label.

Do Your Homework

Now that you realize that taking supplements requires a consumer-beware approach, where should you turn for guidance and sound advice? Start with the supplements facts label. Look here to find a complete list of the ingredients found in the supplement (including the breakdown of "magic formulas"), the nutrients that these ingredients provide, and how these amounts compare with established daily values (DVs). You can also determine which part of the plant is used in an herbal or botanical supplement. Checking the bottle for a USP stamp of approval lets you know that the supplement will dissolve properly in your body, but it doesn't tell you how effectively it will be absorbed (see figure 5.2).

You won't want to rely solely on the label or the health claims plastered all over the packaging. Unlike conventional foods, dietary supplements have no standard serving size. Dosage amounts and schedules have been left to the discretion of manufacturers (the people who want to sell the product), so you need to remember this age-old advice: More is not always better. Some nutrients and substances don't have established daily intakes, so you'll need to stay alert for current information from reputable sources on safe doses.

Make Sure That It Is Legal, Safe, and Effective

When it comes to deciphering health claims, a healthy dose of skepticism and a bit of common sense can help steer you through the maze. You want to consider whether the supplement in question is legal, safe, and effective. Common sense tells you that securing this information requires looking past the promotional literature, advertisements, and anecdotal reports put out by the manufacturers. Because of gaps in the DSHEA, companies commonly exaggerate claims and rely on deceptive marketing techniques to sell products. Typical approaches used include presenting information that may not be accurate or that has been

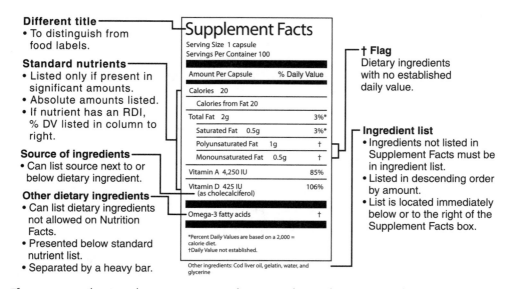

Figure 5.2 The Supplement Facts panel on a product indicates it is a dietary supplement, not a food or over-the-counter medicine.

Reprinted, with permission, from *SCAN'S PULSE*, Fall 1998, Vol. 17, No. 4, official publication of Sports, Cardiovascular, and Wellness Nutritionists (SCAN), The American Dietetic Association, Chicago, IL.

taken out of context; failing to provide scientific research when asked (it's "ongoing" or not available to the public); relying on testimonials from athletes and authority figures (for example, "research scientists"), who are most likely paid to endorse the product; and conducting and reporting their own research without having it published in journals where other scientists have a chance to evaluate it. Incidentally, obtaining a patent means that the product is unique, not necessarily safe or effective.

If you're a top-notch competitive athlete (including masters) subject to drug tests, you'll want to make sure that you don't take a prohibited substance that can disqualify you from further competitions. From an ethical standpoint, you too may be interested in this information, as were many of the purists I met in the mountaineering community while I lived in Boulder, Colorado. Stay abreast of updated guidelines and the latest list of banned substances by contacting your appropriate sports governing body, the National Collegiate Athletic Association, or the United States Olympic Committee. Although the scientifically challenged may find the information opaque, the world's leading authority is the World Anti-Doping Agency (www.wada-ama.org).

You may not like what you find though. You'll discover that some ingredients, such as DHEA and ma huang (Chinese Ephedra), are specifically banned. Other than that, you're on your own when it comes to dietary supplements. Because no governing sports body can guarantee the purity or potency of all the supplements available, anything you take is at your own risk. Many athletes in various sports have been tripped up by supplement manufacturers who contaminate nutritional supplements by adding banned substances, such as prohormones, to boost their effectiveness.

The reminder "Let the buyer beware" should be printed on every nutrition supplement package. Why? When it comes to the possible side effects of using a supplement long-term, you may be part of an ongoing study for the supplement manufacturer! Don't assume that you can resolve safety issues by buying high-priced versions or sticking with "natural drug-free" herbal remedies. To begin with, you may not even be getting what you pay for. For example, one study found that 60 percent of 64 "pure" ginseng products were worthless because they were so watered down with cheaper herbs.

Herbs fall under the same regulations in the United States as do other dietary supplements, which means that they may not be adequately tested to determine how safe or effective they are, especially if taken for longer periods than experts recommend.

For the most part, herbal dosages are recommendations from manufacturers or based simply on historical use. By the way, the dosage listed usually applies to men, so children and women will likely need less. As with all supplements, don't be afraid to call the manufacturer and ask about clinical trials, manufacturing practices, and their use of standardized extracts. Remedies composed of a single herb are generally considered safer than herbal mixtures. Be sure to consult with your doctor about any herbal products that you use, especially if you're pregnant or trying to become pregnant, have a health problem, or take prescription medications.

Banned Substances in Nutritional Supplements: Athletes Pay the Price

Triathlete Kelly Guest, the number-two-ranked male triathlete in Canada at the time, nearly had his competitive career ended by a contaminated dietary supplement. He tested positive for a banned substance and was sent home from the 2002 Commonwealth Games before competing. His suspension also cost him a chance at the Athens Olympics the following month. Guest tested positive for the steroid nandrolone, registering one nanogram, or one-billionth of a gram, over the allowable limit. Subject to Canadian rules in place at the time, he was handed a four-year suspension, a virtual death sentence for a competitive athlete.

Many in the sports world believed that the small amount of the substance detected indicated that Guest had ingested the substance inadvertently and that he not only deserved to be reinstated but also probably never should have been suspended in the first place. A year later an adjudicator, Graeme Mew, ruled that Guest did not knowingly take a banned substance but that he still bore any consequences because he chose to take unregulated nutritional supplements after having been warned of the risks by the Canadian Centre for Ethics in Sport (CCES). Mew was quoted as saying, "I accept that Kelly Guest did not knowingly cheat. . . . If I were able to base my decision upon issues of honesty, integrity, sportsmanship . . . I would have no hesitation in finding in Guest's favour."

During this time, the World Anti-Doping Agency, which governs athlete suspensions worldwide, revised its regulations to establish a two-year maximum for a suspension on the first offense (lifetime ineligibility for a second offense). Guest, at age 27, passed new drug tests, and the CCES reinstated him. His two years of hell were over. Guest has gone on to pursue a successful career as a professional triathlete.

Adapted from Morris Dalla Costa, 2004, "Guest's two years of suspension hell almost over," *London Free Press*. Available: http://www.canoe.ca/Slam040708/col_dallacosta-sun.html.

Now comes the big question: How can you tell whether a supplement does what it claims to do? In other words, will you have more energy, lose weight, run faster, jump higher, and throw farther? Now is the time to pull out that healthy dose of skepticism that I mentioned earlier and remember the counsel "If it sounds too good to be true, it probably is." Be leery of general, broad claims, such as "slows aging" or "speeds up your metabolism," that promise to have a positive effect on a complicated, multifaceted process in the body. Also be alert to "miracle," "secret," and "effortless" effects. Does it make sense, for example, that you could eat all you want and lose weight at the same time? When "scientific" mumbo jumbo appears, read it more closely. For example, aren't you a bit curious about the percentage of people who "may" be deficient and why you "may" be deficient rather than "are" deficient? Contact the manufacturer for more information about alleged benefits and request copies of, or references to, scientific articles reviewed in reputable medical journals.

Bottom Line

I'm not saying that supplements can't work. For some people, some of the time, to some degree, they can. After all, when it comes to the human body and enhancing athletic performance, the science often falls into a gray area. Just keep in mind that we each represent an experiment of one, which may help explain why you don't notice any appreciable benefits from a supplement that a training buddy (or an elite athlete) raves about or why you don't seem to get the same boost from an old favorite that you've taken for years.

You may also simply believe that a product works. Perhaps you started taking a supplement during a period of natural improvement that occurred because of other factors such as improved training or better mental preparation. Maybe you simply experience a psychological lift (known as the placebo effect) when you take a certain product. This mental boost alone can be enough to power you to better performance. Of course, if prudent scientific evidence exists (such as the research that supports using sports drinks during exercise to maintain your blood sugar), or you're diagnosed with a nutrient-specific deficiency (iron-deficiency anemia, for example), then taking a supplement will most likely help.

Even if certain substances are shown to be of some benefit in improving athletic performance, keep the gains in perspective. Your inherited talent, mental attitude, training methods, eating habits, and equipment choices all play a far greater role in your success than could any dietary supplement. Maybe you even excel in spite of something that you take! You can't go wrong covering all these bases before you seek a safe, legal supplement.

Finally, make sure that you're willing to pay the price for taking supplements—literally and figuratively. I know that it's tempting to take supplements for a chronic health problem or for an injury that standard medical treatments fail to solve. Be prepared, however, to feel disappointed and even less hopeful every time you invest in a supplement that doesn't do what it claims to do. You may even become less motivated to seek any kind of help. If you continue to exercise and rely solely on a supplement to cure your illness or injury, you must consider the opportunities that you forfeited to try something else, such as another treatment plan, further medical help, or simply rest and time off. Even if you're just looking for an edge, don't let taking supplements keep you from doing what you might really need to do, such as revamping your training program or learning some basic cooking skills.

Solving Peak Performance Challenges

6

Just when you think you have everything under control, something pops up that snaps you back to reality—a tree root, a flat tire, a broken ski binding. The new obstacle may also be one of the common nemeses discussed in earlier chapters that athletes face every time they head out the door to exercise such as dehydration, glycogen depletion, or bonking due to low blood sugar. On the other hand, the problem may be something that you're not as familiar with, such as anemia or recurring muscle cramps. A food allergy or intolerance may threaten to slow you down too. On top of that, female endurance athletes face some particular challenges, such as feeling bogged down certain times of the month and dealing with the physical and emotional changes associated with pregnancy. In any case, specific nutritional strategies can help you get back on track quickly.

Muscle Cramps

If you've ever suffered with a muscle cramp, you know that they always seem to strike just when you need to make your push toward the finish line. Unpredictable in nature, a cramp is a muscle contraction gone out of control, locking the muscle into a sustained and painful

"It wasn't until I got to the Olympic Training Center that I had any serious testing of my iron levels done. They couldn't believe how low my ferritin stores were for an endurance athlete. Training 25 to 40 hours a week at altitude pushes them even lower. I make a conscious effort to eat red meat several times a week and I take a liquid iron supplement twice a day, otherwise my levels drop right back down. It definitely helped me in Hawaii, and I'm going to stay on top of it as I train for the Olympics. Taking too much iron can be dangerous, though, so my brother (a physician) monitors my blood once a month."

—Tim DeBoom,
three-time Hawaii Ironman winner

125

spasm. The exact cause of muscle cramps and how best to treat them remain unclear. Calf muscles seem to be most susceptible, but a cramp can be in any muscle in the body.

Overexertion, or working a muscle to the point of exhaustion, is the most likely culprit, but predisposing factors such as dehydration, an electrolyte imbalance, or a mineral deficiency may play a contributing role. Undoubtedly, athletes tend to suffer muscle cramps more easily when dehydrated, so don't overlook an obvious solution. Start out well hydrated, drink as much as you can reasonably tolerate during prolonged exercise (ideally two to eight gulps or ounces, or 60 to 250 milliliters, every 15 to 20 minutes), use a sports drink if you're going longer than 60 minutes, and be sure to rehydrate afterward.

One way to monitor your fluid needs during exercise is by noting your ability to urinate. No hard and fast guidelines exist for how often you should urinate during prolonged exercise. If you find yourself not urinating for more than a few hours at a time or you can't urinate for several hours following exercise, you need to pay more attention to your fluid needs during exercise. Don't forget that you can lose two quarts (liters) of sweat per hour during vigorous exercise in the heat. Avoid becoming progressively dehydrated day to day, especially when training in warm conditions, by checking your weight before and after you exercise. Assume that all the weight you lost is fluid that you need to replace that day. Rehydrate by drinking at least 2.5 cups of fluid for every pound (1.3 liters for every kilogram) of body weight lost.

Besides drinking enough fluid, be sure to get enough electrolytes, such as potassium and sodium, in your daily diet. Potassium and sodium help maintain water balance in the body, and the electrical charges that they carry help trigger muscles to contract and relax. A potassium–sodium imbalance may lead to muscle cramps. Although you lose both potassium and sodium in sweat, you should have enough body stores of both to cover these losses. Most sports drinks intended for use during exercise, as well as foods typically eaten during ultralong events, provide both sodium and potassium.

Your best defense against muscle cramps is to eat potassium-rich foods daily and use the saltshaker liberally, especially if you sweat profusely, train in a hot environment, or are involved in ultraendurance events. Potassium-rich foods, such as pinto and kidney beans, potatoes, tomatoes, spinach, cantaloupe, orange juice, bananas, dried fruit, milk, and yogurt make good choices. Potassium supplements shouldn't be necessary, and they can be harmful if you consume large doses over a short period.

If you're in good health and don't have a family history of hypertension (high blood pressure), don't let the popular guidelines calling for a restriction on dietary sodium trip you up. These guidelines target the general population, with the hope of reducing high blood pressure in sedentary and overweight people. As an endurance athlete, you may end up in the medical tent on race day if you subscribe to a salt-restricted training diet. Muscle cramps, especially if accompanied by fatigue and lethargy, can be due to a sodium deficit that develops during prolonged exercise. In fact, many exercise physiologists and nutritionists feel that sodium depletion is the major predisposing factor behind cramping during athletic performances, especially in warm weather.

Keep the saltshaker handy at the dinner table and answer salt cravings when they arise by consuming salty foods, such as pretzels, salsa and chips, pickles, soup, tomato juice, and canned foods. If you participate in ultraendurance events and suffer from recurring muscle cramps despite a daily liberal salt intake, you may need to experiment with salt or electrolyte tablets. Keep in mind that unless you take these tablets with ample fluid, you run the risk of causing gastrointestinal problems and dehydration.

A calcium deficiency is often blamed for muscle cramps too. Calcium, the most abundant mineral in the body, plays an essential role in normal muscle function. But a calcium imbalance is unlikely to cause muscle cramps, because the body tightly regulates calcium levels in the blood. It does so by releasing calcium from the bones when enough dietary calcium isn't available, so sufficient calcium always remains available for normal nerve conduction and muscle contraction.

Nevertheless, some athletes may see their cramps disappear by boosting a calcium-poor diet with foods rich in calcium. To see whether consuming more calcium makes a difference, consume at least two to three servings of calcium-rich foods daily. Dairy foods or other calcium-fortified foods, such as orange juice, soy milk, and tofu, make good choices. If you're unable to consume enough calcium through your food choices, round out your diet with a supplement. If nothing else, it will help protect your bones from becoming depleted.

In the end, if none of these nutritional strategies helps in resolving muscle cramps, a physical therapist can help you explore potential biomechanical causes of muscle cramps, such as a leg-length discrepancy. A lack of flexibility or physical conditioning can also precipitate muscle cramps, so consult an athletic trainer or coach regarding proper stretching and training techniques.

Runner's Diarrhea

Any athlete may suffer from diarrhea and other intestinal problems during or after workouts or long races. Runners, however, appear to be more affected by diarrhea and cramping than other athletes are. Studies reveal that between 19 and 26 percent of marathon runners experience running-related diarrhea. Besides the lack of adequate blood flow to the gastrointestinal (GI) tract during exercise and exercise-induced changes in GI hormones and the nervous system, runners suffer from another abuse. The repetitive and jarring action of running may cause injury to the walls of the large intestine or colon, leading to diarrhea and GI blood loss.

Although diet and medications can certainly be factors in causing runner's diarrhea, drinking plenty of fluids before and during exercise is the best defense against runner's diarrhea and other more serious GI problems, such as "athletic colitis." Experiencing bad diarrhea during exercise but not at other times might indicate that your colon becomes irritated because blood flow during exercise is inadequate. During prolonged exercise, your body diverts blood away from the colon to active muscles and to the skin to disperse heat. Being dehydrated aggravates the situation because your reduced blood volume means that even less blood is available to the large intestine. The lack of blood flow can sometimes cause severe damage to the walls of the colon.

One elite female runner and two elite triathletes (one female and one male) have had parts of their colons surgically removed because of exercise-induced bowel problems. Concentrate on drinking fluids in the early stages of long races. As dehydration progresses, it becomes increasingly difficult for your body to absorb the fluids that you do drink.

Look at your diet too. Eating high-fiber foods, such as bran cereals and whole-grain products, too close to the time that you exercise (especially if you're nervous or anxious) can also cause diarrhea. Insoluble fiber causes the colon to retain water and soften bowel movements, which can result in diarrhea during the stress of competition. Caffeine is known to have a laxative effect, and artificial sweeteners, such as sorbitol and aspartame in candy and diet sodas, can cause diarrhea as well. Develop and stick to a prerace diet of foods that you have tested and know that you can tolerate. Check with your physician about the possibility that giardiasis (an infection of the small intestine caused by a parasite), medications, or herbal supplements are causing diarrhea during exercise. Your health care provider can also advise you on the use of antidiarrheal medications during prolonged exercise.

Iron-Deficiency Anemia

Iron-deficiency anemia, characterized by a low blood iron level, will slow even the fittest and best conditioned endurance athlete. Iron, although present in the body in relatively small amounts, plays a crucial role in the transport of oxygen. The body requires iron to form both hemoglobin and myoglobin. Hemoglobin, found in red blood cells, binds with oxygen in the lungs and then transports it (through the blood) throughout the body. Myoglobin, located in muscles, combines with oxygen and stores it until needed. If you suffer from anemia, your muscles receive less oxygen and, consequently, produce more lactic acid. As lactic acid builds up in your muscles, you fatigue prematurely when you exercise. Other possible signs and symptoms of iron-deficiency anemia include muscle burning and shortness of breath during exercise, nausea, frequent infections, sensitivity to the cold, respiratory illnesses, and a pale, washed-out appearance. Student–athletes should also know that anemia can compromise their ability to think and carry out mental tasks.

Most of the iron in the body is incorporated into hemoglobin (60 percent) and myoglobin (10 percent), with a small amount (2 percent) involved in other intracellular components and enzymes. About 30 percent (less in women) is stored as ferritin, primarily within the bone marrow, liver, and spleen. If iron is lacking in the diet, the body draws from its iron stores (ferritin). When this reserve is depleted, the formation of hemoglobin is affected. Red blood cells cannot carry the oxygen needed by cells, and consequently your capacity to work out or race drops off or reaches a plateau. Before you register an outright low blood iron level and are diagnosed with anemia, however, you may be slowed by low iron reserves (ferritin).

Iron Needs and Losses

Women have higher daily iron needs (18 milligrams) than do teenage males (11 milligrams) and adult males (8 milligrams) because they lose iron through menstrual bleeding. If you suffer from recurring bouts of anemia, the first step is to take a closer look at your diet. A diet low in iron-rich foods is the primary cause of most iron deficiencies, particularly among active women. Even women who make smart food choices often have difficulty meeting their daily iron requirement. Female athletes who place a premium on having a lean physique by dieting or restricting calories will find it virtually impossible to consume enough iron. Vegetarian athletes, male or female, also have a higher risk of developing anemia. The iron in plant foods is not as efficiently absorbed as the iron in red meat, poultry, or fish.

Menstrual blood loss is the second biggest cause of low iron levels in women. Female athletes lose iron-rich hemoglobin each month if they menstruate regularly. This loss can vary substantially depending on the duration and heaviness of the menstrual flow.

Endurance athletes lose iron through various other avenues as well. Iron is lost through GI bleeding that occurs with prolonged exercise, especially if diarrhea or cramping occurs during exercise. Less blood flows to the GI tract during exercise, especially during intense efforts, as more blood flows to active muscles. The lack of blood flow and nutrients in the lining of the GI tract causes cells to die and slough off. The result is occult, or hidden, blood in bowel movements. Some athletes suffer with bloody diarrhea occasionally, but in most cases they are probably not even aware of GI bleeding and this mode of iron loss. Dehydration, an inevitable consequence of participating in endurance events, exacerbates GI bleeding by further reducing the blood flow to the GI tract. Taking aspirin or nonsteroidal anti-inflammatory medications (Advil, ibuprofen, naproxen sodium, and so on) may also increase GI blood loss.

Iron losses through sweat and urine are usually negligible, but these losses can add up with prolonged exercise. For example, the physical jarring that the bladder endures during prolonged exercise, coupled with dehydration, can result in urinary blood losses. Daily exercise, especially if you're racking up the miles, also appears to impair the absorption of iron from the GI tract. Normally, the body absorbs more iron in response to an iron deficiency. In athletes, this compensatory response appears to be blunted. One study, for example, found that iron-deficient runners absorbed only 16 percent of dietary iron as compared with the 30 percent absorbed by nonathletes.

Iron depletion can also result simply from the slow loss of iron due to the chronic injury to red blood cells. The repetitive trauma of hard foot strikes in high-impact sports such as running, for example, destroys red blood cells. Athletes involved in swimming and other nonrunning sports, however, can have exercise-induced anemia, leading to the theory that muscle contractions, acidosis (a decrease in blood pH), or the increase in body temperature associated with exercise may also damage red blood cells. Your liver recycles released hemoglobin from damaged red blood cells up to a point. Beyond that, the hemoglobin is excreted into the urine, thereby compromising your iron status.

Monitoring Your Iron Status

The loss of iron is divided into three stages according to the effect on the ability of the body to make normal red blood cells. In stages 1 and 2, only ferritin, the iron reserves of the body, falls. Stage 1 (iron depletion) is characterized by a serum ferritin level of less than 12 nanograms per milliliter, indicating almost completely depleted iron stores. If this iron depletion continues for several months, stage 2 (iron-deficient erythropoiesis) can result, in which iron transport throughout the body and the production of red blood cells are affected. During both stage 1 and stage 2, a blood test will reveal a low serum ferritin level, but hemoglobin and hematocrit (percentage of red blood cells in the total blood volume) values will remain essentially normal. The mild anemia associated with stage 2, therefore, typically goes undetected. Stage 3 (iron-deficient anemia) results when the lack of iron stores literally compromises the ability of the body to produce normal red blood cells. A blood test will now show below-normal levels of hemoglobin and hematocrit, which will result in a formal diagnosis of iron-deficient anemia.

The normal range for hemoglobin in teenage and adult females is 12 to 16 grams per deciliter. For hematocrit, the normal range is 37 to 48 percent. For teenage and adult males, normal values for hemoglobin range from 13 to 18 grams per deciliter. For hematocrit, the normal range is 45 to 52 percent. Athletes who live and train at higher altitudes typically have more red blood cells, resulting in slightly higher hemoglobin and hematocrit values. Being dehydrated when you have your blood drawn can also produce elevated levels.

When it comes to interpreting serum ferritin values, the general rule in the sports world is that levels below 12 micrograms per milliliter indicate completely depleted iron stores in the bone marrow, whereas values between 12 micrograms per milliliter and the lower limit of the normal range represent minimal iron stores. Diagnostic laboratories typically define normal, or adequate, iron stores as more than 20 micrograms per milliliter, whereas most exercise physiologists and exercise science researchers define serum ferritin levels of 35 micrograms per milliliter as the lower limit of normal for athletes.

You can easily monitor your iron status through specific blood tests that check your hemoglobin, hematocrit, and serum ferritin levels. Hemoglobin and hematocrit are typically included in routine blood work during a yearly physical. Unless you have a sports-savvy physician, though, you'll most likely have to request to have your iron stores, or serum ferritin, checked.

To get the most out of monitoring your iron status, you must first determine your baseline values. Anemia is defined by a hemoglobin or hematocrit value that falls below the normal range. Normal and abnormal values overlap significantly, though, and you should compare your test results only to your personal baseline range. For example, during my career as a competitive distance runner I kept copies of all my blood work, and I've discovered over the years that I perform poorly when my hemoglobin dips below 14 because my baseline runs closer to 14.5 grams per deciliter. A reading of 13 grams per deciliter, however, may not signal anemia for an athlete who has a lower baseline.

Unfortunately, most athletes typically have blood work performed only when they aren't feeling or performing well. This practice means it may take a series of blood tests over time, correlated with physical symptoms and your training and racing performances, to determine your ideal normal range. If you can swing it, have blood work performed when you're at the top of your game too.

Treating Iron-Deficiency Anemia (Stage 3)

If you're diagnosed with iron-deficiency anemia (stage 3), treatment usually consists of 50 to 100 milligrams of elemental iron, two to three times a day. To reduce possible side effects, such as nausea, diarrhea, or constipation, gradually increase the amount that you take from once a day to three times a day as your tolerance increases. Ferrous sulfate, available in a liquid form, is absorbed better than most other varieties. Slow-release products can help reduce constipation.

To enhance the absorption of iron supplements, take them on an empty stomach with 500 milligrams of vitamin C or a glass of juice rich in vitamin C. Be sure to take calcium and iron supplements a few hours apart, because calcium interferes with iron absorption. Allow at least four to six weeks before you have your blood work repeated to confirm that your hemoglobin level is improving. By eight weeks the anemia is usually corrected, although every athlete responds differently. You may need to continue with iron supplements for as long as six months to replenish your iron stores, as evidenced by normal ferritin levels. Be sure to do this under the care of a physician.

Treating Iron Depletion

Athletes with low-normal or decreasing levels of serum ferritin, despite a hemoglobin reading in the normal range (stages 1 and 2), should consider iron therapy too. Anemia impairs athletic performance by reducing the delivery of oxygen to tissues, but iron depletion can diminish your performance by a different mechanism. Iron-dependent metabolic processes at the cellular level, such as energy production in the mitochondria, may become impaired as your iron stores drop.

Studies of the effects of iron supplementation on performance in athletes with low iron stores have produced conflicting results. No improvements in $\dot{V}O_2$max have been shown, but other indicators of improved endurance, such as improvements in treadmill times and lower lactate levels during submaximal exercise, have been recorded. My personal experience and that of endurance athletes with whom I've trained suggest that low iron stores can hinder performance well before an athlete is diagnosed with anemia. As with hemoglobin, an individual threshold, or optimal level of iron storage, most likely exists for every endurance athlete. While living in Boulder, Colorado, my serum ferritin levels fell to 21, most likely because of training at altitude. Although the physician considered this level normal, I began supplementing with iron. Another blood test three months later revealed that I had boosted my iron stores to almost twice that amount. More importantly, the chronic muscle soreness that I had been experiencing cleared up in just a few weeks.

Whether it helps immediately, boosting low (less than 12 micrograms per milliliter) and borderline-low ferritin levels by controlled iron supplementation can prevent outright anemia from developing. The recommended treatment is 50 to 100 milligrams of elemental iron a day (taken with vitamin C) for one to three months, after which you should have your serum ferritin levels rechecked. (Too much iron can be toxic for your liver.) Many times, the hemoglobin level will also increase, indicating that a mild anemia was already present although the initial hemoglobin level was technically in the normal range. Ideally, you want to maintain your iron stores as high as reasonably possible, as evidenced by serum ferritin readings of 50 micrograms per milliliter for women and 70 micrograms per milliliter for men.

Carefully plan your blood tests around your exercise. Your ferritin value can be artificially elevated for 48 to 72 hours following a prolonged bout of exercise such as a marathon or half Ironman (one to two weeks following an ultra) or if you're fighting an infection or experiencing inflammation. High-intensity training tends to decrease ferritin levels gradually, so keep this in mind as you interpret your values.

Preventing Anemia and Iron Deficiency

Emphasizing iron-rich foods in your diet will help prevent an iron deficiency from turning into anemia. The iron in animal foods, particularly from red meat, is more absorbable than the iron in supplements or plant foods (for a list of iron-rich foods see "Best Bets: Iron" in chapter 1). Cooking in cast-iron skillets will also help you maximize your iron intake, as will eating a food rich in vitamin C (fruits, vegetables, or juices) along with iron-containing foods. Female athletes who don't eat meat should consider taking a multivitamin with iron or a low-dose iron supplement (18 milligrams per day).

Because iron deficiency is so common, especially among female athletes, screening for it at least once a year makes sense. Be sure to request a serum ferritin blood test along with the routine tests that look at hemoglobin and hematocrit levels. Keep a log of your blood test results and record other pertinent data, such as the type and amount of training that you were doing, racing performances (if applicable), and comments on your general state of health.

Although you may be tempted to diagnose and treat yourself when you feel rundown and tired, don't start taking appreciable amounts of iron without first seeing a physician. Certain people are susceptible to iron overload, or hemochromatosis, which can lead to serious and irreversible damage to internal organs. Besides, taking iron supplements when you don't have an iron deficiency won't boost your performance, and consuming too much iron can impede the absorption of other minerals, such as zinc.

Understanding Sports Anemia

Incidentally, a low hemoglobin may not always represent a problem, as is the case in dilutional pseudoanemia. Commonly referred to as sports anemia, dilutional pseudoanemia is the natural dilution of hemoglobin that occurs when endurance exercise produces an increase in plasma volume. Plasma, the watery portion of the blood, expands beyond its baseline in response to the exercise-induced release of various hormones. This increase in plasma volume artificially lowers hemoglobin and hematocrit readings.

Because the number of red blood cells remains normal and increases proportionately during exercise as water is lost from the blood in sweat, oxygen-carrying capacity is not compromised. Sports anemia doesn't usually last long. It frequently occurs in athletes who are returning to training after inactivity or increasing their training intensity. Sports anemia doesn't respond to iron supplementation and can be distinguished from iron-deficiency anemia because the lab workup will reveal that the red blood cells do not appear pale or small as they do in true anemia.

Tips for Avoiding a Cold

Your biggest fear may not be hiking through whiteout conditions or descending a steep hill at 40 miles (64 kilometers) per hour on your bike, but simply the thought of catching a cold. As an athlete, you know that a common cold or other upper-respiratory infection can keep you from even getting to the starting line of your favorite activity. What can you do besides pay homage to vitamin C tablets? Plenty.

1. Eat a well-balanced sports diet. Keep your vitamin and mineral reserves at optimal levels so that your immune system will function at its best.

2. Don't shortchange yourself in the sleep department. Disrupted sleep has been linked to a suppressed immune system.

3. Avoid overtraining and chronic fatigue. When in doubt, leave it out, especially if you feel as if you're coming down with something. Give your body a chance to mount an attack without the extra stress generated by intense or prolonged physical efforts.

4. Wash your hands often. Viruses can easily enter your body when you touch germ-ridden hands to your eyes and nose.

5. Avoid large crowds and sick people whenever possible before important events. Consider getting a flu shot if you compete during the winter. You're particularly vulnerable to catching something immediately following a workout or race, so choose your companions wisely!

6. Use carbohydrate-containing beverages before, during, and after intensive training bouts and competitive efforts, which may help lessen the negative effect of stress hormones on your immune system.

7. Don't try to drop weight quickly before a competitive event. Rapid weight loss stresses the immune system.

(continued)

(continued)

8. Keep other life stresses to a minimum. When this isn't possible, recognize that you're vulnerable to colds and infections, and moderate your training accordingly.

9. Experiment with supplements. Despite well-designed studies to the contrary, many athletes continue to believe that the herb Echinacea may boost resistance to colds and flu. Echinacea is most effective when taken at the first sign of symptoms (not beforehand) and then every two hours until symptoms are relieved. Take it for short periods—a few days to a few weeks at most. Continual use can actually suppress your immune system. (Don't take it at all if you're pregnant, nursing, have an autoimmune disease, or have allergies to ragweed.)

10. Sucking on zinc lozenges (the published research was done with zinc gluconate) may reduce the severity and duration of a cold if you take them at the first sign of sniffles. To avoid zinc overload, don't take them for more than a week at a time. Avoid drinking citrus juices and soft drinks, which can interfere with zinc absorption, one half hour before and after taking the lozenges. To reduce feelings of nausea, don't take them on an empty stomach.

11. Taking vitamin C supplements will not prevent you from catching a cold but may help you feel better while you have it. Limit yourself to 1,000 milligrams a day, no more than 500 milligrams per dose. Larger doses might trigger diarrhea or kidney stones in some people. Athletes participating in ultraevents may reduce the oxidative stress to their immune cells by taking vitamin C supplements (about 600 milligrams a day for at least one week before the event).

12. If you do come down with a cold, comfort yourself with an 800-year-old remedy. Remember that a big bowl of hot chicken soup can improve coughing and help clear the lungs.

Adapted, by permission, from D. Nieman, 1998, "Immunity in athletes: Current issues," *Sports Science Exchange* 69(11).

Food Allergies and Intolerances

Athletes often let self-diagnosed food allergies get in the way of eating a well-balanced, healthy diet. After all, about 25 percent of American adults believe that they have a food allergy, but only 1 to 2 percent actually do. A food intolerance, on the other hand, can affect nearly everyone at some point. This next section provides strategies for dealing with both.

Food Allergies

What's the difference between a food allergy and a food intolerance? A food allergy involves the immune system of the body. An allergen, usually a protein, in a food or ingredient causes an allergic person's immune system to overreact.

Perceiving the allergen as being harmful, the body produces massive amounts of immunoglobulin E (IgE), a type of antibody. IgE antibodies circulate in the blood and enter body tissues, stimulating other cells to release powerful substances, such as histamine. The reactions that occur, within minutes to an hour or two later, include tingling or swelling in the mouth and throat, stomach cramps, vomiting, diarrhea, skin rashes or hives, runny nose, sneezing, coughing, and wheezing. In highly allergic people, anaphylactic shock, a severe swelling of the throat, tongue, and airway that obstructs breathing, can occur.

Eight foods cause almost 90 percent of all severe food allergy reactions. In adults, shellfish (shrimp, crayfish, lobster, and crab), peanuts, tree nuts (almonds, cashews, pecans, and walnuts), fish, and eggs top the list. In children, eggs, milk, and peanuts are the main offenders. Soy and wheat round out the list. In general, if you're from a family in which allergies such as hay fever, asthma, or hives are common, you're more likely to be predisposed to developing a food allergy. Although adults rarely lose their allergies, children often outgrow their allergies, especially to milk, soy, and eggs.

Having a food allergy is a rare and serious condition that warrants a proper diagnosis by a board-certified allergist. Try to find one who specializes in food allergies. Keeping a food diary that details the allergic reactions caused by a specific food will provide valuable information, such as how much you can eat before experiencing a reaction and how quickly the reaction occurs after eating the suspected food. To narrow down the cause or help rule out a suspected food allergy, an allergist can perform prick skin tests (PST) or radioallergosorbent tests (RAST) on the blood. Be aware that a positive skin or blood test, by itself, doesn't make the diagnosis of a food allergy. You must have a positive test to a specific allergen and a history of reactions suggesting an allergy to the same food.

Self-diagnosing an allergy can get you into trouble. Avoiding particular foods unnecessarily deprives you of food choices and important nutrients. Incorrect identification of the allergen can also be dangerous. In a true food allergy, even minute amounts of the allergen will cause a reaction. Treatment focuses on avoiding the food after it is identified. (Since 2006 this has become easier to do because all packaged foods must clearly list whether they contain any of the eight major allergens: milk, eggs, fish, shellfish, tree nuts, wheat, peanuts, and soybeans.) Allergy shots, as well as injections of small quantities of extracts from foods that you react to, are rarely effective in relieving food allergies.

Food Intolerances

If you have trouble tolerating a food, it's much more likely that you have a food intolerance. You may suffer from many of the same symptoms caused by an allergy, but your immune system is not involved. Food intolerances tend to come and go in severity and are rarely life threatening. A prime example is lactose intolerance, which occurs when the body lacks enough lactase, an intestinal enzyme that breaks down the sugar in milk. Stomach cramps, gas, and diarrhea signal this problem.

Another important distinction from food allergies is that a food intolerance will often allow you to eat varying amounts of the offending food without experiencing any symptoms. Lactose-intolerance sufferers will often find that they can tolerate milk in different forms, such as yogurt, hard cheese, and ice cream. Using Lactaid tablets, drinking milk with added lactase, or drinking small amounts of milk at meals, not on an empty stomach, can often alleviate the problem too. The good news is that in many cases, your body can learn to adjust to the food as you build up a tolerance to it. For example, routinely drinking 2 to 4 ounces (60 to 120 milliliters) of milk at one meal can condition your body, over time, to handle larger amounts of lactose. (Gluten intolerance or celiac disease, an autoimmune intestinal disease, is an exception because the only effective treatment is to remove all wheat, barley, rye, and oats from the diet. Work with a sports dietitian to design an eating plan that will meet your high-energy needs.)

If you find your list of intolerable foods growing, other factors may be coming into play. Eating certain foods too close to exercise, when you're nervous, or when you're under stress may be causing a reaction. Milk, for example, is routinely blamed for causing cottonmouth—dryness in the mouth accompanied by thick, white saliva. The most likely culprit behind cottonmouth, however, is a combination of emotional stress and the loss of fluids during vigorous exercise and competition. Staying well hydrated before, during, and after exercise—rather than avoiding milk—is your best defense against cottonmouth.

A psychological trigger may be responsible for your food intolerance. You may have experienced an unpleasant event, perhaps during childhood, tied to eating a particular food. Or you may be convinced that eating a certain food was associated with a poor performance in the past. Eating that food then becomes linked with a rush of unpleasant sensations that can resemble an allergic reaction to food.

Finding a Solution

Eliminating a few foods from an otherwise healthy diet shouldn't cause a problem, especially if you eat a variety of foods most of the time. Athletes often temporarily avoid certain foods as they approach an important competition. You may be setting yourself up for nutrient deficiencies, however, if you exclude entire food groups or regularly find yourself able to tolerate only a few foods. If this is the case, seek help from a sports dietitian to help you make food substitutions and plan a well-balanced diet. If your symptoms are linked to food additives, such as MSG or sulfites (common in asthmatics), you should certainly avoid foods containing those substances. Check the ingredient lists on food labels and inquire how foods are prepared when dining away from home.

One way to investigate whether a specific food is the source behind your symptoms is to use an elimination diet. Keeping other factors the same, such as the amount and intensity of your training, eliminate one food at a time for several days. Monitor your symptoms for improvement. To confirm the connection, you need to eat the food again and see whether the symptoms return. Obviously, you can't do this without medical supervision if you've been experiencing severe reactions that you believe are food related. In addition, elimination diets aren't that useful if the symptoms that you experience occur infrequently.

Keep in mind that whenever you push your body to the limit, high levels of epinephrine (adrenaline) can interfere with the normal functioning of the GI tract. The rate at which food empties the stomach can be delayed, increasing the likelihood that you'll experience nausea and indigestion. Mental and emotional stress can also slow the time that it takes for food to leave the stomach. Eating smaller, more frequent meals composed of low-fat, familiar foods can help as you approach a competition or undergo periods of vigorous or stressful training. More often than not, modifying the timing of foods and fluids around exercise can make the difference.

No athlete wants to be slowed by bloating, flatulence, abdominal cramps, or diarrhea. Do your best to avoid abdominal discomfort before important events or races by staying well hydrated and avoiding gas-forming foods, such as carbonated beverages, beans, broccoli, cabbage, onions, and other problem foods that you've identified during training. Establishing a consistent eating pattern and regular bowel habits are your best bet in preventing abdominal and intestinal problems.

Female Athlete Triad

Female fitness enthusiasts, as well as novice and elite female endurance athletes, are at risk for developing a syndrome of interrelated problems known as the female athlete triad. Although not as clearly defined in the opposite sex, male endurance athletes are likely at risk too. The triad is composed of disordered eating, amenorrhea (loss of three or more consecutive menstrual cycles), and compromised bone health, such as stress fractures and osteoporosis. Individually, each of these conditions is worrisome; combined, they can do real damage to your health.

Underfueling, or consuming fewer calories than your body needs to function properly, kicks off the triad. Some athletes end up in an energy (caloric) deficit by inadvertently expending more calories than they consume because of a strenuous training program. More likely, however, underfueling results when physically active girls and women restrict calories in a deliberate effort to lose weight quickly in hopes of improving their appearance or performance. Disordered eating, or unhealthy eating patterns as previously discussed in chapter 3, such as skipping meals, eating as little fat as possible, or periodically overeating and then purging (including exercising compulsively to burn off or cancel out calories), typically set the stage.

In response to the consumption of too few calories, the brain signals the ovaries to produce less estrogen and menstrual periods become fewer and less regular (or don't begin at all in young women). A lack of menstrual periods before age 16 or a loss of regular cycles for at least three consecutive months is called amenorrhea. Studies performed over the last 20 years, by research physiologist Barbara Drinkwater, PhD, and other female athlete advocates, strongly support that menstrual irregularities or even the total loss of the menstrual cycle does not result from the stress of exercise or low body fatness. The cause is low energy (caloric) availability. Amenorrhea can be reversed when an active female adequately keeps up with or replenishes daily the calories that she expends. Note too that you don't have to suffer from a full-blown eating disorder to induce amenorrhea; disordered or dysfunctional eating habits can be enough. Nor does the triad strike only elite athletes. All physically active girls and women who undereat, overexercise, or both are at risk for complications associated with the triad.

The prime danger with amenorrhea is how it affects bones. Hormonal disturbances, such as low estrogen levels, accompany amenorrhea and interrupt the way that bones normally grow and develop. Without enough estrogen, especially during your peak bone-building years (teens and 20s), you lose bone rapidly instead of banking it for the future. Although you may be in your 20s (or look like you are), you could have the bones of a 60- or 70-year-old woman on the inside! This finding is particularly distressing because Drinkwater and others have found that females involved in sports normally present with a 10 to 15 percent increase in bone mineral density compared with their normal peers.

When bones are less dense, you run a higher risk of suffering both stress fractures and soft-tissue injuries. And should you incur osteoporotic fractures (because of brittle bones that break easily), these changes in bone never reverse themselves. Lastly, amenorrhea can interfere with your ability in the future to become pregnant and possibly even put you at higher risk for heart disease.

Athletes, parents, and coaches should know that the American College of Sports Medicine considers amenorrhea to be the most recognizable symptom, or red flag, of the triad. Although certain medical conditions, such as hypothyroidism (an underactive thyroid), can cause amenorrhea, female athletes and those around them often view the absence of periods as a benign side effect of hard training. A 2004 survey undertaken by psychologists Roberta Sherman, PhD, and Ron Thompson, PhD, cochairs of the Athlete Special Interest Group of the Academy of Eating Disorders and consultants to the department of intercollegiate athletics at Indiana University for the past 15 years, confirms this sentiment. Of the almost 2,900 NCAA coaches of female athletes (representing 23 different sports) who responded, 37 percent viewed amenorrhea as normal. Fewer than half of the coaches considered amenorrhea to be abnormal and in need of medical treatment. In reality, a knowledgeable physician should evaluate any active female with amenorrhea to determine the cause of the amenorrhea. The same advice applies to stress fractures, another easily recognizable sign of the triad.

Understand as well that not all three components—disordered eating, amenorrhea, and bone problems—need to occur simultaneously for the triad to be diagnosed. Rather, physically active females tend to slide in and out of the triad, depending on how well they are doing at that time in achieving energy balance (calories consumed at least equal to calories expended). Active girls and women who present with one aspect of the triad should always be screened by a credible sports-minded health professional for the other two.

In 2005 the International Olympic Committee (IOC), which is responsible for the overall health and welfare of competitive athletes worldwide, took a more active stance regarding the female athlete triad. Speaking directly to the athletic community (sports medicine doctors, coaches, athletic trainers, and so on), the IOC released a first-time position stand that outlines practical and definitive steps to take in recognizing, treating, and most importantly, preventing the triad (see "Selected Resources").

Questions still remain about whether a female can catch up if she misses the window of opportunity to attain her genetic potential for peak bone mass (puberty to adulthood, from ages 10 to 12 through 16 to 18). Oral contraceptives given to halt further bone loss do work, but they must be viewed as a stopgap measure because this intervention is not enough to build new bone in a female diagnosed with amenorrhea. Rather, the female with amenorrhea must work, supported by a treatment team (physician, sports dietitian, and possibly a therapist), to restore her natural menstrual cycle through good nutrition. Medications to promote building new bone (that is, Fosomax) are for postmenopausal women only, and women of childbearing age should not use them. Animal studies have shown that because of their long half-life, these drugs can cross the placenta and be absorbed by the fetus.

Incidentally, male athletes can be at risk for stress fractures and osteoporosis as well. Consuming too few calories, especially in conjunction with endurance training, can lower testosterone levels. Insufficient testosterone (analogous to low estrogen levels in females), besides reducing fertility and sex drive, puts bones at risk.

Rarely are dietary changes alone enough to reverse the triad. Lifestyle changes are necessary. If you have been diagnosed with amenorrhea, reduce your training by 10 to 20 percent, increase the calories that you consume, and gain a modest amount of weight (2 to 3 percent of your body weight, or as little as 5 pounds, or 2.3 kilograms, can make a difference) until you regain a normal menstrual cycle. Resistance training can help strengthen bones too. Developing new skills and strategies to manage daily stress is necessary as well. If you've been amenorrheic for a year or longer, a bone-density scan will let you know where you stand in regard to bone loss. If you're unwilling to make lifestyle changes or if making changes doesn't help your menstrual periods return (especially if you have a history of stress fractures or you've been amenorrheic for six months or longer), consider estrogen replacement therapy. Oral contraceptives are generally the recommended method.

When it comes to your diet, work on smoothing out erratic eating habits into a schedule of eating wholesome meals and snacks. If you find yourself constantly obsessed with food, you're probably trying to eat too few calories. If you've been avoiding eating meat, particularly red meat, you may want to reconsider. We don't know why meat seems to protect women's menstrual periods, but it does. Aim to include two to three small servings (3 ounces each, the size of a deck of cards) of red meat per week. Remind yourself that fat is an integral part of any athlete's diet and eat at least 20 percent (45 to 60 grams for most active women) of your calories from fat. You need extra calcium and vitamin D at this point (1,200 to 1,500 milligrams of calcium and 400 to 800 IU of vitamin D daily), so choose foods rich in calcium and vitamin D. Add a supplement to make up the remainder. Keep in mind that just taking calcium supplements isn't enough to counteract the lack of estrogen associated with amenorrhea or prevent further bone loss. After your menstrual periods resume, however, the extra calcium can help you build (up to age 30) or maintain your bone mass.

Eating Disorders in Endurance Athletes

Numerous studies suggest that athletes suffer a high risk of developing a full-blown eating disorder, such as anorexia nervosa, bulimia nervosa, or EDNOS (Eating Disorder Not Otherwise Specified). (See "Common Warning Signs of an Eating Disorder," page 145.) Athletes most at risk include those involved in "appearance" sports (such as gymnastics or skating), sports in which low body weight is considered advantageous (distance running and cycling), and weight-category sports (wrestling and rowing). A study of elite British teenage runners is a typical example. Seventeen of these 35 girls are believed to have suffered some form of eating disorder. Only four progressed through the ranks and made it to the senior national team.

Despite popular opinion in the sports world, eating disorders are not confined to female athletes. Males do suffer less from eating disorders than females do, representing at most 10 percent of all reported cases. Anorexia nervosa, however, is more likely to occur in male athletes than in other males. Moreover, male athletes can become just as addicted to exercise, even in the face of illness or injury, as some female athletes do. Current statistics may underestimate the problem, however, because few studies to date on male athletes have used the well-established criteria set forth by the American Psychiatric Association to diagnose varying degrees of eating disorders. On top of that, because eating disorders are perceived as a feminine disease, male sufferers typically seek help less often.

Nevertheless, male athletes can be just as preoccupied with their body size and shape as many women are. One study examined eating, weight, and dieting practices in 162 competitive collegiate rowers: 82 heavyweights (56 women, 26 men) and 80 lightweights (17 women, 63 men). Lightweight rowers must meet weight restrictions as part of the sport. The findings (based on self-reported anonymous questionnaires) reveal that although female rowers exhibit more disordered eating behaviors overall, male rowers also suffer with significant eating and weight concerns.

In this sample, roughly 12 percent of males (and 20 percent of females) reported having binge eating episodes at least twice a week. Binge eating is defined as the discrete consumption of large amounts of food coupled with a sense of loss of control and followed by emotional distress. Moreover, male rowers reported cutting weight (intentional rapid weight loss) more times per season than females did (4.3 times versus .4 times), and they reported the frequent use of extreme methods to lose weight. Fifty-seven percent of males reported fasting (compared with 25 percent of females), and 2.5 percent reported vomiting (compared with 13 percent of females). Male lightweights, in particular, are at risk for potential psychological and medical problems. They reported greater weekly and seasonal fluctuations in weight, cut weight more frequently, and were most likely to fast to lose weight compared with heavyweights or lightweight females.

Before heading to the 2004 Olympic Games in Athens, Britain's leading middle-distance runner, Commonwealth 1,500-meter champion Michael East, sounded the warning in a July newspaper article. He claimed that many of the country's top male athletes were risking their health by starving themselves in an attempt to run faster. Why? East claims that they were doing so in a desperate attempt to recreate the glory days of the 1980s when Sebastian Coe, Steve Ovett, and Steve Cram led the world at middle-distance running. Bruce Hamilton, the British Olympic team's doctor, echoed East's concern. Hamilton agreed that disordered eating is common among male athletes and that inadequate dietary intake over time compromises all body systems, leaving runners prone to stress fractures, infections, and other problems.

As an athlete, male or female, committed to doing well in endurance sports, you're probably accustomed to doing things in the extreme—for example, rising religiously at five o'clock to train before putting in a full day at work, compiling a decade-long streak of never missing a training day, or spending a rainy Saturday running 30 miles (48 kilometers) instead of going to the movies with friends. Not surprisingly, you could also be extreme in your attitudes and beliefs about body weight and eating behaviors, variables that certainly hold the promise of improving your performance. Being competitive and compulsive (friends and family may have even referred to you as obsessive) contributes to your success as an athlete, but it's the very personality type that can lead to an eating disorder.

Causes of Eating Disorders

Eating disorders are complex in nature. They arise from a combination of factors: family problems, long-standing emotional or psychological issues, major life transitions (for example, reaching puberty or going off to college), possible biochemical imbalances, and societal pressures to be thin or have the perfect body. An eating disorder serves as a coping mechanism, although an unhealthy one. People manipulate food and their bodies as a way to cope with feelings and emotions that they don't know how to deal with in a healthier way.

Simply being involved in a particular sport, by itself, rarely causes an eating disorder. We know this to be true because not every athlete who participates in a "high-risk" sport develops an eating disorder. Experts in this field have two theories to explain the high incidence of eating disorders associated with certain sports, such as gymnastics and long-distance running. First, people who have an eating disorder or are at risk of developing one seem to gravitate toward these sports. Second, being involved in these sports triggers, or precipitates, the development of an eating disorder in someone who is vulnerable or predisposed.

People who develop eating disorders typically share some underlying traits: They often feel unworthy or inadequate; have an intense need to be accepted;

suffer from depression, anxiety, or other psychological illness; and lack the skills to cope with emotions and personal issues. Athletes, even the great ones, can suffer with these issues too. Being involved in an endurance sport can further complicate the picture. You have a heightened awareness of your body (including perceived imperfections), and as a driven and disciplined competitor, you believe that you can always achieve more and do better (the win-at-all-costs attitude). On top of that, you may feel a loss of control over your daily activities as well as your goals. Besides pleasing yourself, parents and family members, friends, teachers, and bosses, you must also answer to coaches, teammates, sport associations or governing bodies, and perhaps even the media. Athletes who suffer with eating disorders typically speak of their weight as the only thing in life that they can control. Ironically, these athletes end up being controlled by the very thing that they desperately want to take charge of.

Anorexia Nervosa

Anorexia nervosa is characterized by self-starvation and significant weight loss, usually with an expressed goal of wanting to lose even more weight. Times of transition in early adolescence through early adulthood (12 to 24 years of age), such as puberty, going to college, a divorce in the family, or the death of a significant loved one, can precipitate anorexia in a vulnerable person. People with anorexia tend to be perfectionists with unrealistic goals, and much of their behavior can be viewed as compulsive or ritualistic.

The criteria for being diagnosed with anorexia include

- refusal to maintain weight at or above a minimally normal weight for height and age,
- intense and irrational fear of weight gain or becoming fat even though underweight,
- distorted body image (for example, feeling fat even when emaciated or believing that one area of the body is too fat even when obviously underweight),
- in females, loss of three consecutive menstrual periods when otherwise expected to occur, and
- extreme concern with body weight and shape (distorted body image).

The possible health complications of anorexia nervosa range from mild to severe enough to be life threatening, especially in physically active people. They include

- slow pulse and low blood pressure,
- hair loss,
- severe loss of body fat and muscle wasting,
- cold intolerance,
- lanugo (fine hair on face and arms resulting from the body's attempt to provide insulation),

- muscle weakness and fatigue or extreme hyperactivity,
- anemia,
- amenorrhea (loss of menstrual periods) and infertility problems,
- stress fractures or osteoporosis,
- overuse injuries,
- inability to concentrate and depression,
- insomnia,
- irregular heartbeat or other abnormalities, and
- laxative dependence.

Bulimia Nervosa

Bulimia nervosa is a secretive cycle of binge eating (although men often binge eat with others around) followed by purging. College-age women are particularly at risk; estimates are that one out of every five (20 percent) suffers from bulimia. Those with bulimia nervosa typically experience (and complain about) frequent or extreme fluctuations in weight, but they cannot be identified solely by their weight because they can be fairly thin to normal to overweight. Excessive exercise, frequent trips to the bathroom after eating, laxative abuse, and strict dieting are potential signs to look for when someone is maintaining a low weight despite eating large amounts of food at one time.

Criteria used to diagnosis bulimia nervosa include

- repeated episodes of binge eating (rapid consumption of large amounts of food in a discrete period of time) and purging, two or more episodes per week for three months or longer,
- feeling out of control during a binge,
- purging after a binge (by self-induced vomiting; use of laxatives, diuretics, or diet pills; fasting, strict dieting, or vigorous or excessive exercise) to prevent weight gain,
- frequent dieting (restrained eating), and
- persistent overconcern with body weight and shape.

The possible health complications of bulimia nervosa range from mild to severe enough to be life threatening. They include

- swollen glands and sore throat,
- dental and gum problems,
- inflammation or tears of the esophagus,
- muscle cramps or weakness,
- edema or complaints of bloating,
- fatigue,
- electrolyte imbalances and dehydration,

- menstrual irregularities or amenorrhea,
- frequent stomach cramps, constipation, or diarrhea,
- laxative dependence,
- irregular heartbeat or other abnormalities,
- depression or social withdrawal, and
- insomnia.

Anorexia Athletica

You may think that many of the athletes you coach, train with, or compete against are excessively concerned with their eating habits and weight. This obsession may not be healthy, but it doesn't mean that they all have eating disorders. Some athletes eat poorly simply because they lack knowledge about what to eat. A growing body of evidence suggests, however, that more and more athletes (especially females) are suffering from a less severe or subclinical eating disorder called anorexia athletica. Although such athletes may not meet the strict medical criteria of being anorexic or bulimic, they nevertheless have serious eating problems and body-weight concerns (see EDNOS). Dieting and maintaining a low body weight start out as the means to an end, improving athletic performance, but somewhere along the line losing weight becomes itself the goal.

Currently, researchers are looking at this phenomenon in female athletes, but considerable carryover applies to male athletes. One male recreational-level triathlete I counseled was weighing himself several times a day, although he appeared to be at a healthy weight. When I questioned him about it, he replied that he was assessing whether his training program was working. Eventually, however, he expressed his true concern. He desired to lose five pounds from around his midsection. He was irritable and tired all the time from restricting himself to three small meals a day, although he worked a full day and trained daily. He repeatedly proclaimed, "If I didn't have to eat, I wouldn't." After spending time with him, it became apparent that losing weight had taken precedence over his future performance, because he lacked the desire and energy to maintain his weekly training program.

Female athletes suffering from anorexia athletica have an intense fear of gaining weight or becoming fat although they're underweight (5 to 15 percent below what is normal for their height) or have an extremely low body-fat level. These women generally don't suffer from the severe emotional distress seen in those who have anorexia and bulimia. Nevertheless, they view their bodies in a distorted way. They maintain their below-normal weight for at least a year by restricting the amount of calories that they eat (about 80 percent or less of what they expend), severely limiting food choices or food groups, and exercising excessively (beyond what is necessary for success or as compared with other athletes of similar fitness levels). Periods of binge eating followed by various purging methods, such as self-induced vomiting and the use of laxatives, are also typically part of the picture.

What Does "Eating Disorder Not Otherwise Specified" (EDNOS) Mean?

Many fitness and sports-minded people who struggle with food, weight, and body image concerns fall under the EDNOS diagnosis, as defined by the American Psychiatric Association, a serious medical condition that requires professional help:

- All the criteria for anorexia nervosa are met except the loss of regular menses (for females) or, despite significant weight loss, the person's weight is in the normal range.
- All the criteria for bulimia nervosa are met except that the binge eating and inappropriate compensatory mechanisms (purging) occur less than twice a week or for a duration of less than three months.
- The regular use of inappropriate compensatory behavior by a person of normal weight after eating small amounts of food (for example, self-induced vomiting after eating two cookies).
- Repeatedly chewing and spitting out, but not swallowing, large amounts of food.

Surprisingly, most of these athletes manage to maintain their weight (albeit low), although they eat far fewer calories than they expend. We cannot tell for sure, but it appears that the combined effects of chronic dieting and exercise may induce the body to conserve energy (calories) or become more efficient at using the available energy. This circumstance could spell trouble in the future if these athletes resort to more extreme dieting measures to maintain their weight or lose more. Even more important, research on elite female endurance athletes continues to point to prolonged dieting as the most important trigger for developing a full-blown eating disorder.

We're not sure about all the implications of anorexia athletica. Although many athletes can perform well initially—after all, that's the allure of losing weight—we know that they cannot do so forever. Even in the short term, those with anorexia athletica may be compromising their true potential. If such a person is chronically low in energy and other nutrients, she or he is more likely to suffer from dehydration and electrolyte imbalances, chronic fatigue, anemia, and upper-respiratory infections, and will recover more slowly from injuries, including stress fractures.

Common Warning Signs of an Eating Disorder

Some common warning signs indicate that eating and weight-related concerns dominate and rule an athlete's life. These warning signs include a marked increase or decrease in weight not related to a medical condition; intense preoccupation with weight and body image (that is, frequent comments about weight or shape); compulsive or excessive exercising beyond purposeful training; development of abnormal eating habits (refusing to eat with others, maintaining a list of forbidden foods, engaging in bizarre food rituals such as moving food around the plate with utensils without actually taking a bite, and so forth); self-induced vomiting (bathroom visits after meals); periods of fasting; abuse of laxatives, diet pills, or diuretics; and amenorrhea. A vegetarian eating style may also be a red flag for eating disorders, particularly among young, athletic women (see chapter 7).

Weight-preoccupied athletes tend to be highly self-critical; appear anxious, irritable, or depressed; and often withdraw from people and activities that they normally enjoy. Fatigue or denial of obvious fatigue, dizziness, chills, abdominal discomfort upon eating, insomnia, shin splints, and stress fractures are all typical day-to-day complaints. Bulimia, a secretive cycle of binge eating and purging, can be harder to identify because an athlete doesn't typically lose excessive amounts of weight or experience amenorrhea as do athletes who suffer with anorexia. Some signs that do indicate bulimia include "chipmunk cheeks" (from swollen glands), bloodshot eyes (from the force of vomiting), knuckle scars, and worn-off tooth enamel (discovered during dental visits).

If you or someone you know suffers from anorexia or bulimia nervosa, understand that it is a serious medical condition that can have irreversible consequences. One study found that 53 percent of patients with anorexia nervosa also have osteoporosis—a condition characterized by brittle bones that fracture easily. The consequences can be even worse. An estimated 1,000 women die each year of anorexia nervosa. Together, anorexia and bulimia cause more deaths than any other psychiatric disorder. Obviously, many of the previously mentioned behaviors or signs, by themselves, do not prove that the person is suffering from an eating disorder. Nevertheless, because the best chance of a complete recovery lies with early intervention, ignoring a potential problem isn't wise. For more information on national organizations that provide help, see "Selected Resources."

Seeking Help

What should you do if a training partner, teammate, or someone you coach is struggling with weight and body-image problems? Don't wait for the person's performance to fall off, for a serious medical problem to prove you right, or even for blood tests to show a problem (because they typically don't). Seek help immediately from someone you trust who is qualified to provide help. A sports medicine physician, a sports dietitian (a registered dietitian who specializes in sports nutrition), or a sport psychologist or therapist who specializes in eating disorders are all good bets. The more serious the eating disorder is, the more likely it is that a team approach (physician, sports dietitian, and therapist) will be needed to promote a complete recovery.

Be sure that you approach friends, teammates, or athletes under your guidance privately and tactfully. Don't mention their weight, talk about calories, or tell them to "just eat normally." Rather, express your concern about their health. Tell them what you see as they train and perform that frightens or disturbs you—for example, skipping meals, having lapses in concentration at work or school, experiencing frequent colds and nagging injuries, not being able to complete workouts or finish strongly, withdrawing from teammates and social activities, or not having fun while pursuing a fitness or athletic goal. Don't judge or criticize their behaviors. Concentrate on the emotional struggle that they are caught up in. Your goal or responsibility is not to change their behavior, not to fix the problem, but to get them into treatment.

Don't be surprised if the person turns down the help that you offer or avoids the issue. Denial is a primary defense mode that people with eating disorders use to protect themselves. Athletes caught in the throes of an eating disorder cannot simply "give up" their distorted beliefs or change their behavior over-night. The person must first learn to communicate in a healthier manner (using the voice, not his or her body) and develop new coping skills to deal with unpleasant emotions and situations. Routinely express your concerns and offer to accompany the friend, teammate, or athlete under your guidance to seek medical help or attend a support group. Many athletes find that approaching a sports dietitian, just for a simple nutrition checkup, to be a nonthreatening first step. If the person refuses to seek professional help during a negotiated time span, share your intention to approach someone else, such as a coach, parent, or spouse, if this is appropriate. Obviously, coaches can insist that an athlete get a complete eating disorder evaluation from a knowledgeable team of sports-minded health professionals before allowing him or her to continue to train or compete. Never forget the fact that although people do recover from eating disorders, they rarely do so without professional help.

Preventing Eating Disorders in Athletes

The best treatment for eating disorders is prevention. Be sure to promote (and model) the message that food is fuel and that a serious athlete respects his or her body by eating the necessary calories and nutrients. Emphasize strength and stamina, not "ideal" body weight. The next best step to take in preventing eating disorders is to intervene early before an athlete's distorted beliefs about food, weight, and body shape and size become firmly entrenched. If you're involved with athletics in any way, you need to send a clear message that the person's physical and mental health always takes precedence over sports performance. Don't minimize or ignore the early warning signs of disordered eating and compulsive exercise. Eating disorders, after all, don't happen overnight. An athlete doesn't simply "catch anorexia" or wake up one morning with a "case of bulimia"—the red flags have been waving for a while. Treat an athlete who struggles with weight or body image issues as you would an injured athlete. Provide the same medical help and guidelines for participation.

If you're a parent or a coach, you especially need to take a closer look at your own attitudes regarding weight and body shape. Body-image distor-tions and disordered eating usually go hand in hand and are pervasive in the sports world. Do you constantly diet to try to obtain an unrealistic perfect figure? Are you perpetuating the oldest myth in the book that the thinner an athlete is, the faster he or she will be? Do you use terms such as *good* and *bad* to describe foods or to describe athletes after they've eaten them? If you must weigh athletes under your guidance, do so in private and set a healthy weight range that includes a minimum weight as well as a maximum weight.

Female fitness buffs and athletes (and coaches who work with them), in particular, need to realize that we are all genetically different, including how much weight or body fat we are predisposed to carry. If you're an athlete who struggles with disordered eating, concentrate on feeling good about yourself. Start by accepting your body type and shape. Although you'll probably never completely ignore the pressure to want to look different, you can work on how your body image influences your current behaviors, and more important, the rest of your life.

Special Concerns for Female Athletes

Female athletes may face unique challenges including premenstrual syndrome, pregnancy, and breast-feeding. The following sections provide nutrition strategies that will help female athletes manage premenstrual syndrome, as well as advice on how to feel your best and remain fit and active while pregnant or breast-feeding.

Premenstrual Syndrome

If you feel that your ability or desire to train or perform suffers at certain times of the month because of your menstrual cycle, you're not alone. One likely cause is premenstrual syndrome (PMS), a condition that affects 90 percent of women to some degree, especially those in their 30s and 40s. Although exercise can help curb the symptoms of PMS, an athlete in touch with her body may be more aware or more sensitive to monthly hormonal fluctuations.

Women of all athletic abilities can suffer from PMS, a complex of emotional, behavioral, and physical symptoms that occurs in some women one to two weeks before the onset of menstruation. The symptoms vary widely among women but tend to fall into four categories: anxiety (mood swings, irritability, sense of being out of control), cravings (increased appetite, craving for sweets or salty foods, fatigue, headache, dizziness), edema (weight gain, breast swelling or tenderness, abdominal bloating), and depression (forgetfulness, crying, insomnia). With PMS, the symptoms resolve quickly (within four days) after the onset of menstrual bleeding. During the teenage years and early to mid-20s, symptoms may be minimal and barely noticeable. As you get older, the symptoms may gradually become worse from year to year or rapidly increase in intensity following the birth of a child.

The exact cause of PMS remains unclear. An imbalance in one of the two female hormones, estrogen and progesterone, or an imbalance of the ratio between these hormones, as well as alterations in brain chemicals, appears to play a role in susceptible women. Not all women suffer to the same degree with premenstrual symptoms. Athletic women may feel particularly hampered by

physical symptoms, such as fluid retention, weight gain, and breast tenderness.
Many also complain of feeling clumsy,
less coordinated, and more susceptible to
muscle or skeletal injuries. Mood swings,
uncharacteristic fatigue, or the energy
lows associated with PMS can also make
it feel hard just to get out the door.

Diet and Supplements

Although nutritional issues alone most
likely don't cause and can't cure PMS,
modifying your diet may help alleviate symptoms. No single treatment has
proved effective for all women, so you
may need to try various strategies to find
relief. In some cases, it may take a few
menstrual cycles to see any effects.

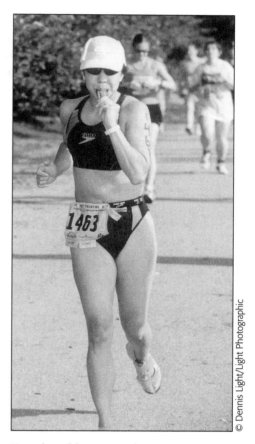

Female athletes need to eat smart to
achieve their athletic goals: eat to train,
don't train to eat.

- Eat small, frequent meals based on
  complex carbohydrates during the
  two weeks before your period is
  due. Going long periods without
  food causes your blood sugar to
  plummet, which accentuates many
  of the symptoms of PMS. Eating
  six small meals a day, about three
  hours apart, will help keep your
  blood sugar level on a more even
  keel. Include plenty of complex
  carbohydrates, such as pasta, baked potatoes, cereal, crackers, bread,
  rice dishes, and vegetables. Choose whole-grain versions rather than
  sugary foods.

  When blood sugar levels get too low, adrenaline is released, which may
  interfere with the normal metabolism of progesterone. In addition, the
  extra adrenaline can make you feel more anxious, tense, or aggressive.
  Eating complex carbohydrates also increases the production of serotonin,
  a brain chemical that leaves you feeling satiated, as well as less depressed
  and less irritable.

- Limit your consumption of simple sweets. Resist the urge to self-regulate
  your mood or energy level with sugar. Simple sugars found in baked
  goods, soda, and candy can cause rapid swings in blood sugar levels.
  You may feel better and temporarily have more energy only to find
  yourself in need of another sugar fix a short while later. Enjoy these
  foods in moderation at mealtimes, not on an empty stomach.

- Stay well hydrated. Dehydration can make PMS symptoms worse,
  especially feelings of fatigue. Limit or avoid alcoholic beverages.

© Dennis Light/Light Photographic

- Avoid caffeinated beverages and other sources of caffeine. Try to eliminate, or at least substantially cut back on, the caffeine in your diet throughout the entire month. We don't know for sure why it may contribute to PMS, but as a stimulant, caffeine also induces the release of adrenaline. Many women find that eliminating caffeine is particularly helpful in alleviating breast tenderness or pain.

- Monitor your sodium intake. The traditional advice has been to cut back on sodium (10 days before your period) so that you retain less water, which may help some women alleviate the bloating, tender breasts, and headaches associated with PMS. Hormonal fluctuations, however, most likely induce the body to retain water (whether or not you eat salty foods) and even cause some women to lose sodium before their periods. Increase your sodium intake slightly to see whether doing so makes a difference, particularly if you typically crave salty foods.

- Boost your calcium intake. During certain phases of the menstrual cycle, fluctuations in calcium-sensitive hormones that regulate calcium levels may set off a host of PMS symptoms by interfering with the brain chemical serotonin. If you don't get 1,200 milligrams of calcium a day by eating calcium-rich foods (see "Best Bets: Calcium" in chapter 1), boost your intake to the recommended level with a daily calcium supplement (in divided doses of 500 to 600 milligrams at a time). Daily calcium supplementation has shown promise in reducing symptoms of mild to moderate PMS, including generalized aches and pains, food cravings, water retention, depression, and mood swings. You may need two to three menstrual cycles to see positive effects.

- Boost your magnesium intake. Magnesium also plays a role in the synthesis of brain chemicals, so make sure that you regularly eat plenty of magnesium-rich foods. Good sources include legumes, whole grains, dark green leafy vegetables, nuts and seeds, tofu, and seafood. Supplemental doses (200 milligrams) may help some women with mild symptoms of PMS, such as bloating.

Here is some advice on other popular treatments for PMS:

- Use caution with vitamin B_6 supplements. Vitamin B_6 is involved in the synthesis of brain chemicals, such as dopamine and serotonin, and in the way that the body metabolizes hormones. Some women report relief of PMS symptoms with supplementation, although most studies do not find it superior to a placebo or sugar pill. Doses as low as 200 milligrams a day, taken for an extended time, may cause irreversible nerve damage, including tingling or numbness of the hands or feet and difficulty walking.

  To derive the possible benefits, eat foods rich in vitamin B_6, including whole grains, soybeans, soy milk, potatoes, salmon, poultry, spinach, broccoli, bananas, and cantaloupe. If you choose to take a supplement, take an entire vitamin B complex containing no more than 50 milligrams of vitamin B_6. Take doses over 100 milligrams a day only under the supervision of a physician.

- Many women find relief from female problems by turning to herbal remedies. Black cohosh and chaste berry tree are purported to reduce PMS by balancing hormone levels, Saint-John's-wort supposedly does the same by acting as a natural antidepressant, and valerian root may reduce PMS by serving as a mild tranquilizer and sleep aid. To reduce possible side effects, try one herbal remedy at a time. Check with your physician first, especially if you take any medications, including oral contraceptives, estrogen, or antidepressants.

Managing Your PMS Symptoms

When it comes to PMS, your best bet is to establish healthy eating patterns, modify your training and racing schedules as needed, and seek healthy ways to manage daily stress. Avoid remedies that promise to cure PMS if you abstain from eating long lists of offender foods, such as refined white sugar, white flour, and so on. Such an extreme diet is not proved effective, is difficult to follow, and can create more anxiety than it's worth.

Keeping a daily chart of your three to five most severe symptoms will help you recognize the effects of PMS on your appetite and athletic performance. Record the absence or presence of your symptoms, their severity, and the day of your menstrual cycle (day 1 starts with menstrual bleeding.) Ovulation (approximately days 12 to 14 of a normal menstrual cycle), for example, boosts a woman's daily energy needs by 100 to 200 calories. You'll be less anxious, less irritable, and less prone to food cravings if you're aware that an increase in appetite is natural and normal at this time.

If self-help techniques, such as healthy nutrition habits, dietary supplements, and a stress management program, prove to be ineffective, explore other treatment options with your physician. Oral contraceptives or antidepressants may also be indicated to help alleviate the emotional and physical symptoms associated with PMS.

Nutrition and Pregnancy

Even when you plan to become pregnant, your game plan may not include sitting around for nine months waiting for the baby to arrive. Many female athletes desire, and are able to retain, a high degree of fitness during pregnancy. Returning quickly to competition following the birth of a child is also a powerful motivator for many female endurance athletes. Listening to your body and maintaining healthy eating habits before, during, and after your pregnancy is key to ensuring a healthy baby and a healthy, fit mom.

Prepregnancy Diet Concerns

Paying attention to your diet before you plan to conceive can reduce your risk of having a baby born with a birth defect that affects the brain or spinal cord (neural tube defects), such as spina bifida or anencephaly. The first eight weeks after conception are the most crucial time in your baby's development. By the eighth week, the developing fetus has a complete nervous system, a beating heart, a fully formed digestive system, and the beginnings of facial features. Neural tube defects occur during the first month of pregnancy when the neural tube is forming. As many as half of all pregnancies are unplanned, so many women, including female athletes, don't realize that they are pregnant at this time. Weight gain can be minimal during these first few weeks, and a woman may attribute a late or missed menstrual period to hard training efforts or the stress associated with competitions.

Consuming 400 micrograms a day of the B vitamin folate or folic acid will help your developing baby form and develop new and normal body tissues. (Folate is used when the vitamin is found naturally in foods; folic acid is used when it is found in supplements.) Natural sources of folate include legumes, such as lentils and dried beans, leafy green vegetables (especially spinach and broccoli), whole grains, orange juice, and some fortified breakfast cereals. Grain products, such as breads, pasta, rice, cornmeal, and enriched flours, are now being fortified with small amounts of folic acid too. Nevertheless, most women do not consume adequate amounts of folate in their diet.

If you're contemplating pregnancy, see your doctor before you try to conceive and begin taking a prenatal vitamin–mineral supplement as directed to obtain the folic acid that you need. Because many pregnancies are unplanned, the March of Dimes, a research organization that studies birth defects, recommends that all women of childbearing age, whether planning to become pregnant or not, take a multivitamin with 400 micrograms of folic acid daily and eat folate-rich foods. (Excessive levels of vitamin A can be toxic to a developing baby. Avoid taking a daily multivitamin containing more than 5,000 IU of vitamin A.)

Abstaining from alcohol makes sense too. No safe level of alcohol consumption has been determined for pregnant women. Consuming limited amounts of alcohol after conception but before becoming aware that you're pregnant shouldn't cause distress. Regularly consuming alcoholic beverages, however, does affect the developing fetus. Having one to two drinks per day can result in a smaller baby. Drinking greater amounts can lead to birth defects associated with fetal alcohol syndrome. The earlier you eliminate alcohol, the better off your baby will be.

Dealing With Morning Sickness

Weight gain, food cravings, fatigue, and morning sickness are issues that all pregnant women have to deal with. Most female athletes are prepared to slow down as they gain weight throughout their pregnancy. You may even be looking forward to satisfying a craving or two. You may not be prepared, however, for the slowdown caused by morning sickness and fatigue during the first few months of your pregnancy.

Morning sickness, characterized by nausea with or without vomiting and fatigue, affects 50 to 90 percent of pregnant women to some degree. Despite being studied for at least four thousand years, the exact cause of morning sickness remains a mystery. Fluctuating hormonal levels, dehydration, and a trigger of some sort most likely combine to produce the next round of nausea.

Because every pregnancy is different, what triggers morning sickness will also vary from woman to woman. You'll have to experiment to find what works for you in reducing or alleviating the symptoms of morning sickness. Some age-old remedies that have stood the test of time include keeping soda crackers near your bed to nibble on before you get up and not brushing your teeth right after eating. You may find that eating a snack before you go to bed or when you awaken during the night may ward off nausea in the morning. A heightened sense of smell is typical during pregnancy, and smells or odors may play a large role in triggering bouts of morning sickness. Try to sleep with the window open. Avoid cooking odors, perfume, aftershave, and cigarette smoke. If the smell of some foods makes you sick, avoid them.

Be prepared to eat small meals every two to three hours to keep your blood sugar from getting too low, which may induce nausea. Don't worry about craving or only being able to tolerate junk food during bad periods of morning sickness. The goal is to find foods that you can eat and keep down. Your favorite workout food, the one you can stomach during a hard effort or in the middle of a race, might just do the trick. Concentrate on eating nutritious foods after the nausea and vomiting pass. Eating typically causes you to drink more, which will help you avoid becoming dehydrated. Drink beverages slowly and between meals to combat nausea. Of course, you'll want to pay particular attention to drinking enough fluids before, during, and after exercise.

Weight Gain and Energy Needs

You may be surprised that eating for two requires only an extra 300 calories a day, primarily during the second and third trimesters. That's not much—in fact, three glasses of low-fat milk will do the trick. As you reduce your training, you may not even need to eat any extra food to meet your energy needs. Let your rate of weight gain be your guide. You'll want to gain 25 to 35 pounds (11 to 16 kilograms) during your pregnancy to reduce the chance of complications, such as having a baby that weighs too little or is born prematurely. Pay particular attention to eating two to three hours before you exercise, as well as immediately afterward, to minimize exercise-induced falls in blood sugar. Keep supplemental carbohydrate (for example, sports drinks, energy gels, and energy bars) on hand to ingest during exercise as needed, even during short sessions when you typically wouldn't need anything.

Gaining less than 5 pounds in the entire first three months can be perfectly normal. Typical gains are about a pound per week after that. Athletic women may easily gain more than the recommended range, particularly if you're lean and enter your pregnancy with a low body-fat level. If that's the case, don't worry about what the scale says. If you're eating healthy foods and continuing with your exercise routine (with modifications as necessary), your baby will profit from the extra weight that you gain.

Nutrient Needs and Food Cravings

During pregnancy, you need more of certain nutrients. Besides folic acid, active women need to pay particular attention to getting enough calcium, iron, and protein. Your calcium needs jump to 1,200 milligrams a day, or the equivalent of four servings of dairy foods (see "Best Bets: Calcium" in chapter 1). As your baby's bones calcify, calcium moves out of your bones and across the placenta. Without adequate calcium stores, you run the risk of weakening your bones. This increases your risk of developing a stress fracture when you return to training, and for developing osteoporosis earlier in life.

Pregnancy doubles your iron requirement to 30 milligrams a day, because you need to make hemoglobin for extra red blood cells for yourself and the developing fetus. Along with the inevitable loss of iron that occurs with blood loss at birth, your iron stores will also be used to create your baby's iron stores. Because many female athletes, particularly those involved in endurance sports, have low iron stores, you should have your iron status checked early in your pregnancy and at regular intervals thereafter. Although pregnant women commonly experience fatigue, especially during the first trimester, developing iron-deficient anemia only makes matters worse.

You also need an extra 10 grams of protein every day—the amount supplied by one glass of low-fat milk and a piece of whole-grain bread. Although most female athletes can easily meet their increased protein needs through food alone, supplementing with calcium and iron makes sense. Incidentally, individual food cravings do not typically reflect any particular nutrient deficiency. Go ahead and appease your cravings within reason. Food aversions and cravings probably arise during pregnancy because of changes in your sensitivity to tastes and smells.

Foods to Avoid While Pregnant

Food safety during pregnancy is simple. Just be careful about ingesting anything that you wouldn't serve your baby. Besides alcohol, watch out for caffeine, artificial sweeteners, contaminants from pollution or bacteria, and herbal supplements. Restrict your daily intake of caffeine (considered a necessary substance by many athletes!) to 300 milligrams or less, about the amount in two cups of brewed coffee. Some studies suggest that drinking more than that may increase your risk of giving birth to an underweight baby. Although artificial sweeteners appear to be safe for pregnant women to consume, relying on natural sweeteners, like sugar, honey, or molasses, is a safer route to follow.

Skip soft cheeses such as feta, blue cheese, Brie, Camembert, and Mexican-style cheeses during your pregnancy. These items, as well as hot dogs, luncheon meats, and cold cuts, can be contaminated with a bacteria called listeria, which causes a flulike illness. Transmitted across the placenta, listeriosis food poisoning can lead to premature delivery, miscarriage, stillbirth, or serious health problems for your newborn child. Because of the risk of bacterial contamination, you should also stay away from raw or undercooked meat, poultry, and shellfish; sushi; unpasteurized milk or juice; and raw eggs found in homemade ice cream, eggnog, and raw cookie dough. Because of their potential mercury content, restrict your intake of tuna and swordfish to twice a week.

As for herbal supplements, few if any of these products have been tested for safety during pregnancy or lactation. If you're considering taking herbal supplements during your pregnancy (or while breast-feeding), consult with your physician first.

Breast-Feeding

Breast-feeding, not pregnancy, is the time more aptly referred to as eating for two. Your body requires an additional 600 or more calories a day to produce enough milk. Studies have shown that most breast-feeding women who exercise seem to increase their daily food intake spontaneously by 400 to 500 calories to cover their increased energy needs. The rest of the energy comes from fat stores accumulated during pregnancy for that purpose.

Dieting or excessively restricting your calories to speed up the process of returning to your prepregnancy weight doesn't make sense. You'll end up irritable and low on energy just when you need it the most during the first few months when you're fighting off the effects of sleep deprivation and adjusting to a new schedule. Don't try to lose more than one to two pounds per week. You took nine months or more to gain the weight, so you will likely need at least nine months to lose it, although regular exercise can speed up the timetable.

To keep up with your baby's demand for milk, you'll need to consume enough calories, adequate carbohydrate, and plenty of fluid. Plan to have a minimeal each time that you nurse, such as a piece of fruit or half a sandwich, plus at least 8 ounces of fluid, such as water, milk, or juice. A poor diet is more likely to decrease the quantity, not the quality, of the milk produced. If you're having trouble producing enough milk, reevaluate your food choices and boost your calorie intake. (A baby who gains 4 to 8 ounces a week the first month, and 1 to 2 pounds per month the first six months, is getting enough milk and gaining weight appropriately.) Your calcium needs remain high (1,200 milligrams per day) during lactation, and you should continue to monitor your iron stores (serum ferritin) and supplement with iron as needed.

Dehydration can be a problem until you recognize how much your fluid needs have increased. Drink enough so that you feel you have to urinate every time you feed your baby. The clearer your urine, the better hydrated you are. Don't plan to exercise strenuously if your urine isn't clear. Dark, concentrated urine indicates that you're already in a dehydrated state.

Intense exercise efforts affect the composition of breast milk by decreasing immunoglobulin A, a substance important for a healthy immune system, and by increasing the amount of lactic acid that appears in breast milk. The increase in lactic acid causes a sour taste that your baby may find unpleasant. Within 60 to 90 minutes after exercise, however, breast milk returns to normal, so these changes don't appear to be significant. If your infant appears to react to your breast milk following exercise, try breast-feeding your baby before you head out to train.

7

Endurance Eating for Vegetarians

"At 165 to 170 pounds, I'm not going to get by on 2,000 calories a day. During peak training times, I may eat 8,000 to 10,000 calories. I have not been sidelined with an injury for more than a few days in nine years—and that's not only due to smart training. A lot of injuries that athletes suffer are because of the quality and quantity of food they consume."

—Scott Jurek, the course-record holder and seven-time defending champion of the Western States 100-Mile Endurance Run and the course-record holder and defending champion of the Badwater Ultramarathon

Endurance sports and vegetarianism have much in common. Both endeavors require you to be both an artist and a scientist. Guidelines exist for each discipline, but there's more than one way to get the job done. And although you can certainly jump recklessly into either venture, a little planning goes a long way when it comes to achieving success.

If you choose a vegetarian sports diet while training for and competing in endurance and ultraendurance events, you can obtain all the nutrients that you need. But you must be as committed to meeting your nutritional needs as you are to fulfilling your athletic goals. By reading this chapter, you will become more knowledgeable about the nutritional issues associated with a vegetarian diet and how best to meet your nutrient needs from plant sources. Nonvegetarian athletes will also benefit by learning how to incorporate more plant foods into their diets.

Defining Vegetarianism

You haven't eaten red meat in years but still occasionally enjoy chicken and fish. Your training buddy drinks milk and eats cheese, but avoids eggs and meat of any type. So who's the vegetarian? Actually, vegetarianism means different things to different people. Vegetarian practices run the gamut from simply eliminating red meat to excluding all animal products, even foods derived from animal sources, such as honey and gelatin.

Athletes cite different reasons for reducing or eliminating animal products from their diet. You may want to improve your health, boost your performance, follow spiritual guidelines, protect the environment, abide by your love of animals, or have some other reason for following a vegetarian eating style.

The following terms describe the general categories of vegetarian diets:

- Vegans (or strict vegetarians) eat only plant foods, such as grains, beans, fruits, vegetables, nuts, and seeds, and consume no animal products (meat, fish, poultry, seafood, eggs and egg products, and dairy foods, such as milk and cheese).

- Lacto-vegetarians eat dairy and plant foods, but eliminate all meat, poultry, fish, seafood, and eggs.

- Ovo-vegetarians eat eggs and plant foods, but avoid meat, poultry, fish, seafood, and dairy foods.

- Lacto-ovo vegetarians include eggs, dairy, and plant foods in their diet, but exclude all meat, poultry, fish, and seafood.

- Semi- or partial vegetarians refuse red meat but occasionally eat chicken, fish, and seafood along with eggs and dairy foods.

Rewards and Risks of a Vegetarian Diet

With careful planning a vegetarian eating style can improve your health and your performance. Simply eliminating animal foods without finding appropriate substitutes, however, results in an unbalanced diet that does more harm than good. As a vegetarian athlete you must put more thought and planning into your daily food choices to incorporate alternative sources of key nutrients such as calcium, iron, zinc, and protein. Otherwise, your health and performance will suffer.

Rewards

For the most part, opting for a vegetarian eating style is a healthy path to follow. Health experts continually urge us to eat more plant foods and fewer animal products, which lack fiber and tend to be high in fat and cholesterol. Think about the basic messages contained in MyPyramid. The recommendation for someone who requires 2,000 calories a day includes 6 ounces (90 grams of carbohydrate) of bread, cereal, rice, and pasta (at least half from whole grains), 2 1/2 cups of vegetables, and 2 cups of fruit, accompanied by 3 cups (750 milliliters) of milk and 5 1/2 ounces (40 grams of protein) of meat, poultry, fish, dry beans, eggs, and nuts. Adding it all up, the pyramid prescribes more plant-food servings than it does animal foods. Planning meals around grains, beans, soy foods, vegetables, and fruit definitely supports optimal health. Studies show that compared with the general public, vegetarians have lower rates of hypertension and certain cancers, as well as much lower risk of developing heart disease and diabetes. Eating a plant-based diet can also make it easier to maintain a healthy weight.

A plant-based diet also supplies plenty of carbohydrate that helps replenish glycogen stores—a prerequisite if you work out daily, train more than once a day, or want to keep moving for hours on end. Endurance athletes need to consume approximately 60 percent of their daily calories from carbohydrate-rich foods. Foods from the grains group, fruit and vegetable groups, as well as beans, soy foods, milk, and yogurt fill the bill. If you're filling up on these foods, you're most likely already adopting a vegetarian or near-vegetarian diet. You should be able to obtain the rest of the nutrients that you need, including enough high-quality protein, if you eat a variety of foods daily and make some savvy substitutions for the foods that you eliminate.

Risks

Despite all the benefits associated with a vegetarian eating style, I find it difficult to comment specifically about whether endurance athletes perform better on meatless diets. The vegetarian theme includes too many variations. Many athletes eat healthy, well-balanced vegetarian diets, but others struggle with vegetarian meal plans that are too restrictive. The bottom line is that you shouldn't automatically assume that your health or performance will improve simply because you eliminate red meat or other animal products. A vegetarian lifestyle, in fact, has been linked to menstrual abnormalities, and in some athletic women, vegetarianism may even be a red flag that signals an eating disorder.

I've counseled a number of semi- or near vegetarians who make poor food choices and end up with diets low in protein, iron, zinc, and calcium. How does this happen? Try this diet on for size: no red meat; few if any eggs, dairy, or soy foods; and limited amounts of fish, poultry, and beans. Survival depends on eating lots of bagels, salad, pasta, energy bars, and desserts or snack items. You're likely to end up in this rut if you make little effort to shop and prepare snacks and meals, if you aren't keen on trying new foods, or if you live in a carnivorous (meat-eating) household and routinely eat only the starchy parts of family meals.

Consuming the nutrients and calories that you need to partake in endurance endeavors becomes more difficult as you eliminate foods and food groups. Vegan diets pose the greatest challenge. Eliminating two food groups increases the risk for deficiencies, especially of some key nutrients such as vitamins B_2 and B_{12}, iron, zinc, and calcium. Endurance athletes often struggle to meet their high calorie needs on vegan diets as well.

Special Nutrient Concerns for Vegetarians

Vegetarians typically define themselves by the foods that they don't eat. You will commonly hear a vegetarian say, "I don't eat meat," but how often do you hear one say, "But I do eat bok choy, tofu, and garbanzo beans"? To reap the benefits of vegetarianism, you need to seek alternative sources of nutrients for the foods that you choose to eliminate. The easiest way is to focus on including a variety of foods in your daily diet, such as whole grains, dark green leafy vegetables, and soy foods.

If you're curious about how your vegetarian eating style stacks up, ask yourself a couple of questions: Do you, or are you willing to, explore new foods to meet your nutrient needs? Do you, or are you willing to, plan meals and snacks to meet the high energy needs of being an endurance athlete? If you can answer yes to both questions, you're on your way to eating a healthy, well-balanced vegetarian diet.

Calories, Carbohydrate, and Fat

Vegetarian athletes typically have little problem eating enough carbohydrate. Breads, cereals, pasta, rice, fruits, vegetables, beans, lentils, some soy foods, milk, and yogurt all supply carbohydrate. By their nature, vegetarian diets rank higher in complex carbohydrates and fiber and lower in saturated fat and cholesterol than diets containing meat. Eating enough whole grains, however, can be a challenge for some vegetarians. Developing a taste for barley, brown and wild rice, bulgur, couscous, kasha (buckwheat), millet, and quinoa is particularly important for vegetarian athletes. Besides supplying complex carbohydrates, these foods provide protein, iron, zinc, and other trace minerals. An easy first step is to switch to eating whole-grain cereals and whole-wheat bread, crackers, and pasta.

Your daily fat requirement (at least 20 percent of total calories) doesn't change if you follow a vegetarian diet. In fact, many vegetarians assume that eliminating animal products ensures a low-fat diet. Don't count on it. You can easily rack up fat calories if you rely too heavily on nuts and seeds, cheese and other whole-milk dairy foods, and high-fat snack and convenience foods. If this is an area that you need to work on, read food labels and choose low-fat alternatives whenever possible. If you rely on nuts and cheese for protein, consider leaner options, such as dried beans and peas, lentils, and soy foods. Don't forget that you can always cut back on how much or how often you eat a particular food.

Plant foods are bulkier and usually lower in calories than animal foods, so some athletes end up feeling full before they consume enough calories. Vegan diets, in particular, are high in fiber and low in fat. If you're having trouble consuming enough calories, don't skip meals or snacks (plan to eat six or more times a day), and concentrate on including plenty of high-calorie, nutrient-dense foods such as nuts and seeds, nut butters, fruit juices, dried fruit, and dairy foods. Cooking with small amounts of fat or oil will also help boost your calorie intake. Desserts and snack foods supply loads of calories. Just be sure that you first eat foods that are more nutritious.

Protein

Getting enough protein is a concern for many vegetarian athletes. Because endurance athletes have higher protein needs, sprinkling a few chickpeas on a salad or crumbling a little tofu into a vegetable stir-fry won't get the job done. Most female endurance athletes need 65 to 90 grams of protein a day; active males typically require 95 to 120 grams daily.

Keeping up with your protein needs requires a two-pronged approach: Eat a variety of plant foods daily and consume enough calories to maintain your weight. Consuming too few calories means that protein gets used for energy rather than for building, repairing, and maintaining body tissues, including muscle. If you continue to eat poultry, fish, eggs, and milk products, getting enough high-quality protein shouldn't be a problem. Animal foods provide all the essential amino acids (which must be derived from the diet because the body cannot make them) that we consistently need to have on hand. The body constantly recombines amino acids to create the new proteins that it needs. Plant sources of protein, such as grains, dried beans and peas, nuts, seeds, and vegetables, are considered lower-quality because they contain low levels of one or more essential amino acids. Soybeans are the exception. They contain certain amino acids in higher amounts than found in other beans, so ounce for ounce, soybean protein is equivalent in quality to animal protein.

In the old days, vegetarians were advised to combine specific plant foods, such as rice and beans, within a meal. Eaten together, these foods would complement each other by providing all the essential amino acids needed to build new complete proteins. Today we know that combining plant foods at the same meal isn't necessary. The body can assemble its own complete proteins from a small pool of free amino acids that it maintains for this purpose. If you are a vegetarian, however, this system is effective only if you eat a variety of plant foods, as well as enough calories, every day. Of course, bean burritos, lentil soup with corn bread, and peanut butter sandwiches made with whole-wheat bread taste good, so you still have a valid reason for eating these combinations.

To boost your protein intake and avoid the carbohydrate-overload trap, consciously include a protein-rich food at all your meals and snacks (see table 7.1). Lacto-ovo vegetarians, for example, can add milk products (regular or soy) or eggs to any meal or snack. Eat hot or cold cereal with milk, dunk a bran muffin into yogurt, snack on a slice of cheese pizza, or prepare french toast for breakfast. Another good strategy is to make sure that you don't eat your grains plain. Smear nut butters, low-fat cottage cheese, or hummus on a bagel. Vary your pasta toppings by using canned spicy beans one night and a vegetable and tofu stir-fry another. Keep in mind that anything made for pasta can just as easily be spooned over brown rice or instant couscous or rolled in tortillas.

Vegetarians who eliminate animal foods without substituting traditional vegetarian staples have the most trouble meeting their protein needs. A good rule to follow is to eat legumes (dried beans and peas and lentils) and soy foods

Table 7.1   Protein Content of Commonly Eaten Foods

Food	Typical serving	Protein (grams)
Meat (red meat, poultry, fish)	3 oz (85 g) cooked	21–25 g
Cottage cheese	1/2 cup	13 g
Milk or yogurt	1 cup (250 ml)	8 g
Cheese	1 oz (28 g)	7 g
Egg	1 medium	6 g
Lentils	1 cup cooked	18 g
Beans	1 cup cooked	12 g
Edamame (boiled soybeans)	1 cup cooked	22 g
Soy nuts	1 oz (28 g)	11 g
Soy milk	1 cup (250 ml)	10 g
Tofu	3 oz (85 g) (1/5 block)	10 g
Peanut butter	2 tbsp	8 g
Nuts or seeds	1 oz (28 g)	5 g
Bread	1 slice	3 g
Pasta or grain	1 cup cooked	6 g
Potato	1 small	2 g
Starchy vegetables (peas, corn, winter squash)	1/2 cup cooked	2 g

daily. Quick-fix beans (precooked canned varieties) and meat substitutes made from soybeans provide an easy and simple way to get the protein that you need. Choose hearty soups and stews made with lentils, split peas, and beans. Try baked beans on your next baked potato or serve a quick meal in a can such as vegetarian chili. When it comes to soy foods, experiment with different forms. Serve meat substitutes (check the freezer section in natural food stores and the health food section of grocery stores) and use textured vegetable protein in dishes that traditionally call for meat, such as chili and tacos.

Keep in mind that animal foods provide a more concentrated dose of protein than plant foods do. A typical small hamburger or chicken breast (3 ounces, the size of a deck of cards) supplies 25 grams of protein. You'll have to eat a generous cup of cooked beans plus a cup of cooked grain or two cups of pasta topped with 3 ounces of tofu to match that. You can determine the amount of protein in the foods that you typically eat by checking the nutrition facts label on food packages. Be certain to compare the serving size against the portion that you actually eat.

To estimate your daily protein requirement in grams, multiply your weight in pounds by .55 to .75 (in kilograms by 1.2 to 1.7). Athletes who eat primarily vegetarian foods should select the higher end of the range, especially those who participate in ultraendurance events.

Adding More Soy to Your Diet

You've heard all about the wonders of soy, but how do you actually eat the stuff, or at least sneak some into your diet? This list contains some simple suggestions to get you started.

1. Drink soy milk (fortified with calcium and vitamin D) and use it in place of skim milk in recipes for soups, muffins, pancakes, waffles, and pudding.
2. Create smoothies by blending fresh fruit (bananas and strawberries work well) with vanilla-flavored soy milk.
3. Add diced firm tofu or chunks of tempeh to your favorite spaghetti sauce, chili, vegetable soup, stew, stir-fried dish, and casserole.
4. Combine soft tofu with cottage cheese or ricotta cheese in lasagna and stuffed shells or use it as a cheese substitute in pasta dishes.
5. Blend soft tofu into low-fat sour cream for a baked-potato topping or use it instead of sour cream or yogurt.
6. Crumble tofu into scrambled eggs during the last minute of cooking.
7. Snack on roasted soy nuts (found in most supermarkets).
8. Prepare tempeh on the grill. Steam it first, marinate in barbecue sauce, and then grill until brown. Add cubes of firm or extra-firm tofu to shish kebab.
9. Add soy protein isolate (powder) to milk shakes, fruit smoothies, and fruit juices or sprinkle it on hot cereal for an added protein boost.
10. Try tofu dogs (soy hot dogs), veggie patties (soy-based burgers), and other meat alternatives; replace ground meat with textured vegetable protein in tacos, spaghetti sauce, and chili.

Refer back to table 7.1 for the protein content of some commonly eaten foods. Use this list as a reference to keep track of your daily protein intake.

Iron and Zinc

Athletes who eat a meatless diet run a greater risk of getting too little iron and zinc. Even marginal deficiencies can hamper your performance. With an iron-poor diet, you won't form enough hemoglobin and myoglobin, the oxygen-carrying molecules in the blood and muscles, which will leave you feeling weak and fatigued. Female athletes, in particular, are at greater risk for low iron levels because of smaller reserves and greater losses through menstruation. Athletes need adequate zinc to fight off infections and help wounds and injuries heal.

Absorbability is a key issue when it comes to getting enough iron and zinc. About 20 to 30 percent of the iron in meat (heme iron) is absorbable, compared with only 2 to 8 percent in plants (nonheme iron). The zinc from animal sources is generally more absorbable too because fiber and compounds called phytates found in whole-grain foods can interfere with zinc absorption.

All types of meat, not just red meat, contain the more easily absorbed heme iron. You'll benefit by including poultry (especially the dark meat), fish, and seafood in your diet. Don't rely on dairy foods or eggs to come through in this department because both are poor sources of iron. Some good plant sources of iron include fortified breakfast cereals; wheat germ; dried beans, peas, and lentils; leafy dark green vegetables like spinach, kale, and collard greens; tofu and textured vegetable protein; nuts and seeds; dried fruit; and prune juice.

Vitamin C enhances the absorption of iron, so serve foods rich in vitamin C with the iron-rich plant foods listed earlier. Foods high in vitamin C include strawberries, kiwi, cantaloupe (rockmelon), citrus

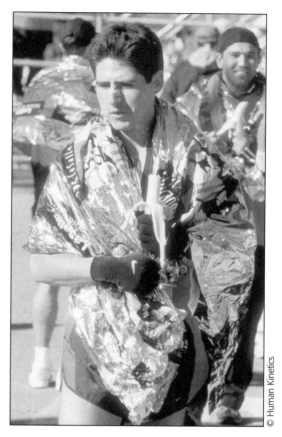

© Human Kinetics

A well-balanced vegetarian diet provides the calories and nutrients needed to reach the finish line.

fruits, red and green peppers, broccoli, and tomatoes, to name a few. For example, drink a glass of orange juice with a bowl of iron-fortified cereal or cook beans in a tomato sauce. Cooking in a cast-iron pot or skillet will also raise the iron content substantially because the mineral leeches into the food. Meat contains a compound, the MFP factor, that promotes the absorption of nonheme iron too, so have your iron-rich vegetables and any meat you may eat together.

Animal foods (especially oysters) contain abundant amounts of zinc, whereas plant foods provide only moderate amounts. You need to make an effort to include several servings of zinc-rich foods in your diet every day. If you consume enough protein, you're most likely getting enough zinc. Significant plant sources of zinc include lentils, beans, whole grains, whole-wheat bread, wheat germ, nuts, soy and dairy foods, and some fortified breakfast cereals.

Don't be too quick to reach for supplements that provide beyond 100 percent of the RDA for iron and zinc. Clearly, if iron-deficiency anemia is a problem, additional iron will help. You should start, though, by monitoring your iron levels through routine blood tests that look at your hemoglobin, hematocrit,

Vegetarian Calcium Sources*

1 cup (250 ml) of milk

1 cup of fortified soy milk or rice milk

1 cup of yogurt

1.5 oz (42 g) cheese

1 cup of tofu (made with calcium sulfate)

1 1/2 cups of cooked dark leafy greens—kale, collard, turnip greens

2 cups of cooked bok choy

3 cups of cooked broccoli

1 1/2 cups of canned baked beans

1/2 cup of soy nuts

11 dried figs

3 tbsp of sesame seeds

4 oz (115 g) of canned salmon or sardines (with bones)

1 cup of fortified orange juice

fortified breakfast cereals (varies)

*Contains at least 300 milligrams per serving.

and serum ferritin (storage form of iron) levels. Too much iron can interfere with the absorption of zinc and copper, and cause constipation. Over-supplementing with zinc may cause a relative deficiency in other minerals, such as copper, because they all compete for absorption. Eating plant foods rich in iron and zinc, however, won't cause any problems. Play it safe—make the effort to include good meatless sources of iron and zinc.

Calcium and Vitamin D

Besides building strong bones and teeth, calcium helps your muscles to contract and relax, your nerves to send messages, and your blood to clot properly. Vitamin D aids in the absorption of calcium and phosphorus, nutrients essential for healthy bone tissue. Your daily calcium needs vary depending on your gender, age, and (for women) your menstrual status. Shoot for at least 1,000 milligrams a day. If you eat dairy foods, you can get plenty of calcium from fat-free and low-fat milk, yogurt, and cheese. Plant foods that contain calcium include dark leafy greens (such as kale, mustard, collard, and turnip greens), bok choy, broccoli, beans, dried figs, soy nuts, sunflower seeds, and other calcium-fortified foods, such as orange juice, cereal, breakfast bars, tofu (processed with calcium sulfate), and fortified soy or rice beverages. If you occasionally eat animal foods, canned sardines and salmon (be sure to eat the bones) are a good source of calcium too.

Check the nutrition facts label on your orange juice, soy and rice beverages, and tofu. If you're relying on these foods for calcium, select calcium-fortified varieties and tofu prepared with calcium sulfate. Green leafy vegetables can provide adequate calcium, but you'll have to eat enough of them to make it count. For example, you need to eat three cups of broccoli or one and a half cups of kale to equal the calcium in one glass of milk or one cup of yogurt. (Don't forget, at 300 milligrams a cup, you need the equivalent of at least three glasses of milk a day to reach your daily goal of 1,000 milligrams of calcium.) If you think that calcium supplements are the answer, be aware that a diet low in calcium is also likely low in protein and vitamin D. Calcium supplements won't help with that. To increase absorption, take calcium supplements with meals, in doses of 500 milligrams or less at one time, and not along with an iron supplement.

Few foods are naturally high in vitamin D. Our bodies usually make enough when our skin is exposed to sunlight (at least 15 minutes several times a week.) Fortunately, athletes routinely spend a great deal of time outdoors wearing little clothing! Keep in mind that your skin becomes less efficient at making vitamin D as you age, and sun exposure may not be adequate in northern climates during the winter months. Good food sources of vitamin D include fattier fish (like salmon), egg yolks, and fortified foods such as milk, butter, margarine, breakfast cereals, and soy beverages. Vegans should consider a vitamin D supplement (200 IU per day; over age 50, 400 IU per day; over age 70, 600 IU per day).

A Day in the Vegetarian Life

Here is a nutrition-packed, one-day vegetarian menu. Preparation time for each meal is under 10 minutes.

Breakfast

1 cup of quick oatmeal, topped with 1 cup of fat-free vanilla yogurt and 2 tbsp of raisins

2 slices of hearty grain bread with 1 tbsp of peanut butter

8 oz (250 ml) of orange juice

Lunch

1 garden burger on a whole-grain bun, with sliced tomato and onion

1/2 cup of pasta and bean salad

Handful of baby carrots dipped in yogurt salad dressing

Snack

1 cup (250 ml) of calcium-fortified soy milk

1 soft pretzel

Dinner

1 cup of black bean chili, over top of 1 cup of cooked Mexican-style rice and corn mix

Dark green salad with 1 tbsp (15 ml) of low-fat dressing

1 cup of frozen yogurt with 1/2 cup of fresh or frozen strawberries

Tally for the day:

Calories: 2,660

Protein: 100 g (15%)

Carbohydrate: 400 g (60%)

Fat: 74 g (25%)

B Vitamins

If you eat a well-balanced vegetarian diet, full of whole grains, enriched grains, legumes, nuts, seeds, fruits and vegetables, and plenty of calories, you should have no trouble meeting your need for thiamin, riboflavin, niacin, vitamin B_6, and folic acid. Vitamin B_{12} is needed to maintain healthy red blood cells and nerve fibers. Vitamin B_{12} is a unique vitamin, produced by bacteria in the soil and in animals. Unless they are in the habit of ingesting soil along with their greens (as animals do), most people meet their needs by eating animal foods, so you're covered if you consume eggs, dairy products, fish, or poultry. Deficiencies are rare, even in vegetarians, because the daily requirement is small (2.4 micrograms a day), and the human body carefully hoards and guards its supply.

The only plant foods that are reliable B_{12} sources are fortified foods such as soy milk, soy burgers, and certain breakfast cereals (such as Total or Product 19). Nutritional yeast (Red Star brand T-6635), not regular baking yeast, is also a reliable source. Don't count on tempeh, spirulina, sprouted legumes, miso, sea vegetables, or umeboshi plums; these foods don't contain the active form of vitamin B_{12}. Vegans who don't routinely eat fortified products should take a supplement because subtle neurological damage can occur before you know that you have a deficiency.

Special Health Concerns for Vegetarians

A meatless diet does not guarantee good health and better performance. Unless you stick to some basic guidelines and stay abreast of your calorie and nutrient needs, you may encounter some difficulties. Two particular problems that may slow vegetarian athletes are amenorrhea (in women) and disordered eating habits.

Amenorrhea and Vegetarianism

Female athletes who adopt vegetarian diets may be at higher risk for amenorrhea, a medical condition characterized by low estrogen levels and loss of menstrual periods. Women who follow a plant-based eating style typically have lower levels of hormones that affect menstruation, such as estrogen and prolactin, than do nonvegetarian women. These hormonal levels appear to be altered by some component characteristic of a vegetarian diet; possibilities include high fiber intake, low fat content, or the presence of weak plant hormones. Because amenorrhea is also linked with extreme or extensive exercise, the problem may be compounded among vegetarian athletes. High rates of amenorrhea have been reported in vegetarian athletes, particularly in runners. In one study, vegetarians made up 25 percent of the runners with amenorrhea but only 11 percent of the runners who had regular menstrual periods.

If you develop amenorrhea, don't ignore it. You're three times more likely to develop a stress fracture, and low levels of estrogen at any age can cause premature bone loss. Look at your current eating habits. You often need to gain only 2 to 3 percent of your body weight (2 to 4 pounds for a 120-pound woman) to restart your menstrual periods.

As an endurance athlete, you can easily burn off large amounts of calories through exercise, so you may develop amenorrhea because of an energy imbalance. You simply don't consume enough calories to sustain your high energy expenditures. If you feel that your current vegetarian eating style doesn't keep up with your calorie needs, eat more fat (at least 20 percent of your total calories) and protein and cut back on fiber-rich foods that fill you up quickly. If possible, cut back on how intensely you exercise and reduce your training volume by 10 to 20 percent, even more if you're trying to conceive.

Be certain that you consume adequate protein. The research suggests that athletes with amenorrhea tend to have diets low in protein compared with athletes who menstruate regularly. Some studies show that adding meat (red meat in particular) has a protective effect on menstrual periods, although it's unclear why. Obviously, it's a matter of personal choice whether you include or exclude meat in your diet. Depending on your long-term goals, you may want to reevaluate the effect that including small portions of meat several times a week could have on your health and performance.

Disordered Eating and Vegetarianism

Some vegetarian athletes, male and female, inadvertently consume too few calories to sustain their high energy output. Others, however, consciously restrict the foods that they eat under the guise of vegetarianism. In other words, they choose (or choose to continue) a vegetarian eating style as a way to control their eating habits and cope with pressure to be thin. These people may feel better about themselves or superior to others when they eat differently, or they may feel "more perfect" when they don't eat certain foods.

Some hallmark behaviors to look for are vegetarians who narrow their protein choices to a few "acceptable" items; avoid fat by shunning nuts and seeds, nut butters, dairy products, and other higher-fat items; and skip meals or elect not to eat in social settings rather than prepare or search out vegetarian fare. If you, or someone you train with or coach, pursue vegetarianism primarily as a politically correct means to lose weight or achieve a lean appearance, heed the warning signs. Such harmful and ineffective eating behaviors set you up for anemia, stress fractures, and possibly a full-blown eating disorder.

Parents and coaches of teenage athletes need to be vigilant when it comes to young people and vegetarianism, the reasons that teens give for renouncing foods, and the effectiveness with which they replace those foods with healthy substitutes. Girls, in particular, may adopt vegetarianism as a socially acceptable way to mask their disordered eating habits.

Researchers at the University of Minnesota surveyed high school students across Minnesota and found that teenage vegetarian girls are twice as likely

Quick Vegetarian Snacks and Meals

Whole-grain pancakes

Whole-grain muffins or cookies

Graham crackers, rice cakes, whole-grain crackers, tortillas

Instant macaroni and cheese, couscous with lentils, polenta, or mashed potatoes

Instant brown rice or other grains

Bagels or whole-grain bread with nut butter

Oatmeal or cold cereal with milk

Dried fruit—raisins, apricots, dates, figs, papayas, apples

Frozen juice bar

Bean taco, burrito, or enchilada

Lentil or split-pea soup

Fruit shakes or smoothies

Low-fat cottage cheese

Yogurt (dairy or soy)

Canned beans, vegetarian chili

Ethnic frozen meals—Mexican, Chinese, Thai, or others

Tofu hot dogs

Veggie burgers

Quick mixes of tabouli, hummus, refried beans, or black beans

Roasted soy nuts or other nuts

Vegetable pizza

to diet, four times as likely to induce vomiting, and eight times as likely to use laxatives as are their meat-eating peers. These findings support a reverse study of 116 patients who suffered with anorexia nervosa (self-induced starvation): 54 percent avoided red meat, although only 4 percent had done so before the onset of their eating disorder.

One of my clients, a 13-year-old who adopted a vegetarian diet at age 5, played soccer, swam, ran, and participated in gymnastics during a typical week. When a swim coach at a summer camp delivered the erroneous message that athletes should avoid eating fat, my client began to count calories and fat grams, skip meals (saying that she was not hungry or that the vegetables tasted terrible), and exercise twice a day. After she lost 10 pounds and her menstrual periods stopped, her parents took action.

Upon meeting her, I found that besides not eating meat, she didn't like fish, rarely drank milk, ate eggs only if they were prepared for her, and wrinkled her nose at the mention of beans or tofu. Obviously, she wasn't doing too well at covering her protein, iron, and calcium needs. She also wasn't consuming enough calories to balance those that she burned through exercise. Fortunately, a strong desire to continue at her sports activities motivated this teen to gain weight.

A vegetarian diet can be either a healthy way to eat or a haphazard eating style that comes up short in many key nutrients. To reap the benefits of vegetarianism, you must be willing to do two things: stock your kitchen with some vegetarian staples (and know how to prepare them!) and invest some time and energy exploring new foods that will help you meet your nutrition needs.

Adapted, by permission, from S.G. Eberle, 1997, "The vegetarian runner," *Marathon and Beyond* 1(5): 69-77.

Learning From the Best: *Vegetarian or Vegan Eating for Endurance Athletes*

Scott Jurek, a two-time Ultrarunner of the Year and a vegan, contends that following a vegetarian, even vegan, eating style doesn't have to be complex or life consuming. What it takes is planning and being willing to solve problems—to figure out what you need to do and to be creative about doing it. Read on for his tips on how to excel at meeting your nutritional needs as a vegetarian or vegan endurance athlete.

1. Think about quantity as well as quality. The biggest downfall of vegetarian and vegan endurance athletes, especially ultra athletes, is often just not getting in enough calories. If you're a vegetarian who eliminates and doesn't replace, that is, you don't look for alternative sources, you will suffer the consequences of consuming too few calories. Although eating as clean as possible is important, this does not mean starving yourself.

2. Plan your protein. As recommended, Jurek relies on heavy hitters—tofu, tempeh, and legumes, a serving of each at least once a day. Smoothies also contribute valuable protein in the form of soy yogurt and added hemp or brown rice protein powder. Jurek cautions athletes not to rely on heavily processed soy protein powders.

3. Don't fear fat. Endurance athletes don't need to shy away from fat. Jurek meets his high energy needs by getting 20 to 25 percent of his daily calories from healthy fats—avocados, olive oil, almond butter, and almonds being his favorites.

4. Don't make excuses, even on the road. At home, keep quick-fix staples on hand. When feasible, take a small cooler with you when traveling (as Jurek routinely does). Be creative when dining in restaurants, such as asking for a commonly stocked alternative protein source such as extra nuts and seeds on the side or canned garbanzo or kidney beans. Look for these items on salad bars too. Asian restaurants are the best bet for dense protein foods such as tofu. Jurek also travels with protein-rich energy bars, such as Nectar bars and Larabars, as well as freeze-dried or dehydrated tofu, dehydrated hummus and instant lentil, and split-pea or other dried legume soups. These items travel well, and you can eat them after your restaurant meal or easily prepare them at the table by requesting hot water.

5. Embrace food. Jurek loves to eat and prepare food. He relishes the psychological boost that comes from knowing that he has taken the time and energy to fuel his body adequately. He challenges endurance athletes to think of food as a life source, allowing them to do what they love to do.

6. Fuel up during supported races. Vegetarians and vegans will find plenty of options for race foods among what is typically offered at aid stations. Almost all drinks and foods are vegan and therefore provide exactly what an endurance athlete needs—a steady supply of carbohydrate. For concentrated liquid calories, Jurek drinks soy protein-based products such as Balanced Total Nutritional Drink and Power Dream Soy Energy Drink. During ultraendurance races, calorie-rich energy bars help too.

8

Planning Meals for Endurance Athletes

Unless you've been hibernating the past several years or training in isolation, you probably have plenty of nutrition knowledge. Most of the sports-minded people I meet have more than enough information, but they still claim that they don't know how to eat. When it comes to making smart and healthy choices from day to day, the key is to translate what we know to be true into practical and useful eating habits that we can do (and keep doing). For example, whether you need to reduce or expand your food selections to meet your daily needs (including calories), eating regular meals and snacks is the easiest way to get the job done. You'll also boost your metabolism and have more energy during the day when you need it most. Besides, ignoring your hunger and skipping meals just makes it harder because doing so usually leads to making poor choices or overeating at the next meal.

If you eat at least three times a day, you need to make a decision about what to eat more than a thousand times a year. I find that active people, even elite athletes, are too caught up in *what* to eat and would benefit tremendously from putting more of their energy into *how* to eat. What you choose to eat will vary from day to day and situation to situation. You may plan to eat chicken at dinner only to arrive at your friend's house to find sirloin steak being served. A slice of pizza may be the best choice at two o'clock, before an after-work run, but not at four. Eating a bagel some mornings might be enough; other mornings it won't be. Downing a few energy gels and an energy bar or two may be the most supportive thing you can do on a Saturday ride but not be a wise choice for a weekday afternoon.

In other words, eating a smart sports diet is both a science and an art. Although recommendations about what to eat do exist, they are situational. Just as you decide what shoes and clothing to wear on a long bike ride or what pace to maintain in the first half of a race, you must choose foods based not only on your current needs, but on longterm goals, as well. No one else, including the latest diet guru, can tell you what to eat, nor can you determine beforehand exactly what and how much you will need to eat on any given day to get the job done. For people used to tracking the seconds with stopwatches, measuring distances to the 10th of a mile, and following workout plans determined by others, eating smart may be challenging, confusing, and even anxiety provoking. But it doesn't need to be.

Five Guidelines on How to Eat

To provide some structure (and much needed calmness regarding food), I've developed some guidelines for athletes on how to eat. These guidelines work whether you are eating in (at home) or out, at work (or at school), or while on the road. They are designed to help you eat consistently in a way that leaves you physically ready and mentally prepared to embrace and enjoy your workouts, your relationship with food, and your life in general.

#1: Plan to eat every three to five hours while awake

First, don't let yourself get too hungry. Plan to eat every three to five hours while you're awake to keep your blood sugar (fuel for your brain) from dipping too low. If you allow yourself to become too hungry, you won't perform to your full potential. You're also apt to toss your good intentions out the window and simply eat whatever food is in sight, which may not be the healthiest fare. Eating every few hours will also help you maintain a healthy weight because doing so keeps you from back-loading calories—not eating enough during the day when you need the energy the most (and are most likely to burn off the calories) and then shoveling in calories over a few hours between dinner and bedtime. Besides, if you don't start eating early in the day, you will find it nearly impossible to get in all the nutrients that you need. Are you realistically going to have three cups of vegetables, two pieces of fruit, and three cups (750 milliliters) of milk (or the equivalent) at dinner alone?

#2: Eat from at least three food groups at mealtimes

The timing of these meals is up to you, because it depends on your schedule and other commitments for that day. But eating three well-balanced meals is a given. When planning meals, even as you wait in line at your favorite eatery or stand in front of the refrigerator with the door open, remember this guideline: Eat from at least three food groups at every meal. (You don't have to stop there—challenge yourself to include servings from four or even five food groups.) Some athletes take this concept a step further by creating their own meal plan. To do this, take the recommended servings that you need from MyPyramid and divide them up among three meals and however many snacks you typically eat (two to three for most endurance athletes). Having a written plan of action will help you keep your eye on the big picture.

Eating breakfast improves your ability to perform at school and work and is essential for maintaining a healthy weight. Making time to eat lunch can reduce stress, enhance productivity, and recharge you for the afternoon, especially if you train at the end of the day. Preparing a gourmet meal for dinner isn't necessary or required, but sitting down is. You deserve a break at the end of a long day and need to refuel for the next one. Besides, sitting down for dinner is an enjoyable way to reconnect with family and friends. Remember, many poor training days can be linked to poor eating days.

Here are some quick fixes to help you eat regular meals:

- Choose to eat breakfast. If you've gotten out of the habit (and that's what it is) or conditioned your body not to be hungry, rethink the importance of this meal. If you're not hungry, check out your current eating habits. You're most likely eating too much or too late at night. Stop eating an hour earlier at night. Keep cutting down the time until you are hungry enough to eat breakfast. Anything goes for this meal from traditional breakfast foods to leftovers. The ultimate quick breakfast is a glass of juice, a glass of milk, and a bagel.

- Make lunch a priority. Again, anything goes. Brown bagging has the advantage of always being available, especially if you can't get away from your desk or other commitments. Pack your lunch the night before and keep stashes of nonperishable items (instant oatmeal, peanut butter, crackers, dried soup, dried fruit, energy bars, and so forth) in your briefcase, locker, or desk drawer for the days that you forget to bring a lunch. Drink liquid lunches, such as meal replacement supplements or instant breakfast drinks, when you're really pressed for time or need more calories. If you eat out or at a cafeteria, do your best to make wise choices. Concentrate on eating carbohydrate-rich lunches, not fat-laden meals. Compensate at other meals or snacks for what you don't eat or can't get at lunch.

- Sit down for dinner. This guideline applies even when eating out. Keep MyPyramid in mind and aim to fill out the food groups as you would at home. By choosing the restaurant or eatery carefully, you'll have plenty of options. If you use some creativity, even convenience-store cuisine can offer acceptable fare. Although some endurance athletes can afford higher-fat items, the list in appendix D ("Eating on the Run: Dining Out") emphasizes higher-carbohydrate, lower-fat selections for those who eat out regularly.

To help meet the challenge of what to eat for dinner when eating in, save time and mental energy by planning ahead. This approach will help you be more creative when it comes to deciding what to eat. Eating the same few foods or too much of any single food can be boring and get you into trouble. Furthermore, if you get too hungry or don't have the right ingredients on hand, you'll end up doing what you always do—grabbing whatever is the easiest.

Quick Meal Planning When Eating at Home

1. Work out a system beforehand. Plan five simple meals for the upcoming week, concentrating on what the main entree will be. (Between leftovers and eating out, you should be covered.) At dinnertime, simply select one. Some athletes do well with a set routine, for instance, chicken every Monday, pasta on Tuesday, fish or seafood on Wednesday, and so on. To add variety, prepare the entree a different way or vary the side dishes that you serve it with (for example, couscous or instant stuffing instead of rice).

2. Keep staples on hand to throw together quick, nutritious meals: milk and cereal, scrambled eggs and toast or toaster waffles, baked potato (use the microwave) topped with beans or cottage cheese, pasta and meat sauce, bean-based soup and sandwich, canned chili and crackers, and so on. Round out your meal with some fresh, frozen, or canned fruit, juice, or vegetables (raw or cooked).

3. Keep a running list of items that you need to restock your staples or to prepare special meals. Take it with you when you shop. A well-stocked kitchen is the key to preparing tasty, time-saving meals. Shop at a familiar store so that you can locate items quickly. (For staples to keep on hand, see appendix D: "Eating on the Run: Stocking Your Pantry.")

4. Buy part of dinner and prepare the rest. For example, buy a rotisserie chicken or meat loaf and add your own healthy sides, such as instant mashed potatoes and microwaved or steamed vegetables without sauces or butter. Alternatively, take advantage of prepared foods, such as boneless, skinless chicken breasts, cubed or sliced cooked turkey, skinned fish filets, peeled shrimp, canned beans, instant-cooking grains, salad-bar produce or salad in a bag, and grated cheese.

5. Have fun at mealtimes. Experiment by buying one new food from the grocery store each week or try a new recipe once a month. Don't get bogged down by thinking that you have to create an entire new meal; just make one new item and serve it with some familiar standbys. Experiment. Keep the best and toss the rest.

6. Cook for more than one meal. Cook meals in bulk on the weekends and then date and freeze them in family-size or individual-size containers.

(continued)

(continued)

Alternatively, prepare at least enough at dinnertime so that you have leftovers to eat at another meal the following day.

7. Stock your kitchen with all or some of these time-saving devices: a sharp knife, cookware that can go from freezer to microwave, small electric or hand-operated food chopper, blender, vegetable steamer (no pots to watch), rice cooker, toaster oven (toasts, bakes, or broils small amounts of food), microwave, and a Crock-Pot or slow cooker (requires more preparation time in the morning but dinner is ready when you arrive home).

#3: Eat a protein-rich food and/or some healthy fat at every meal

Carbohydrate supplied by the foods that we eat provide energy, but not even athletes can live on carbohydrate alone. Including protein (to the tune of at least 15 to 25 grams, which you can obtain from 2 to 3 ounces of meat, poultry, or fish, or the equivalent in soy foods, eggs, or dried beans) at mealtime sustains us, but it's fat that really satisfies. If you fill up on carbohydrate you can find yourself either eating too much or being hungry again in an hour or two. For most busy and active people, this approach isn't desired or practical. To meet your daily nutritional requirements and keep a steady blood sugar level for a more reasonable period, make sure to include a protein-rich food at mealtime, especially lunch and dinner. One way to remember this is with the phrase "Don't eat your grains plain." Smear your bagel with peanut butter, toss baked beans over noodles, or throw seafood or chicken into your favorite sauce and pour it over pasta, rice, or couscous.

Fat, however, is what really satisfies us—both physically and mentally. Judicious use of healthy fat (see chapter 1 for a review) is much more productive in the long run than trying to avoid all fat or not paying any attention at all to what type or how much you eat. Because it digests much more slowly, meals (and snacks) that contain fat slow the rise and fall in blood sugar that occurs after we eat. This means that we feel full longer and can last four to five hours before needing (at least physiologically) to eat again. Fat also makes the foods that we eat taste good, satisfying our taste buds and our brains. Extras or fun foods like sweets, chips, and french fries also provide fat and play an important role in a smart sports diet. For more on that, keep reading.

#4: Design snacks that include at least one food from a food group

Do your body a favor and think of snacks as minimeals or opportunities to get the nutrients that you need. (Selecting foods that are more nutritious is particularly important if you tend to graze throughout the day instead of eating defined meals.) For active people who juggle workouts around their other commitments, well-designed snacks or minimeals are often the only way to accomplish the job. As much as possible, snack on foods that come from the five food groups. Select at least one food from a food group, or even better, put together foods from two different food groups, such as whole-wheat crackers and cheese or yogurt and fruit. See "Performance-Enhancing Snacks" for more ideas.

Save fun foods like cookies, cake, chips, and ice cream to have at mealtimes. You can easily overeat these foods on an empty stomach (especially if you've gotten too hungry), and they can crowd out healthier fare. In addition, active people and athletes often worry about the fat or nutrient content the whole time that they are eating a fun food. They continue to focus on the food instead of how they feel, diluting the pleasure of eating these foods. They may miss the "I'm full" signs and eat too much. Build sweets and treats in at mealtimes (you know that you're going to eat them anyway). By slowing down and allowing

Performance-Enhancing Snacks

Peanut butter and jelly or banana sandwich (half or whole)

Trail gorp (nuts, raisins, dried fruit, and so on)

Instant oatmeal with dried apricots

Cereal or low-fat granola with fruit and yogurt

Banana, pumpkin, or date bread and a carton of milk

Cookies (oatmeal raisin, fig bars, vanilla wafers, gingersnaps, animal crackers, or graham crackers) and milk

Low-fat cheese and crackers or rice cakes

Tuna fish and crackers

Pita bread with low-fat cheese

An English muffin or bagel topped with peanut or other nut butter

Low-fat muffin with milk, yogurt, or juice

Rice cakes or crackers and hummus

Slice of pizza (thick crust and vegetable toppings)

Baked potato topped with salsa, cottage cheese, or low-fat cheese

Cup or bowl of soup and crackers

Three-bean, pasta, or potato salad (with low-fat dressing) and a roll

Raw vegetables dipped in low-fat salad dressing or salsa

Nonfat refried beans or salsa and baked chips or crackers

Piece of fresh fruit and pretzels or low-fat popcorn

Fresh fruit dipped in yogurt or chocolate-flavored syrup

Frozen fruit juice bar or low-fat frozen yogurt

Angel food cake with fresh berries or a dollop of yogurt

Half a papaya or cantaloupe filled with yogurt or cottage cheese

Breakfast drink or shake made with low-fat milk, ice cream, or yogurt

Fruit smoothie (fruit, yogurt, and milk or juice)

Meal replacement drink

yourself to savor the foods that you want to eat, you're much more likely to indulge in an appropriate amount. Also, keep in mind the 80-20 rule. If you're making smart choices most of the time (eight out of ten or 80 percent of the time), then go easy on yourself the rest of the time (20 percent).

Fill in or round out your diet with energy bars, but don't make them the main part of it. At their best, energy bars supply a convenient dose of energy. They work well as an easily digestible preworkout or prerace meal, as fuel during exercise (as tolerated), and as a way to help replenish muscle glycogen stores following exercise. You might also rely on energy bars (meal replacement

Do Energy Bars Fit Into a Smart Sports Diet?

Run this diet by your taste buds: carrot cake for breakfast, an almond brownie for lunch or an afternoon snack, and a chocolate praline following your evening workout. This regime is possible—thanks to the endless array of energy bars available to athletes. You may even believe that energy bars (also called sports or endurance bars) are, well, real food.

Containing more than simple and complex carbohydrates, energy bars typically include varying amounts of protein, fat, vitamins, and minerals, as well as antioxidants, herbs, and other potentially performance-enhancing substances (although little evidence exists that these substances have any effect on athletic performance). You may also be consuming items that you don't want, such as caffeine, palm kernel oil (a saturated fat common in coated bars), or high-fructose corn syrup (a refined sweetener).

The food pyramid was designed with real foods in mind. From that perspective, energy bars don't fit neatly into any food group. Despite being fortified with vitamins and minerals, most carbohydrate-rich bars are high in sugar and contain little or no fiber. "Balanced" bars may provide protein but without the accompanying iron and zinc found in protein-rich foods. Some bars really aren't much different from a candy bar or a bunch of fat-free cookies combined with a vitamin pill.

Having an occasional energy bar, even up to one a day, isn't likely to do you any nutritional harm (if you can afford the calories). Most will count as at least one serving in the grain group, and if they contain protein, 7 grams is the equivalent of 1 ounce of meat. Beyond that, think about energy bars as extras. They are a sports food or a fuel supplement to an otherwise healthy diet based on real food. Consider that foods are more than just the sum of their parts. The nutrients in food work together to produce an effect greater than that which a single nutrient could produce. It's not exactly clear what quantity or combination of nutrients the body requires. On top of that, some potential health boosters, like the phytochemicals (plant chemicals that may help the body ward off aging and disease) found in fruits and vegetables, haven't yet been fully identified, so they can't possibly be in your favorite bar. For those reasons, routinely replacing meals or snacks with processed foods doesn't make sense for your health or your performance.

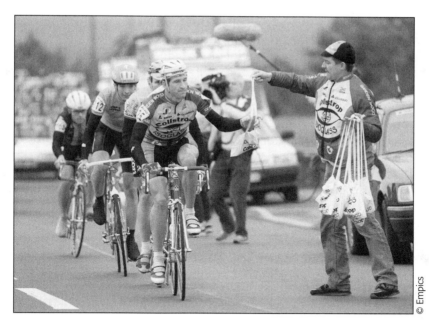

Consistency in fueling and training will help you move past the starting line toward a successful finish.

products too) as a backup, perhaps on busy days or while traveling when you would otherwise miss or skip a meal or snack. To be sure of what you're getting and what you're missing out on, check the nutrition label and ingredients list of whatever bar you choose. Many bars lack substantial amounts of some key nutrients that athletes are often low in, such as vitamins A and C, calcium, iron, and fiber.

#5: *Drink a healthy beverage with every meal or snack*

As an athlete, the time to think about being well hydrated is not right before you head out the door. Make life easy. Attend to your fluid needs throughout the day simply by drinking a healthy beverage with every meal or snack. You might drink water, or, depending on the situation, you might choose 100 percent juice, low-fat milk, herbal tea, or a sports drink. (See chapter 1 for a review of healthy beverages.)

Sample Meal Plans for Endurance Athletes

Look at the following sample meal plans to view how an endurance athlete can enjoy a variety of tasty foods and fulfill his or her nutritional requirements on a typical training day. When you exercise—first thing in the morning, at lunchtime, or after work—will determine exactly what foods are best to eat when. But eating well-balanced meals, supplemented by healthy snacks, remains constant. What varies is the amount of food that you eat at a sitting and the actual time that you choose to eat your meals and snacks. For instance, you may eat breakfast, and at lunchtime, the baked potato wedges and only half the sandwich. If you've already worked out (or time allows for adequate digestion), saving the other half for a midafternoon snack makes sense, especially if you tend to eat dinner late or special circumstances call for a late dinner.

Notice also that active people and athletes at all calorie ranges (especially those racking up long distances) need to spend some of their extra or additional calories on foods and drinks appropriate for use during and after exercise. The goal isn't to skimp on necessary sports drinks and energy gels (or other sports food needed for fuel) during or after training bouts so that you can spend the calories on extra sweets, alcohol, and foods high in fat like french fries and cream cheese. Remember, athletes who eat in a way that leaves them physically ready and mentally prepared are the ones consistently able to work out or train at a high level.

Sample Calorie Meal Plans for Athletes

2,200-CALORIE SPORTS PLAN

Breakfast

> 1 cup (250 ml) of orange juice
>
> 1 cup low-fat milk
> or 6 oz (170 g) of low-fat flavored yogurt
>
> Black coffee or tea

> *Breakfast burrito*
>
> 1 flour tortilla (8 in., or 20 cm, diameter)
> 1 scrambled egg (in 1 tsp of low-fat soft or tub margarine)
>
> 1/3 cup of black beans
> 2 tbsp of salsa

Note: Orange juice, milk, or yogurt can be saved for a midmorning snack.

Lunch

> Water or unsweetened beverage
>
> 3/4 cup of baked potato wedges
> with 1 tbsp of ketchup

> *Roast beef sandwich*
>
> 1 whole-grain (2.5 oz, or 70 g) sandwich bun
> 3 oz (85 g) of lean roast beef
> 2 slices of tomato
>
> 1/4 cup of shredded romaine lettuce
> 1.5 oz (42 g) of part-skim mozzarella cheese
> 1 tsp of yellow mustard

Dinner

> 1 cup low-fat milk
> 1/2 cup of flavored white rice
> with .5 oz (14 g) of slivered almonds
>
> 1 cup of steamed broccoli
> 1 cup of low-fat ice cream

Stuffed broiled salmon filet

3 oz (85 g) of salmon, cooked

1 oz (28 g) of bread stuffing mix

1 tbsp of chopped onions

1 tbsp of diced celery

2 tsp (10 ml) of canola oil

Snacks/Extras

1 cup of cantaloupe

Energy bar (200 calories)
  or 4 cups of rehydration sports drink
  or 3 fig bars and 4 oz (112 ml) of 100% fruit juice

Total: 2,235 calories, 109 g protein (20%), 325 g carbohydrate (58%), 55 g fat (22%)

2,600-CALORIE SPORTS PLAN

Breakfast

1 cup of orange juice

1 cup of low-fat milk
  or 6 oz (170 g) of low-fat flavored yogurt

Black coffee or tea

Breakfast burrito

1 flour tortilla (8 in., or 20 cm, diameter)

1 scrambled egg (in 1 tsp of low-fat soft
  or tub margarine)

1/3 cup of black beans

2 tbsp of salsa

Note: Orange juice, milk, or yogurt can be saved for a midmorning snack.

Lunch

Water or unsweetened beverage

3/4 cup of baked potato wedges
  with 1 tbsp of ketchup

Roast beef sandwich

1 whole-grain (2.5 oz, or 70 g) sandwich
  bun

3 oz (85 g) of lean roast beef

2 slices of tomato

1/4 cup of shredded romaine lettuce

1.5 oz (42 g) of part-skim mozzarella
  cheese

1 tsp of yellow mustard

Dinner

1 cup of low-fat milk

1/2 cup of flavored white rice
  with .5 oz (14 g) of slivered almonds

1 cup of steamed broccoli

1 cup of low-fat ice cream

Stuffed broiled salmon filet

4 oz (112 g) of salmon, cooked

1 oz (28 g) of bread stuffing mix

1 tbsp of chopped onions

1 tbsp of diced celery

2 tsp (10 ml) of canola oil

Snacks/Extras

1 cup of cantaloupe

Energy bar (200 calories)
or 4 cups (1 liter) of rehydration sports
drink
or 3 fig bars and 4 oz (112 ml) of 100%
fruit juice

1 tbsp of peanut butter

1 oz (28 g) of whole-wheat crackers
or 2 full graham crackers

1 cup (250 ml) of 100% fruit juice
or 5 oz (140 ml) of wine

Total: 2,641 calories, 124 g protein (19%), 381 g carbohydrate (58%), 69 g fat (24%)

3,000-CALORIE SPORTS PLAN

Breakfast

1 cup of orange juice

Black coffee or tea

Breakfast burrito

1 flour tortilla (8 in., or 20 cm, diameter)

1 scrambled egg and 2 egg whites
(in 1 tbsp of soft or tub margarine)

1/2 cup of black beans

2 tbsp of salsa

Midmorning snack

1 cup of low-fat milk
or 6 oz (170 g) of low-fat flavored yogurt

1 cup of cold whole-grain cereal
or 1 packet of instant oatmeal

Lunch

Water or unsweetened beverage

3/4 cup of baked potato wedges
with 1 tbsp of ketchup

Handful of baby carrots

Roast beef sandwich

1 whole-grain (2.5 oz, or 70 g) sandwich
bun

4 oz (112 g) of lean roast beef

2 slices of tomato

1/4 cup of shredded romaine lettuce

1.5 oz (42 g) of part-skim mozzarella
cheese

1 tsp of yellow mustard

Afternoon snack

1 cup of cantaloupe

1 tbsp of peanut butter

1 oz (28 g) of whole-wheat crackers

Dinner

1 cup of low-fat milk

3/4 cup of flavored white rice
  with .5 oz (14 g) of slivered almonds

1 1/2 cups of steamed broccoli

Stuffed broiled salmon filet

5 oz (140 g) of salmon, cooked

1 oz (28 g) of bread stuffing mix

1 tbsp of chopped onions

1 tbsp of diced celery

2 tsp (10 ml) of canola oil

Snacks/Extras

1 energy bar (250 calories)
  or 16 oz (500 ml) milk shake (made with skim milk)

2 cups (500 ml) of rehydration sports drink

1 energy gel
  or 8 oz (250 ml) of 100% fruit juice
  or 2 cups (500 ml) of rehydration sports drink
  or 1 medium banana

Total: 2,993 calories, 157 g protein (21%), 418 g carbohydrate (56%), 77 g fat (23%)

3,500-CALORIE SPORTS PLAN

Breakfast

2 cups (500 ml) of orange juice

Black coffee or tea

Breakfast burrito

1 flour tortilla (8 in., or 20 cm, diameter)

1 scrambled egg and 2 egg whites
  (in 1 tbsp of soft or tub margarine)

1/2 cup of black beans

2 tbsp of salsa

Midmorning snack

1 cup of low-fat milk
  or 6 oz (170 g) of low-fat flavored yogurt

1 cup of cold whole-grain cereal
  or 1 packet of instant oatmeal

Lunch

Water or unsweetened beverage

3/4 cup of baked potato wedges
with 1 tbsp of ketchup

Handful of baby carrots

Roast beef sandwich

1 whole-grain (2.5 oz, or 70 g) sandwich
bun

4 oz (112 g) of lean roast beef

2 slices of tomato

1/4 cup of shredded romaine lettuce

1.5 oz (42 g) of part-skim mozzarella
cheese

1 tsp of yellow mustard

Afternoon snack

1 cup of cantaloupe

1 tbsp of peanut butter

1 oz (28 g) of whole-wheat crackers

Dinner

1 cup of low-fat milk

1 cup of flavored white rice
with .5 oz (14 g) of slivered almonds

2 cups of steamed broccoli
with 2 tbsp (30 ml) of regular salad
dressing

Stuffed broiled salmon filet

5 oz (140 g) of salmon, cooked

1 oz (28 g) of bread stuffing mix

1 tbsp of chopped onions

1 tbsp of diced celery

2 tsp (10 ml) of canola oil

Snacks/Extras

1 energy bar (250 calories)
or 16 oz (500 ml) milk shake
(made with skim milk)

2 cups (500 ml) of rehydration sports drink

1 energy gel
or 8 oz (250 ml) of 100% fruit juice
or 2 cups (500 ml) of rehydration sports drink
or 1 medium banana

1 beer (12 oz, or 355 ml)
or 6 oz (175 ml) of wine
(~150 calories)

Total: 3,502 calories, 163 g protein (19%), 482 g carbohydrate (55%), 92 g fat (24%)

PART II

Condition-Specific Nutrition Plans

9

Shorter-Range Events

"If you have leaned down for a race, you will always feel heavy going into a competition. The best triathletes in the world all feel this way. That 'feeling' is your body allowing its glycogen stores to fill before race day. If you eat normally and hydrate leading up to a race, your taper will make you feel this way. You may be unnerved, but reassure yourself that everything is going to plan."

—Mark Fretta, four top-15 finishes in International Triathlon Union (ITU) World Cup events, which put him atop the world rankings

Perhaps you're just getting started as an endurance athlete, or maybe you've figured out that you excel at the "shorter end" of endurance-related sports and activities. Whatever the reason, having a defined goal, whether it is tackling local hiking trails or putting it on the line in a 10K road race or a sprint triathlon, can be motivating and keep life interesting. Despite popular opinion, having a well-thought-out nutrition plan is still very much part of the equation for achieving success in these shorter endurance ventures. And, if you have any plans to participate or compete in longer endurance events and races, you'll need to begin to practice and hone your nutritional strategies during these higher-intensity, shorter-range efforts.

This chapter will help you explore or work at excelling in higher-intensity, shorter-range endurance events and races,* such as the following:

Running: 5K, 8K, 10K, and 10-mile road races or these distances as a single leg of

---

*Note: keep in mind that this designation is somewhat arbitrary in terms of times and distances because time of physical exertion in endurance events and races depends on fitness level and experience—what might be a shorter-range effort for a highly trained competitive endurance athlete could be a long-distance effort for a fitness enthusiast.

a team relay race, shorter trail races (those that take up to two hours to complete)

Duathlon or triathlon: sprint distance, Olympic distance

Cycling: short amateur and pro-am road races and time trials (lasting two to three hours or less), standard cyclo-cross and mountain bike races (lasting two hours or less), the cycling leg of a triathlon or mountain bike team relay race, organized rides taking two to a leisurely four hours to complete

Multisport or adventure racing: short two- to three-hour multisport adventures, undertaking a single leg of an adventure team relay race

Hiking or trekking: forays of up to four hours, especially if at a moderate to fast pace, such as fast-packing

Winter sports: recreational cross-country ski and snowshoe outings and races lasting one to three continuous hours, shorter Nordic ski races (lasting 75-90 minutes or less)

What separates these shorter-duration events and races from merely going out for a run (or ride or swim or ski) or from long-range and ultraendurance events and races is the shorter duration and the intensity or pace that you plan (hope) to undertake and maintain. If you're a serious competitor, you'll be putting in hours of training or working out for a race or activity that will take a fraction of that time to complete. Training specifically for the activity is essential, and race-day strategy, including going out at the proper pace, is extremely important. Keep in mind that carbohydrate provides most of the energy used by working muscles and that a faster pace (especially going out at a fast pace, settling in, and then picking up or kicking in to finish strongly) dictates that both anaerobic and aerobic energy systems be in play. (See chapter 2 for a review of energy systems.)

Just as important, you may simply want to enjoy yourself as much as possible while you're out there and get to the finish. Let's face it—some active people and recreational athletes never quite get in all the recommended hours or miles of training, and thus undertake athletic challenges that exercise scientists would categorize as being beyond what they have physiologically prepared for. In this case, paying attention to your nutritional needs before and during the event or race is crucial to your ability to enjoy yourself and finish (and avoid becoming sick or injured). Being physically underprepared coupled with making poor nutrition decisions is not a winning combo.

Preevent Nutrition Game Plan

If you're going into the race or event having followed a smart sports diet during the training period, you should have more than adequate glycogen stored in your muscles (up to 300 to 400 grams of glycogen, or 1,200 to 1,600 calories) and liver (100 grams, or 400 calories) to fuel the anaerobic and aerobic demands placed on working muscles during the actual race. In other words, before shorter-range endurance races, especially those lasting 90 minutes or less, you don't need to carbohydrate-load or superload the muscles with glycogen as do marathoners, Ironman triathletes, or cyclists who are attempting a century ride (100 miles).

Some athletes, however, do run the risk of gradually depleting glycogen stores while preparing for competitions and never allowing their muscles to regain their full potential supply. Athletes most at risk are those involved in heavy training who don't adequately rest before races, those who follow low-carbohydrate diets, or those who are overly concerned about maintaining a desired weight. In these circumstances, an athlete may enter a shorter-range endurance competition with glycogen stores insufficient to sustain an all-out competitive effort. Remember, you burn proportionately more carbohydrate as your pace quickens and as oxygen becomes less available to working muscles (and carbohydrates are the only fuel that you can burn during flat-out efforts). Likewise, you'll burn more carbohydrate during fast starts, surges, ascents of hills, and sprints to the finish line. (Review chapter 4 on how to maintain adequate glycogen stores in your muscles from day to day.)

One to Two Days Before the Event and Dinner the Night Before

Your overall nutritional goal is to top off fluid and glycogen stores by eating snacks and meals composed of familiar foods that you like and drinking a healthy beverage along with each meal and snack (see chapter 8).

As for dinner the night before, no one magical or preferred prerace dinner exists. The only rule is to stick with familiar foods that you enjoy. This is not the time to be adventurous! You don't want to be up all night making trips to the bathroom. Although you most likely will naturally tend toward carbohydrate-rich foods like pasta, rice, tortillas, and potatoes, keep in mind that athletes have competed successfully after eating all kinds of foods. (For carbohydrate-rich meal ideas, see table 4.2 in chapter 4.) You don't need to stuff in carbohydrates at this time! Eat at a reasonable time for you, consume appropriate-sized portions, and know that you can eat again, if need be, before bedtime (for example, milk and cereal or an energy bar).

Some athletes become obsessed with having the perfect prerace meal or the same one every time. To keep your stress level in check, become comfortable with a variety of acceptable foods or meals, especially if you travel to races and events, because there is no guarantee that you will always be able to get the same foods. Remind yourself that this "last supper" is only one of many factors that go into your preparation for the next day's event or race.

Last, but not least, prepare and pack any nutrition essentials that you plan to consume during the event or race such as sports drinks, energy gels and bars, and foods that have previously passed the test in training (as well as a recovery drink or bar and food for afterward). Double-check that any equipment you plan to use, such as hip packs or bum bags, water bladders, and gel flasks, is in good working order. Make up drink bottles (or another system of hydration) the night before so that you can just grab them in the morning (and so that during warm weather you can freeze bottles beforehand).

Morning of the Event

Eat breakfast. No matter how early you plan to hit the trail or how early the gun goes off, eat something. You might choose something as simple as toast with jam or honey, a glass of juice, or a banana. If need be, get up early, eat, and go back to bed. Eating breakfast tops off your liver glycogen stores (your "brain fuel"), which have become depleted overnight, and settles your stomach, meaning that you won't be distracted by or become anxious about hunger pains and falling blood sugar as you wait to begin. Liquid breakfasts, such as a meal replacement beverage (see chapter 5), are good for sensitive or nervous stomachs, as well as for those with long drive times to get to the starting line. To avoid surprises, stick with foods that you are used to eating.

You will need to time when you eat breakfast so that you don't end up stranded in the bathroom beforehand or feel uncomfortably full while racing. Athletes vary widely in what they can tolerate, but resist the urge to skip breakfast altogether, especially if you will be on the go at a moderate to fast pace for more than an hour. In general, the more time you have beforehand, the more solid food you should be able to tolerate and the more you can (and most likely will need) to eat. No concrete recommendations exist, but most people do well with .5 grams of carbohydrate (two calories) per pound of body weight (1.0 gram carbohydrate or four calories per kilogram) if they eat one hour before the event (for example, a canned liquid meal or energy bar that provides 100 to 300 calories) or up to 2.0 grams of carbohydrate per pound four hours before (for example, a hearty breakfast that holds you). Keep in mind that liquid foods clear the stomach faster than solid foods do.

Drink plenty of familiar (well-tolerated) fluids such as water, sports drink, fruit juice, and milk up to two hours before the start. Doing so will give you time to urinate any excess. If you choose not to eat breakfast, drinking carbohydrate-containing beverages such as sports drinks or juice becomes even more important, and, if you're used to having tea or coffee in the morning, don't skip it today. Five to 15 minutes before the start, drink another cup of water or a sports drink. (For energy gel users, this is the time to consume a packet with a few gulps of water.)

Treat any sports foods that you will use during the race or event like you would any other piece of equipment that you rely on. First, don't leave home without it. Second, don't wait to the last minute when you're nervous or excited to figure out what you need to do. Double-check that your bottles are on your bike or in your knapsack, that fluid is flowing easily through the bladder hose, or that your hip pack or bum bag is loaded with an energy gel or two. You can also carry single energy gel packs in a pocket or pinned to the inside of your shorts, or tucked into your cycling shorts or sports bra.

During the Event

During these relatively shorter events and races, your main job is to monitor your fluid needs and prevent dehydration, which can lead to a more dangerous situation, such as heat exhaustion. Elite runners, sprint triathletes, and time trial cyclists often will not drink during shorter endeavors. Most competitors, however, as well as completers, either will need to drink or would benefit greatly from drinking during shorter events and races. The benefits of drinking during the event are particularly significant for heavy sweaters, underprepared athletes, and those who are competing at altitude or in warmer or more humid conditions than they're accustomed to.

Remember, this isn't about what you can do, such as ride 30 miles or race a 10K, without "needing" any water. This is about working with your body to be as physically and mentally prepared as possible to enjoy and conquer the upcoming challenge. If you'll be on the move for a couple of hours or longer, maintaining a normal blood sugar level will affect your ultimate success. Shorter-range events and races also provide opportunities to practice techniques and strategies for eating and drinking while on the move that won't be optional if you move up in distance. (For more sport-specific tips and strategies, see chapters 10 through 12.)

Drinking water should be adequate in most situations, especially if you'll be on the move for an hour or less. Don't be afraid, however, to consume a sports drink. No law says that sports drinks can be consumed only if you're going longer than 60 to 90 minutes. In fact, the carbohydrate boost from sports drinks (and gels) may be just what makes the difference (especially if you didn't eat breakfast) in your ability to kick or finish strongly at the end of any shorter endurance race or event. Individual fluid needs vary widely—from a gulp or two to several ounces every 15 to 20 minutes from the time you start.

For events and races lasting longer than 60 to 90 minutes, sports drinks are recommended because they are the most efficient way to consume what you need—fluid and carbohydrate. Supplemental carbohydrate, from sports drinks, gels, and, if appropriate, energy bars and real foods, help you maintain a normal blood sugar level and prevent hypoglycemia, or bonking, as the event or race unfolds. The effort that you are putting out will seem easier and your goal more doable when your brain receives a constant supply of fuel.

Individual needs vary widely, depending on your fitness level, preevent glycogen stores, your pace, the activity, the weather, and course conditions. The general rule is to consume 25 to 60 grams of carbohydrate (100 to 250 calories from carbohydrate) per hour of activity after the first hour.

For most adults, one gulp of fluid roughly equates to drinking about 1 ounce (30 milliliters). Novice competitors need to realize that slowing down, walking,

Sample Carbohydrate Counts

1 cup (8 oz or 8 gulps) of standard sports drink	12 g–15 g
1 energy gel packet	25 g
1 package (1.58 oz, or 45 g) of Sharkies (energy sport chews)	36 g
Glucose tablets	4 g–5 g each
6 Clif Shot Bloks chews	48 g
1 packet (1 oz, or 28 g) of Sport Beans jelly beans	25 g

or even stopping altogether to drink enough fluid is far better than dropping out of the race (or getting injured or feeling miserable the entire time) because of being dehydrated or glycogen depleted. The more comfortable you are drinking on the move, the more likely you are to meet your fluid needs. The only way to become proficient is to practice, practice, practice!

Running Simply grabbing a cup or two off an aid station table isn't good enough; you have to get the fluid down. Practice the following favored technique: Grab a cup, pinch or crush it lightly to form a funnel, and take one or two gulps at a time. In self-supported running adventures and trail races, use bladders, hip belts, or other bottle carriers specifically designed for runners.

Cycling Use your common sense when drinking on a bike. Concentrate on the road, look ahead for hazards, and slow down if necessary. When riding one-handed as you reach for a water bottle (or energy gel or food), keep your bike from veering by gripping the center of the handlebar next to the stem with your stronger arm. Always empty your down-tube bottle first and then switch it with your full seat-tube bottle. Keep in mind that rapid evaporation of sweat can give you the false sense that you're losing only minimal amounts of fluid. The windchill factor that occurs during cycling may prevent you from feeling warm or overheated, which also delays or masks the feeling that you need to drink.

Depending on your goals, as a road cyclist you may need to master drinking in a variety of situations—reaching with either hand; taking bottles from a jersey pocket, another rider, or a support vehicle; while braking, riding in a pack, climbing, riding in a pace line, or at a feed zone.

Some situations, such as mountain bike and cyclo-cross races, favor keeping your hands free. Use a bladder hydration system designed specifically for cyclists. From a safety standpoint, a bladder system is superior because your hand will be off the handlebars for only a split second while you grab the drinking tube. In organized rides, bladders allow you to carry a large volume of your preferred drink to meet your needs between supported rest stops. On rides in which you have access to water along the way, save weight by packing baggies of premeasured powdered sports drink.

Triathlons and multisport adventures Keeping a sleek aerodynamic bike on the road is challenging, especially in windy conditions. Because triathletes spend the largest portion of time in a race cycling, becoming proficient at drinking while on your bike is a priority. Be sure to practice at your intended race pace.

Multisport athletes who use water bottles need to keep them easily within reach—not buried at the bottom of a pack. A hands-free bladder system that is hardy (puncture resistant) and nonrestrictive may be an option.

Hiking and winter sports Although you may not feel thirsty when exercising in cold weather or may want to avoid making pit stops, hydration remains a priority. If using bottles, always keep them easily accessible—not buried at the bottom of your pack. A water-bottle carrier with insulated water bottles (fill with prewarmed drinks in cold weather, if feasible) or a bladder system that is insulated, lightweight, and nonrestrictive is an option. Keep in mind that tubes and valves in fluid-delivery systems designed for winter use can still freeze up in cold temperatures, so old-fashioned insulated water bottles are often the way to go if you expect extreme conditions.

Ski marathoners need to practice the following favored drinking technique. On a slight downhill (a flat section can work too if you can keep moving without using your arms), whip your bottle carrier around to the front, pull the bottle out, and tuck the pole on that side under your arm. The idea is to remain aerodynamic by drinking in a tucked position. Take advantage of your position in a racing pack. If you're in front, gliding and drinking helps prevent people from passing. If you're drafting off others in a pack, you can drink while being shielded from the wind and maintain your pace.

After the Event

Your job isn't quite finished when you cross the finish line. Be mindful of the carbohydrate window and jump-start the recovery process by rehydrating with a carbohydrate-rich beverage (or food) within 30 minutes of finishing. Aim for at least .5 grams of carbohydrate per pound (1.0 grams per kilogram) of body weight. Numerous options in liquid form are available if you don't feel like eating immediately after vigorous exercise: sports drinks (14 to 19 grams per cup, or per 250 milliliters), fruit juice (25 to 40 grams per cup), high-carbohydrate or meal replacement beverages (check the label, some provide as many as 50 grams per serving), milk or fruit smoothies made with milk (12 grams per cup), or nondiet soda (40 or more grams in a typical-sized can).

Jump-start the muscle-building and repair process by consuming, if possible, a small amount of protein (as found in some recovery drinks, energy bars, yogurt, and milk) within this same period. At the very least, include quality protein at your next meal—eggs, meat, poultry, fish, beans, dairy, or soy—within one to two hours of your finish. (See chapter 2, page 41 for review.)

Drinking alcohol following all-out efforts may impede your recovery by hampering your efforts to rehydrate (as a diuretic, alcohol causes your body to lose fluid) and by interfering with the ability of your body to replenish its glycogen stores. Your best bet is to make rehydrating with nonalcoholic beverages your first priority. Beyond that, realize that following an intense physical effort, your body may not be able to tolerate or process alcohol as well as it normally does, so indulge in moderation.

Jot down some notes about the sports drinks and foods that you used—what worked, what didn't, and what you want to try next time.

Learn From the Best: Competing in Shorter-Distance Triathlons

American Mark Fretta, a world-class triathlete, is a fast learner. He needed less than six years to reach the number-one spot on the International Triathlon Union world rankings. Read on as Fretta shares his winning nutritional tips for getting to the finish line as quickly as possible.

1. Listen to your body—it knows best. At one point, Fretta, like many endurance athletes, began drinking a recommended hydration product during races that had the supposedly ideal mix of protein (amino acids) and carbohydrate. Constantly hitting the wall earlier during the run leg of his triathlons, Fretta struggled to figure out the reason. After switching back to a drink with higher carbohydrate and sodium levels, he regained his energy level. He learned, albeit the hard way, that hydration drinks with protein can supply too little carbohydrate, especially on race day.

2. Practice, practice, practice. Even elite athletes had to start somewhere. Fretta admits that while he could ingest almost anything while swimming or cycling, running was a whole different story. He would feel sick at the smallest intake of anything solid or liquid during his runs. Rather than ignoring this crucial facet of racing triathlons, Fretta slowly began to eat and drink small amounts during his run workouts. Sticking with it, Fretta became accustomed to ingesting fluids and energy gels while running. He profits from improved endurance not only on race day but also during workouts.

3. Eat breakfast on the morning of the race. As recommended, Fretta always eats breakfast on race morning. Your body requires a lot of energy to race, and you want to capitalize on every opportunity that you can to top off your glycogen stores. Fretta generally eats the same thing before every race so that he knows what to expect. His choice includes a carbohydrate-rich energy bar, a raisin bagel, and perhaps a small bowl of oatmeal. He avoids meats (and high glycemic index foods like white bread and rice when racing in Asia) but will have a small piece of cheese for some protein. When traveling abroad, he tries to bring these foods with him or buy them when he first arrives.

4. Get in a groove. Boost your confidence and keep race-day jitters under control by establishing a pattern for eating before and during the race. First, experiment and hone your prerace meals. Pizza is Fretta's first choice for dinner the night before a race. Fretta recognizes that pizza is a great source of both carbohydrate and protein (cheese and meats) and maintains that it is also a comfort food. He has even gotten his U.S. national teammates to participate in this tradition when traveling together. Fretta relishes the camaraderie that they share, the fact that they eat a lot (without stuffing themselves), and the great race-day results that their prerace routine has produced. He aims to be done eating this meal at least 14 hours before the start of the race.

Shorter, high-intensity efforts increase the risk that stomach and intestinal problems will occur during the race. Having suffered from such distress in the past, Fretta now accepts this fact and plans accordingly on race morning. Because skipping breakfast isn't an option, he does whatever is required to be finished eating three hours before his race.

During the race, Fretta sets himself up by consuming one PowerGel on the first lap of the bike section of the race and then another one beginning on the last lap of the cycling section. He has figured out that this system, along with the carbohydrate drink that he consumes on the bike, is usually enough

(continued)

to get him through the run. He can then concentrate on running and reduce the chance of gastrointestinal trouble by relying on small amounts of water during the run.

5. Fretta offers three final nutritional strategies for triathletes of all ages and abilities:

- If you have leaned down for a race, you will always feel heavy going into a competition. Fretta insists that the best triathletes in the world all feel this way. That feeling is your body allowing its glycogen stores to fill before race day. If you eat normally and hydrate leading up to a race, your taper will make you feel this way. You may be unnerved, but reassure yourself that everything is going to plan.

- Hydration, especially for a race in hot weather, begins several days before race day. Don't try to catch up the morning of a race. This may lead to hyperhydration and literally cause you to race more slowly! Also, it doesn't matter how short the race is or that you're not among the leaders—you still need to drink during the race. If you sweat, you're losing fluid from your body. If you're losing fluid from your body, your blood volume is decreasing. As your blood volume decreases, your muscles don't receive optimal levels of energy, nutrients, and oxygen. Unless you drink something, you're going to slow down and waste even more time.

- Work hard to get in some calories on the bike. As Fretta knows, you benefit from this extra fuel during the cycling portion of the race as well as during the run. Opt for a hydration drink with carbohydrate or use energy gels, which are quick and easy to digest.

© Getty Images

Mark Fretta understands that success hinges on eating habits that are as well-developed as the muscles and the mind.

Long-Distance Events

10

Participating in endurance sports can be described as addictive. For some, a distance or endeavor that once seemed impossible, perhaps even unimaginable, to complete is now a routine activity that they insist they could almost do in their sleep. Seeking new challenges and conquests, physical or mental, you, too, may be intrigued to move up the endurance ladder and explore what happens as you are on the move for a longer time. Or perhaps, on a whim with friends or in a moment of foolishness, you signed up and told everyone that you're going for the big (in this case, long) one this time—the marathon (26.2 miles, or 42 kilometers), Torture 10,000 (10,000 feet, or 3,000 meters, of climbing in 100 miles, or 160 kilometers, of cycling), or some other "see you in a few to several hours at the finish line" escapade that you or someone else has dared to dream up.

Whatever your goal, either competing in or simply surviving a long-distance endurance adventure or race, you'll need to master drinking while on the move, and most likely eating too. Otherwise, the time that you're out there can pass all too quickly (if you're forced to drop out or stop before you've attained your goal), or it will seem that the end will never, ever come (if you're reduced to a slow, painful I'm-never-doing-this-again crawl).

"I didn't think I was going to make the team. I felt great until about 22 miles. Then I started to feel depleted, and as a veteran of the sport I knew exactly what was happening to me: I was running out of energy. With 3 miles to go I was just hoping that the finish line would come, because I knew it was going to be the longest 3 miles of my career, and it surely was."

—Deena Kastor, prohibitive race favorite entering the U.S. Women's Marathon Trials, holding on to qualify for the Olympic Games, where she went on to win a bronze medal

This chapter is for endurance athletes who choose to move up in distance or for those striving to set a new PR in long-distance endurance events and races,* such as the following:

Running: half marathon and marathon races, trail-running adventures or races taking 2 to several hours to complete, relay races of up to a day long with teams of two or more people

Duathlon or triathlon: long-course events, half Ironmans

Cycling: metric century/century rides especially if hilly; double century rides, road time trials and races lasting 3 to 4 hours or longer ; mountain bike races lasting 3 hours or longer; or 24-hour races with teams of two or more people

Multisport or adventure racing: off-road triathlons and other multisport races lasting 2 hours or longer, 4- to 8-hour multisport recreational adventures, half- to full-day adventure races, solo efforts in shorter multisport races

Hiking or trekking: 4- to 8-hour continuous hikes, treks, or ascents

Winter sports: half- to full-day snowshoeing outings, backcountry ski outings, or marathon ski races such as the Birkebeiner

There is no substitute for putting in the distance or hours of training required to prepare physically, as well as mentally, to succeed at these long-distance challenges. At the same time, you must also prepare your gastrointestinal tract to absorb and digest fluids and fuel during exercise. In other words, it's not enough to know how to run, bike, cycle, ski, or climb. Long-distance endurance endeavors require that you master drinking and refueling while on the move to avoid being forced to slow down (or even drop out) because of dehydration, glycogen depletion, or bonking. You must train your brain so that you drink and eat when you have no appetite, under unpleasant conditions, when things are going well (why bother, what could go wrong?), and when they're not (when stomach distress hits you, for example).

There are no shortcuts. Progress comes only from practicing (including trial and error) to determine which fluids, foods, and equipment work best for you and what techniques you need to master to get the job done. Your job is to research and determine beforehand if (and what) fluids and foods will be provided along the course. Self-supported challenges mean that you alone are responsible for the logistics of meeting your fluid and energy needs. Adventures and races involving friends and teammates add an additional layer of commitment. All team members must take seriously the responsibility to hydrate and fuel themselves. In other words, pick your teammates and adventure partners wisely.

Note: Keep in mind that this designation is somewhat arbitrary in terms of times and distances because time of physical exertion in endurance events and races depends on your fitness level and experience—what might be a moderately long effort for a seasoned competitor or extremely fit outdoors enthusiast could be a day-long endeavor for a recreational athlete or fitness-minded exerciser.

Carbohydrate loading before long-distance events and races is another invaluable tool that long-distance endurance athletes need to explore and practice. Some athletes might also need to experiment with using glycerol, caffeine, or electrolyte (salt) tablets during prolonged exercise. (See chapter 5 for review because the strategies require experimentation in training long before the event or race day.) For many endurance athletes, long-distance events and races also serve as training bouts or stepping-stones for ultradistance challenges and thus provide excellent opportunities to practice and hone refueling strategies.

Despite the long distances involved, the reality remains that some active people and athletes don't manage to accomplish the recommended hours or miles of training and thus undertake athletic challenges that exercise scientists would categorize as being beyond what they have physiologically prepared for. In this case, paying attention to your nutritional needs before and during the event or race is critical to your ability to enjoy yourself and finish (and avoid becoming sick or injured). Being underprepared, coupled with making poor decisions about fluid and fuel needs during long-distance events or races, is disastrous and can even endanger your life.

Preevent Nutrition Game Plan

Your job beforehand is to respect the nutritional aspect of long-distance endurance endeavors and eat in a way that sets you up to be physically ready and mentally prepared for the challenge that lies ahead. In simple language, you must start a long-distance race or event well hydrated and well fueled. If you've trained properly and eat a normal diet the few days before the race or event, you can expect to store roughly 2,000 calories of glycogen (between your muscles and liver), or enough fuel for approximately 90 to 120 minutes of vigorous activity (or a few hours at moderate intensity or pace).

Because working muscles rely heavily on carbohydrate as fuel during these distance endeavors, as well as on the efficient breakdown of fat (which depends in part on the body's having sufficient carbohydrate available; see chapter 2 to review), enhancing or boosting your glycogen stores by carbohydrate loading makes sense. This practice reduces the chance that you will deplete your muscle glycogen stores and hit the wall before you reach the finish line.

Keep in mind that carbohydrate loading does not require eating enormous quantities of food, nor does it mean loading up on high-fat foods. To enter the race or event feeling fresh and well rested, you'll want to taper your training as the day of the event approaches. You'll be expending less energy (calories) in training, so you don't need to eat hundreds of extra calories to boost your carbohydrate intake. Rather, concentrate on increasing the percentage of your calories that comes from carbohydrate-rich foods. Some athletes find it easiest simply to add a serving or two of a high-carbohydrate beverage (see chapter 5).

Because you'll be relying on your body to perform *and* get you back home or to the finish line safely, you also need to know how to avoid bonking (hypoglycemia, or a too-low blood sugar level) and hyponatremia (low blood sodium level) when competing in long-distance events and races. Part of this is knowing what measures to take beforehand to reduce your risk (see chapter 14 for an in-depth review of hyponatremia).

Last, endurance athletes must be aware of the risks of using nonsteroidal anti-inflammatory drugs (NSAIDs, such as ibuprofen and naproxen sodium) during long-distance races or events. Combined with dehydration, taking NSAIDs during prolonged exercise can increase your risk of kidney problems as well as predispose you to hyponatremia. You'll need to pay particular attention to your fluid intake before and during the event or race if you choose to take NSAIDs.

A Few Days to the Week Before the Event

The main goal is to carboload. Ideally, you have found a carbohydrate-loading routine that works for you by experimenting before long training efforts. Understandably, depending on your performance goals and the time of year (or where you are in your season), you may not be able to taper your training fully before every long-distance race or event that you undertake. Boosting carbohydrate intake, however, is helpful, and it becomes more and more essential as you ask your body to perform vigorously past 90 minutes.

As long as you fill up on carbohydrates and not fat, don't be alarmed if you feel bloated or gain a couple of pounds in the days leading up to your event or race. Your body stores a considerable amount of water as it stows away carbohydrate as muscle glycogen. This extra water will help delay dehydration during the event or race.

Drink plenty of familiar (well-tolerated) beverages such as water, fruit juice, sports drinks, and milk with your meals and snacks. Having beverages along with foods helps your body hold on to the fluid longer. To avoid increasing your risk for hyponatremia, avoid the urge to drink too much plain water, especially during the day and evening before the event. Monitor your urine color. It should be pale yellow, not clear like water.

To decrease your risk of hyponatremia further, maintain or increase your intake of salt leading up to events and races in which you'll be continuously on the move for three to four hours (at moderate to high intensity) or longer, particularly if you'll be competing in hot or humid weather or if the conditions will be warmer than those that you normally train in. Add table salt to foods or eat your favorite salty foods, like soup, tomato juice, canned vegetables and chili, pretzels, and pickles.

Female endurance athletes, those at the back of the pack (a slower pace often means more opportunities to drink and thus overhydrate), undertrained athletes (more sodium loss through sweating), athletes troubled with cramping, and those not acclimated to the heat need to be particularly mindful of getting adequate sodium. If you've had problems with hyponatremia or dealing with the heat in the past or have a health problem like high blood pressure, speak with your physician before taking salt (or electrolyte) tablets in the days leading up to (or during) a long-distance event or race.

If the event or race involves travel and meals eaten away from home, be sure to take with you any special or favorite food items that you simply can't do without. Make smart food choices a priority on travel days because all-day travel and eating poorly is a double whammy that can wipe out the fittest athlete. Be prepared by bringing foods that travel well and by stocking up on energy bars and powdered meal replacement products. Consider using a high-carbohydrate beverage or meal replacement product to supplement your carbohydrate needs if time-zone changes or your travel schedule will interfere with your regular eating habits. As much as you can control it, don't try new foods or change your eating habits in the week leading up to a long-distance event or race.

Review your nutrition game plan for the day of the event or race. Early in the week, make sure that you have enough of all nutrition essentials that you plan to consume during the event or race, such as sports drinks, energy gels and bars, and, if appropriate, foods and electrolyte (salt) tablets that have previously passed the test in training. Double-check that any equipment that you plan to use, such as hip packs or bum bags, bladder hydration systems, and gel flasks, is in good working order. Gather and prepare your sports foods and equipment (as well as a recovery drink or bar and food for afterward) no later than the night before. If feasible, fill drink bottles (or another hydration system) the night before so that you can just grab them in the morning (and so that during warm weather you can freeze bottles beforehand).

Preevent Dinner

When it comes to eating the night before a long-distance event or race, rest assured that no magical or preferred prerace dinner exists. The only rule is to stick with familiar foods that you enjoy. This is not the time to be adventurous because you want to avoid making late-night trips to the bathroom. Although you most likely know to feature carbohydrate-rich foods like pasta, rice, and potatoes, keep in mind that endurance athletes have competed successfully after eating all kinds of foods, including pizza, steak, and Mexican food! (For carbohydrate-rich meal ideas, refer back to table 4.2.)

Stuffing yourself with carbohydrate isn't necessary at this time! In other words, don't feel obligated to get your money's worth at the traditional prerace pasta feed. (Serious competitors, in fact, may do well to avoid eating in public places with crowds.) Don't be afraid to include reasonably sized portions of meat or other protein-rich foods as well as some fat at this meal, because these foods have staying power and can help you sleep through the night. Most athletes do fine having a glass of wine or a beer if it's part of their regular routine. Eat at a reasonable time for you, consume appropriate-sized portions, and know that eating again before bedtime (for example, a carbohydrate-rich snack such as milk and cereal or an energy bar) is more productive than stuffing yourself now.

Some athletes become consumed with having the "perfect" prerace meal or eating exactly the same thing each time. Keep your stress level in check by becoming comfortable with a variety of foods or meals, especially if you travel to races and events, otherwise you waste precious mental energy that compromises your performance. The goal is to stay flexible and eat as many different foods as you can. If you firmly believe that certain foods will enhance your performance, by all means, eat them!

Finally, remind yourself that your success the next day hinges on numerous factors and that this "last supper" is only one of them. Focus your mental energy on how you will be fueling yourself *during* the event or race. What you do (or don't do) the next day, when you're on the move for a few to several hours, has a much greater effect on your stamina, your endurance, and the ultimate outcome than worrying about eating the perfect foods the night before.

Continue to drink plenty of familiar (well-tolerated) fluids, but don't overdo it by drinking bottle after bottle of plain water or other sodium-free beverages.

Morning of the Event

Plan to eat a high-carbohydrate breakfast a few hours before the start of your event or race, especially for a late-morning or midday start. Although you may be able to skip breakfast and do well in shorter-range events and races, the odds aren't in your favor as you move up in distance. If you don't eat breakfast, how many waking hours, as well as total hours, will have passed since you last ate? What will happen if the start is delayed?

Eating breakfast helps settle your stomach and ward off hunger pangs as you wait for the race to begin. (Many athletes find that they feel satisfied longer by eating earlier and including higher-fat foods like peanut butter or cheese.) More important, eating breakfast refills your liver glycogen stores (which can be almost gone by morning), which are critical for maintaining a stable blood sugar level during prolonged exercise. These carbohydrate reserves will help power hardworking muscles and fuel your brain so that you can make wise decisions while on the move. If you're simply too nervous to eat the morning of the event or race, drink your breakfast in the form of a breakfast shake or meal replacement product. (As a last resort, eat a substantial late-night snack before going to bed.) No concrete recommendations exist, but most people do well by consuming .5 grams of carbohydrate per pound (1 gram per kilogram) of body weight if they eat one hour before the event (for example, consuming a canned liquid meal or energy bar that provides 100 to 300 calories), or up to 2 grams of carbohydrate per pound four hours before (for example, eating a substantial breakfast that will "hold you").

Keep in mind that liquid foods clear the stomach faster than solid foods do. If coffee or tea is part of your usual preexercise routine, go with it. Most athletes do best sticking with what they know (and ideally have confirmed by experimenting before long training efforts). If in doubt, leave it out.

Continue to hydrate with plenty of water or a familiar sports drink up to two hours before the start. Doing so will give you time to urinate any excess. Five to 15 minutes before the start, drink another cup of water or a sports drink. For athletes who consume an energy gel before the start of a prolonged endeavor, this is also the time (as close to the actual time of the start of the activity) to consume a packet with a few gulps of water.

Before you leave home or for the race, double-check that you have all your nutrition essentials: sports foods, equipment (bottle carriers, bladders, and so on), and recovery foods and beverages for afterward. Set up any transition areas or refueling stations as permitted and make certain that every person who needs to be familiar with the nutrition game plan (teammates, friends, support crew) knows this information.

During the Event

Your job throughout your long-distance event or race is to assess and monitor your fluid, carbohydrate, and electrolyte needs. In other words, give your body what it needs so that your most important piece of equipment, your body, doesn't prematurely limit you or knock you totally out of the race. The general guidelines listed in the following sections are a consensus of scientifically supported recommendations made by credible sports nutrition and exercise science experts, including the American College of Sports Medicine, the American Dietetic Association, and the Australian Institute of Sport.

Fluid

- Drink early and often: Take in 2 to 8 ounces (60 to 250 milliliters) every 15 to 20 minutes of prolonged exercise, starting immediately from the onset (fluid needs are highly individual, depend on a variety of factors, and are best determined in training efforts beforehand).

- Do not rely solely on plain water throughout an entire long-distance event or race.

- Properly formulated sports (electrolyte replacement) drinks are the easiest way to meet fluid and energy (carbohydrate) needs simultaneously. Soda or fruit juice may be an option depending on the activity, the athlete's intensity level, and availability.

- Exercisers and athletes must drink to match their fluid losses to avoid potentially dangerous situations—underhydration leads to dehydration (which increases the risk of heat illness) and overhydration leads to hyponatremia.

- Glycerol users must still replace fluid losses as much as possible by drinking water and fluid replacement drinks throughout the event or race.

- Despite not feeling as thirsty in cold-weather adventures and races or wanting to avoid making stops for bathroom breaks, athletes must keep hydration a priority.

Fuel

- Consuming supplemental carbohydrate during prolonged vigorous exercise lasting longer than 90 continuous minutes preserves glycogen stores and allows the athlete to extend the distance traveled at the desired pace.

- The general recommendation is to consume 25 to 60 grams of carbohydrate (100 to 250 calories from carbohydrate) per hour of activity after the first hour.
- Meet carbohydrate needs with properly formulated sports drinks, energy gels, and other easily digested, well-absorbed, and well-tolerated carbohydrate sources (glucose tablets, sport chews, candy, soda) as well as with well-tolerated solid forms such as energy bars and other carbohydrate-rich foods.
- Waiting too long to refuel, which increases the likelihood that dehydration will occur, adds to the risk of experiencing gastrointestinal problems (cramping, vomiting, diarrhea).

Electrolytes

- Being mindful of sodium intake before prolonged exercise lasting longer than three or four continuous hours, matching fluid intake (drinking) to fluid losses (sweating and urination) during exercise, and consuming a properly formulated sports drink that includes sodium will be adequate to prevent hyponatremia in most exercisers and athletes.
- Female endurance athletes, those at the back of the pack, undertrained athletes, athletes who have troubles with cramping, and those not acclimated to the heat or who have experienced difficulties dealing with the heat in the past are at higher risk of developing hyponatremia during or following prolonged exercise.
- Some people will benefit from ingesting or will require additional sodium during prolonged exercise (for example, table salt, salty beverages and foods, salt tablets).
- Use caution when consuming electrolyte (salt) tablets because stomach distress, vomiting, and diarrhea can occur if you use electrolyte tablets improperly (take them with too little fluid) or take them in a dehydrated state (no firm guidelines exist, so you must experiment to determine your individual needs).
- Consider weight gain during prolonged exercise as a warning sign that you are overconsuming fluid, thereby increasing the risk of hyponatremia.

Sport-Specific Tips

Every sport discipline presents unique challenges for hydrating and refueling while on the move. Watch and learn from experienced veterans and practice at every opportunity. Being foolish or lazy about nutritional needs during a race undermines, and can even negate, your prerace hard work and preparation.

Runners

Water stations in marathons are akin to pit stops in auto racing. Don't even think about bypassing them, especially the early stations. Your running pace will determine which water stops to key on, because you need to drink water or a sports drink every 15 to 20 minutes (aim for 2 to 8 ounces depending on your individual needs). Don't wait until you feel thirsty—once you're dehydrated, you won't catch up. Don't be afraid to drink plain water, but don't rely solely on it throughout the entire race. Sports drinks are undoubtedly the easiest way to meet fluid, carbohydrate, and electrolyte needs simultaneously.

Drink the water offered along the course; don't pour it over your head. Although a quick dousing may temporarily cool you off, pouring water over your head instead of drinking it doesn't make sense. Would you drive your overheated car to the gas station, pull up to the water hose, open the hood of the car, and then spray the water on the overheated engine?

Go with gels. Easy to ingest while running, energy gels are best taken with 4 to 6 ounces of water (not a sports drink) to reduce the risk of stomach upset. Plan to ingest a packet right before an aid station where water is available. Most gels supply 20 to 25 grams of carbohydrate (80 to 100 calories) per packet. If you plan on carrying more than one energy gel packet with you, use one of the convenient palm-sized flasks that clip to the waistband of your running shorts. These refillable flasks can carry and dispense as you desire it up to five servings (packets) or more of gel. Runners who plan to take longer than four to five hours to complete a marathon may consider wearing a waist pack instead to tote energy gels or other well-tolerated solid foods, such as energy bars.

If you're fast enough that you've earned the privilege of picking up water bottles at aid stations designated for elite marathoners, use your imagination and decorate your bottles. You want them to be easy to spot and easy to grab. Don't panic if a bottle is not where you planned it to be. Slow down slightly to try to spot it, but don't waste too much time. Remind yourself that you can get plenty of water or sports drinks along the course. Start grabbing cups of fluid immediately and slow down if necessary to be sure that you consume enough.

During off-road events, set your watch and drink on a preplanned schedule, every 15 to 20 minutes. You may forget to drink in trail races because varying terrain and extreme weather conditions can cause time to pass differently. If you're familiar with what's coming up, planning is easier. If you're a novice or the course is new to you, ask experienced runners. If you find yourself not drinking enough when using a bladder system or a traditional waist-belt bottle carrier, switch to a hand-held bottle carrier.

Don't underestimate your energy needs during self-supported adventures and races. If aid stations are limited or don't exist, prepare and place drop bags beforehand or enlist the help of family, friends, or teammates to resupply you along the way. (If you're on your own during longer training efforts, plan a loop course that brings you past a central resupply point.)

Cyclists and Mountain Bikers

Keep your thinking cap on. As a cyclist, you walk a finer line than most endurance athletes do when it comes to staying on top of your nutritional needs during exercise. Your fluid and energy needs are some of the highest among endurance athletes because of the distance and duration of endurance cycling events. Despite knowing that, cyclists often find themselves caught off guard. Bonking, the depletion of muscle glycogen stores that causes you to slow your pace dramatically, is a prime example.

Keep in mind that rapid evaporation of sweat can give you the false sense that you're losing only minimal amounts of fluid. The windchill factor that occurs during cycling may prevent you from feeling warm or overheated, which can delay or mask the feeling that you need to drink. On top of that, your body weight is supported while cycling, so you don't receive any feedback from ankles or legs being traumatized by pounding. Drafting and coasting allow you to continue to perform at a good pace. In other words, you can easily ignore or underestimate your nutritional needs because you won't feel poorly until it's too late. Anticipate your needs and adhere to a plan.

Be realistic about your fluid losses (urine and sweat) and your fluid intake while on the bike. Ingesting 16 to 20 ounces of fluid per hour during prolonged riding is reasonable for most cyclists under normal conditions. Riding in extreme conditions, such as heat and wind or high humidity, further increases your fluid needs. Your stomach should cooperate and be able to tolerate up to a quart (32 ounces for male riders, less for smaller females) an hour, so aim for two small or one and a half large bottles per hour in extreme conditions. If drinking colder liquids doesn't make you nauseous (because of delayed emptying from the stomach), it can help cool you down and provide a needed boost on a ride in extreme conditions. (Add ice to bottles or freeze half a bottle of water or sports drink the night before and top it off immediately before you get on the bike.)

Keep up with your energy needs while on the bike. Continuously replenish the carbohydrate that you burn. By topping off liver and muscle glycogen stores and eating breakfast, most riders can perform well for the first one and a half to two hours of cycling (for example, the first 30 miles, or 48 kilometers, of a century ride), relying only on an electrolyte replacement drink. If you expect to cycle longer than two hours, plan to refuel while on the bike. To extend your glycogen stores, begin to eat as soon as the event or race starts. Don't wait until you bonk or until your blood sugar bottoms out to try to remedy the situation.

Your calorie needs will vary tremendously depending on a multitude of variables, such as road surface, terrain, weather, wind resistance, speed or intensity, and your fitness level. Figure on about 30 calories per mile (~19 calories per kilometer) as a rule. Keep in mind that your estimated calorie needs increase dramatically as your speed increases (see table 10.1).

Road races Depending on the distance and specifics of each race, you may still be carrying most of your own food (in jersey pockets) and drink. In longer

Table 10.1 Estimated Energy Cost of Road Cycling

Average speed (miles per hour)	Estimated calories (per kg of body weight) needed per hour while riding	For 50 kg (110 lb) cyclist	For 60 kg (132 lb) cyclist	For 70 kg (154 lb) cyclist	For 80 kg (176 lb) cyclist	For 85 kg (187 lb) cyclist
12	5.6	280	336	392	448	476
13	6.2	310	372	434	496	527
14	6.8	340	408	476	544	578
15	7.4	370	444	518	592	629
16	8.1	405	486	567	648	689
17	8.9	445	534	623	712	757
18	9.8	490	588	686	784	833
19	10.7	535	642	749	856	909
20	11.8	590	708	826	944	1003
21	12.9	645	774	903	1032	1097
23	15.5	775	930	1085	1240	1318

Notes: Weight in kilograms = weight in pounds divided by 2.2.

Select your average speed over the duration of the *entire* ride (do not calculate average speed based solely on riding downhill, riding uphill, or riding with a tailwind). Example: 70 kilogram rider who averages 18 miles per hour and completes a century ride in 5.5 hours would require about 3,773 calories or 650 to 700 calories an hour (9.8 cal/kg/hr × 70 kg × 5.5 hours = 3, 773 calories divided by 5.5 hours = 686 calories per hour).

Adapted from http://www.ultracycling.com/nutritional/calories.html.

pro-amateur races (lasting four hours or longer), racers often have food and water distributed to them as they roll through designated feed zones on the side of the road.

Stay with foods that you are used to eating as much as possible. Eat after cresting a hill, not shortly before a substantial climb or while climbing. Eat when you're at the end of a pace line, not in the middle or while pulling.

Sports drinks remain the best choice to meet fluid needs, because they do triple duty by meeting fluid, carbohydrate, and electrolyte needs. If you find that the sweet taste deters you from drinking enough during extended races, carry an extra bottle of plain water and drink alternately from it or use energy gels (begin with one packet taken with a few gulps of water about every 30 to 45 minutes).

Organized and self-supported rides   Wearing a bladder hydration system allows you to carry a large volume of fluid without worrying about the need to stop and possibly lose your group. Be sure to choose a model designed specifically for cyclists.

Always carry something with you, such as prepackaged powdered drink mix and a snack (for example, energy bars or a peanut butter sandwich), in case you don't like what is offered at rest stops or need to refuel before or after a scheduled rest stop. What you take with you will determine how you carry it—jersey pocket, backpack, or taped to your bike.

Eating on the bike becomes even more of a necessity if you are a slower rider because of the longer time that you spend riding.

Stopping to enjoy a real lunch break can provide a psychological boost; just don't gorge yourself because doing so will divert blood away from working muscles to your gastrointestinal tract. (Organized rides often have a boxed lunch that you can buy beforehand.) Save your big meal for the end of the ride.

Recreational riders may choose to stop and eat at organized rest stops provided during century rides and other daylong events. Foods typically provided include fruit (often apples, oranges, and bananas), energy bars, energy gels, granola bars, bagels, peanut butter sandwiches, cookies, and mini candy bars. During longer rides, you might find potatoes, sandwich fixings, and ice cream bars.

Experienced professional endurance racers suggest this no-fail formula for a 150- to 160-pound (68- to 73-kilogram) cyclist who is attempting to finish a hilly century ride in approximately five hours: Start with a Camelbak full of water, one bottle of electrolyte replacement drink, and one bottle of a high-calorie drink, like Spiz (500 calories in 16 to 20 ounces). Carry baggies containing premeasured powder and refill your bottles at every rest stop or along the way as needed. Consume 500 calories or one bottle of your high-energy drink per hour religiously right from the start.

Mountain bike rides and races Set up a drinking schedule and stick to it. Keep it simple. Because you can easily lose track of time when you're undertaking a serious personal effort, especially when it involves traversing challenging terrain and negotiating descents, set your watch to remind you to drink every 15 minutes. Take advantage of any opportunity that you have to down a few sips. For example, drink during easy ascents, when you tend to sit more upright and can more easily steady the bike with one hand.

Depending on the length of the ride or race and the available support, carry extra sports drink powder with you in premeasured amounts. Spend the time to stop and mix up more as needed. Establish good habits now before you venture into ultralength rides. For example, develop a feel for where your water bottle is on your bike so that you don't have to take your eyes off the trail when you reach for it.

Keep your hands free by using a bladder hydration system. From a safety standpoint, a bladder system is superior because your hand will be off the handlebars for only a split second while you grab the drinking tube. Clean your bladder system promptly if you put a drink containing carbohydrate into it. These drinks promote the growth of bacteria and mold, especially in hot weather. To avoid having to do time-consuming cleanups, put only water in the bladder and make the sports drink in your bottles two or three times more concentrated. Then alternate drinking between the two.

Fuel up on real food. Over the long haul, real food is more fulfilling than energy bars and gels. Supplement the calories in your electrolyte replacement drink by eating easy-to-carry finger foods (toss in your jersey pockets) that go down easily, such as raisins, grapes, small baked potatoes (eaten cold), and fig bars. Stick with foods that have worked for you on training rides. In longer races, in which you rely primarily on liquid calories from concentrated drinks, snack on real food for a psychological boost.

In 24-hour mountain bike racing, make food an important part of the experience. Get together with your teammates, figure out what everyone wants, and then shop for it together. On the bike, rely on a sports drink and water. Off the bike, refuel with real food. The key to a strong finish is to drink a recovery beverage (for example, a high-carbohydrate or meal replacement product) immediately after completing each leg to restock your glycogen stores. Follow up with a small meal within an hour.

Triathletes

During a long-distance triathlon, aim to replace at least 30 to 50 percent of the calories that you expend, which for most triathletes translates into a starting point of 200 to 300 calories per hour (some elite athletes can train themselves to absorb more). Most of these calories (70 to 75 percent) should come from carbohydrate—sports drinks, energy gels and bars, and other solid foods that are well tolerated. Consuming items that provide small amounts of protein and fat during half Ironmans can also help sustain you over the long haul.

Swim Because urinating isn't a problem on this segment, hydrate right up to the start of the race. In ocean swims, you'll inevitably swallow some salt water, so be prepared for a burning sensation in your throat. If you swallow enough salt water, your tongue will swell and you may begin the bike ride feeling sick to your stomach. Some triathletes even suffer from seasickness during choppy open-water swims. The best plan of attack is to wear earplugs to combat nausea and know how to breathe bilaterally to minimize the effects of a choppy sea.

Bike Become one with your bike. Triathletes spend the largest portion of time in a race on the bike, so you need to be proficient at eating and drinking on your bike at your intended race pace. During a race, control or slow your pace slightly when you are ready to rehydrate and refuel. Keeping a sleek aerodynamic bike on the road can be challenging as you juggle food and water bottles, especially in windy conditions. If stomach problems have hindered you during the run in previous races, review what you do on the bike. Try backing off from eating during the last half hour on the bike and don't overload your stomach by trying to do everything—gels, bars, and higher-calorie sports drinks that contain protein.This last suggestion is especially relevant to female triathletes.

Run Gastrointestinal distress, such as nausea and bloating, can be common during the running segment. The jostling nature of running and the progressive dehydration associated with several hours of continuous exercise slow the absorption of fluid and nutrients from the stomach. Recognize that an inability to urinate during the running segment is a red flag indicating that you've become too dehydrated. Slow or stop when you approach aid stations to ensure that you consume some fluid and aren't just pouring it on yourself or the ground.

If vomiting ensues during the run, think of it as wiping the slate clean. Slow or stop, regroup, and start over with your rehydrating and refueling efforts. An episode of vomiting is definitely a temporary setback, but you can rebound after you start to absorb the fluid and calories that you need. Sometimes chewing solid food, such as an energy bar or a banana, can help settle a queasy stomach and provide a much-needed mental lift. Some athletes find that chewing on a calcium tablet helps.

Transitions   Relax and take your time as you make the transitions both onto the bike and into the run. Set up your transition area in a logical, organized manner so that you can't possibly exit the transition area without your nutrition essentials. For example, if you're wearing a bike jersey or sport pack to carry food while on the bike, put it on top of your unbuckled helmet or across your bike seat. Obviously, you should prepare bike jerseys and packs beforehand, as well as any bike food holders, such as bento boxes and gel flasks, that you need during the race.

Always keep an extra water bottle handy in the transition area to drink from as you head out on the run. Take advantage of your slower pace as you make the transition into running by using it as an opportunity to refuel. As mentioned before, you may feel better by getting fuel in at the start of the run (for example, by drinking a sports drink) than by cramming food down during the latter stages of the bike portion. (To simulate race conditions, practice your transitions by racing against a friend during training.)

Marathon Skiers

Drink early in ski marathon races, ideally within the first 15 minutes. Choose an electrolyte replacement drink to meet your fluid and carbohydrate needs. You may not feel as thirsty while competing in cold weather or you may want to avoid making pit stops, but keeping on top of your fluid needs remains a priority.

Advances in technology have produced bladder hydration systems with tubes and valves that are less likely to freeze up in cold temperatures, but these systems aren't foolproof. If you've experienced problems before or expect extreme temperatures, wear a water-bottle carrier (with an insulated 16-ounce, or 500-milliliter, water bottle or larger) strapped around your waist instead.

Refuel at every feed station. Cross-country skiing uses the entire muscle mass of the body, so your energy needs are extremely high. You can generally expect a feed every 10 to 15 kilometers in most ski marathon races. Be prepared to slow down to obtain a cup of fluid because volunteers may not be trained to deliver feeds by running alongside you. Save the sports drink that you are toting for between feeds and during rough patches when you need an energy boost. Slower skiers may need to stop and refill their bottles at feed stations or wear a bladder system that allows them to carry more fluid. Foods typically available at feeding stations are sports drinks (water too), hot chocolate, soup, orange slices, energy bars and gels, cookies, and brownies.

Carry energy gels as backup fuel. Store energy gels in a water-bottle carrier that has small pockets or tape a packet to the front of your jersey or the inside of your arm (on top of your jersey). Choose a place on your body that you can easily reach. Consuming energy gels with water is best, so time your intake with a feeding station.

Be aware of the symptoms of bonking. You may feel unusually cold and experience shivering, or you may simply run out of energy. Two warning signs that trouble is just around the corner are experiencing hunger pangs and having overwhelming negative thoughts. Recognize that your brain needs fuel immediately. Consume carbohydrate-rich drinks and foods as soon as possible and pay attention to your hydration and fuel needs for the rest of the race. Two situations that may boost your normal energy needs are hilly courses and extreme weather.

Adventure Races and Off-Road Multisport Adventures

Know where your next drink is coming from. Whether it's an off-road multisport adventure or a one-day adventure "sprint," adequate fluid intake is paramount for survival and success. Try bladders, waist belts, or water-bottle holsters that attach to the daisy chains on the front of a pack's shoulder strap. Keep in mind the ruggedness of the terrain. A bladder system that becomes punctured won't be of much use.

In single-day races, determine how frequently you will pass through staging areas, which in turn will determine how much fluid you need to carry with you on each leg. Figure on a minimum of one water bottle (20 ounces) per person per hour, depending on the activity and the weather. (In self-supported situations, always use iodine tablets or other safety measures to purify water found along the way.)

Drink a sports drink in addition to plain water. The electrolytes that these drinks contain will help prevent muscle cramps and hyponatremia and will stimulate you to keep drinking. The carbohydrate provided by sports drinks will fuel your brain as well as your muscles. This attribute is a definite advantage when adventures and races hinge on navigation skills or your ability to decipher mysterious or special tests throughout the race.

Don't wait until you feel thirsty to drink. Watch for the telltale signs of dehydration: headache, nausea, loss of appetite, personality change (stops bantering or answering questions), infrequent urination (dark color), clumsiness, lack of energy, and inability to tolerate heat or cold. Dehydration increases your risk for heat exhaustion, heat stroke, and hypothermia, all of which can prevent you (and your group or team) from finishing, especially during longer ventures. Stop before dehydration progresses too far. In severe cases, stop, seek shade, and try to rehydrate by sipping small amounts of water or other fluids as tolerated.

Have a plan for refueling. Lack of appetite is the norm during daylong adventures and races. Just because you're hot, sweaty, dehydrated, fatigued, sleep deprived, covered with mud, possibly well off course, and don't feel the least bit hungry, you still must replenish your limited glycogen stores. In single-day ventures, sports drinks, energy gels and bars, and any other carbohydrate-rich foods (bananas, fig bars, breakfast and granola bars, Pop Tarts, bagels, sandwiches, and so on) that you find appealing and have access to should do the trick.

Other Nutrition Truths for Endurance Athletes

You are responsible for experimenting in training (before the actual event or race) to discover and build a repertoire of acceptable foods and drinks, and any other supplements, that you will use to meet your fluid, energy, and electrolyte needs during long-distance events and races. You must figure out the basics—what and how much you need to eat and drink and when you need to eat and drink it. Don't neglect to put your strategies to the test in various weather conditions at your intended race pace or intensity.

- The only way that drinking and eating on the move become automatic on the day of the event or race is by practicing beforehand. Aim to be consistent and stick with what you know. When your favorite or old standby is no longer working, however, you must be willing to try something new. If you're contemplating tackling ultralength challenges, you first need to establish smart drinking and refueling habits in long-distance events and races.

- Consider how your body processes foods during exercise. Blood flow to the gastrointestinal tract falls as your pace or intensity increases, making it harder to digest and absorb foods that you take in. In addition, your ability to consume and absorb calories when running (because of significant jostling of the stomach) is far less (by as much as 50 percent) than when cycling. Rely on simple carbohydrates during high-intensity (closer to your $\dot{V}O_2$max) efforts or when you need a rapid energy boost. Choose electrolyte replacement drinks, energy gels (take with water) and sport chews, glucose tablets, and if tolerated, soda or juice. During longer efforts of moderate intensity, add solid foods and high-calorie liquid drinks to boost your calorie intake and your spirits.

- Refuel frequently instead of eating a large quantity at any one time, which diverts blood away from your working muscles. In other words, spread your hourly energy needs over 15- to 20-minute increments. Don't try to cram it all down on the hour mark. The best sports drinks, high-calorie liquid drinks, energy gels, and energy bars for you are the ones that go down and stay down.

- Hitting the wall means that you have essentially depleted your muscle glycogen stores. Your legs (and other major muscle groups) have gone on strike, even though you may have been consuming adequate fluids and calories. Your training, or lack thereof, improper pacing, and general fatigue can contribute to this phenomenon. You will often be able to continue and finish, albeit not with the desired performance.

- Bonking, when the body completely shuts down because of a severe drop in blood sugar, is a much more serious situation. The glycogen stored in muscles and the liver is essentially gone. Muscles and, more important, the brain are not receiving sufficient fuel. If left untreated, you may become increasingly irritable, confused, and disoriented. You could find yourself sitting or lying down and could possibly lapse into a coma. Stop whatever activity you were engaged in and boost your blood sugar by consuming readily absorbable carbohydrates, such as sports drinks, energy gels, soda, fruit juice, or glucose tablets, if available. Seek or ask for medical attention if necessary.

- The best way to avoid bonking is to create a calorie buffer. Liquid calories in the form of electrolyte replacement drinks and high-energy liquid products are favored because they tend to be well tolerated and require less effort to get down than solid foods do. Large male endurance athletes often have to consciously work to consume enough calories (for example, as much as 500 calories per hour of prolonged cycling as compared to 300 calories per hour for smaller female athletes) to stay in energy balance.

- Athletes who struggle with sensitive stomachs and other gastrointestinal problems are advised to learn beforehand what sports drink will be served during races and organized events. They can then train with that product or, if they will have access to water, carry their own acceptable powdered sports drink in premeasured baggies and reconstitute it along the way.

- The less fit you are, the fewer shortcuts you can take. Knowing what you can survive on and still perform well with comes with experience. If you are less fit or less efficient (a novice rider or trail runner, for example), you need to drink and eat on a regular schedule. Set your watch or bike computer and train yourself to drink every 15 to 20 minutes and refuel every 30 to 60 minutes to keep pace with the energy that you're expending.

Postevent Recovery Plan

Do yourself a big favor and shorten your recovery time by replenishing your glycogen stores as soon as possible following a long-distance event or race. You'll feel more energetic the rest of the day, and your muscles will experience less muscle damage and be less sore in the following days. Train yourself to take advantage of the first 30 minutes (the carbohydrate window) after

Team Up to Work on Fluid and Fuel Plans

In events and races in which you rely on others to finish (relay and adventure races, for example) or to provide safety and companionship (treks and ski adventures), make sure that all group members takes seriously the responsibility to hydrate and fuel themselves. In other words, pick your teammates and adventure partners wisely! It's one thing if you are on your own. You hurt only yourself if you don't drink and eat as needed. If you're part of a group or team, you must be willing to force it down.

1. Make a nutrition game plan together beforehand. Don't wait until you're far from home or falling off race pace to find out that the food and drinks that you've been lugging around and counting on to get the group to the finish line are not acceptable or well tolerated. Discuss food likes, dislikes, and any allergies first and then plan accordingly.

2. Food can make or break the experience. Besides calories, carbohydrate, and electrolytes, the foods that you eat during long group adventures and relay races provide a mental boost and improve morale. Or they should. Include fun foods and, as much as feasible, a wide variety of real foods with different tastes and flavors (especially salty foods because so many sports foods are sweet tasting) so that something will always look appealing.

3. Divvy up the goods. All members of any group or racing team should carry fluids and some essential foods in their pockets, bum bags, or backpacks for convenience and, more important, in case they become separated from the group. Be sure that everyone in the group is eating and drinking. Share fluids and food as needed.

4. Keep an eye on teammates. Obviously, you need to be responsible for staying on top of your personal fluid and fuel needs, but at the same time you must monitor your teammates. In adventure races, for example, the first team to cross the finish line together wins. Teams that lose a member because of illness, fatigue, injury, or a team disagreement are disqualified. Dehydration, depletion of muscle glycogen stores, or a low blood sugar level makes the adventure or race seem even harder than it is. Be particularly sensitive to mood swings or personality changes; a friend or teammate in trouble may become extremely quiet or irritable and argumentative.

crossing the finish line. You may tend to let down after you've completed a challenging goal. Concentrate on quickly replacing fluids and carbohydrate, especially if you have another race in a few days or the following weekend.

Be prepared: Anticipate that you won't feel hungry following prolonged exercise. Begin by drinking carbohydrate-rich beverages, such as sports drinks, fruit juice, milk shakes, smoothies, lemonade, soda, high-carbohydrate beverages, or meal replacement beverages. Ease in carbohydrate-rich foods as soon as you can. If feasible, include a small amount of protein (10 to 20 grams) within this same window to prompt muscle repair. (At the very least, eat a well-balanced meal that includes a quality source of protein within two hours.)

Don't wait until you reach home (or for your appetite to return) to begin replenishing glycogen stores. Postrace activities and long car rides home eat up valuable time. Get in the habit of packing a recovery drink (powder to mix with water or a canned supplemental beverage) and drink it within 15 to 30 minutes of finishing.

Be mindful to avoid rehydrating solely with plain water over the first few hours after prolonged exercise, especially if you aren't consuming any sodium-containing foods. By overdrinking plain water (often in an attempt to feel better because you believe that you're very dehydrated or that you "must be" following prolonged efforts), you may induce hyponatremia (low blood sodium level). Rehydrate instead with a sports (electrolyte replacement) drink or other salty fluids, such as soup or broth.

Drinking alcohol may impede your recovery by hampering your efforts to rehydrate (as a diuretic, alcohol causes your body to lose fluid) and by interfering with the ability of your body to replenish its glycogen stores. Your best bet is to make rehydrating with nonalcoholic beverages your first priority. Beyond that, realize that following a strenuous physical effort your body may not be able to tolerate or process alcohol as well as it normally does, so indulge in moderation.

As soon as possible, jot down detailed notes on the success of your nutrition game plan, including prerace meals—what worked, what didn't, and what do you want to do differently next time.

Counteract losing weight from heavy training demands with a recovery period. Many endurance athletes lose a substantial amount of body fat while meeting the high energy demands of training for long-distance events and races. Give your body a full chance to recuperate, including gaining a modest amount of weight (if necessary), before jumping back into your full training regimen. (Some serious-minded athletes will consciously have to eat in a manner that promotes regaining lost weight.)

Eating smart and indulging within reason (including higher-fat foods and other fun foods) will help you avoid becoming run down or susceptible to injuries and will provide a much-needed mental break as well. This interlude will allow you to return to an ambitious training schedule and healthy eating habits with renewed motivation.

Learning From the Best: Racing a Marathon

Deena Kastor, the first American woman to break 2:20 in the marathon, trains hard and long, consistently logging more than 100 miles a week. Through it all—winning a bronze medal in the Olympics, winning her first major marathon against world-class competition, and setting a new American record (2:19:36, a 5:20 pace), Deena emphasizes the key to her success: Don't be too obsessive in any one direction, don't get in a rut, and don't be afraid to be creative. In her words, find a balance. Read on to find out how she applies this mind-set to decisions about food and nutrition when undertaking a marathon.

Practice makes progress. Kastor empathizes with fellow runners on the challenges of drinking while running at race pace. She reports that she needed a couple of months to become comfortable with grabbing a water bottle while on the go. Kastor says that marathoners shouldn't shy away from drink stops even if they feel foolish or are flustered on race day. Kastor recounts that during the London Marathon she saw the elite runners' fluid station almost too late and literally banged her leg on the table as she grabbed her drink.

Focus on getting in the carbohydrate that you need—no one cares that the drink splashes onto your face or even into your eyes. All runners have fumbled through an aid station or two at some point. The most important thing is to stay conscious of your timing during the race. Replicating what she does during her long training runs, Kastor hydrates and refuels with a sports drink every 20 minutes, right from the onset of the race.

If need be, readjust your attitude about drinking and refueling during the race. For Kastor, a marathon isn't 26.2 miles. It's eight water-bottle stations long. Kastor finds counting down the aid stations a fun and easy way to break up a marathon and make it more manageable. Each drink that she gets down brings her that much closer to the finish line.

Because long training efforts before the actual race are so critical, Kastor encourages runners to make a conscious effort to start out long runs well fueled and to be sure to take in enough energy and fluids along the way. Otherwise, going the distance has little purpose. Instead of getting stronger, you're only getting out of energy (caloric) balance and overstressing your body. When the more popular sports drinks didn't settle well, leaving her feeling bloated, Kastor kept experimenting until she found one that she could tolerate. Instead of being discouraged and disgruntled, runners can make a game of finding an acceptable sports drink—for example, by conducting a taste test in which everyone in the family, even the kids, can get involved. Your system can and will adapt if you stick with it—learn what drink will be available on race day and give yourself plenty of time to get used to it.

Make your prerace meals count. Kastor's joy around food continues right up to the race. The night before the race she finds the best Italian restaurant in town and dines with her closest supporters, even toasting them with a glass of wine. Her focus is on getting in carbohydrate with some easily digested protein, but she doesn't gorge or overdo it. Her favorite meal? Pasta with her favorite sauce (pesto) and fish.

Far more important to Kastor is what and how much she eats the morning of the race. This is the only time during the year that she counts calories. She is adamant

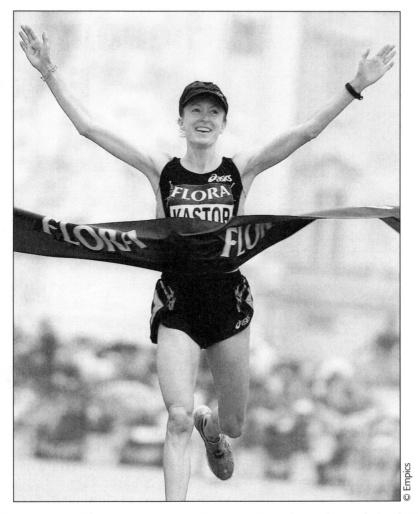

Deena Kastor knows the importance of having a positive relationship with food. Her goal is to show up for the race healthy, strong, and well fueled.

© Empics

about starting out in energy balance, so she consumes 400 to 500 carbohydrate-rich calories, through a bagel, a banana, and a sports drink, to replace the energy that her body burned overnight.

If perfection is your goal, be perfect at balancing it all out. For Kastor, it's simple. What runners need to succeed in the marathon is what all humans need to stay healthy and enjoy life—exercise, food, and rest. She is dismayed by athletes who are ruining the art of perfection by making poor decisions such as fearing food, restricting what they eat, or allowing their training to dominate their family life. To perform, you need quality fuel. Kastor, who professes never to have suffered from prerace anxiety, coaches athletes to make decisions along the way that will lead to their standing on the starting line confident and eager to go. That process includes showing up healthy, strong, and well fueled.

11

Ultraendurance Events

"The hardest part about an ultrarun isn't the running. It's getting my stomach to cooperate."

—Ann Trason, world-record holder in the 40-mile, 50-mile, 100-mile, 100K, and 12-hour runs; 14-time women's winner of Western States 100-Mile Endurance Run

Perhaps you've spent a lifetime pushing the limits. So, why would you stop when it comes to sports? Or perhaps you're driven, even just once, to conquer something that only a select group of hardy souls before you has accomplished. The world of ultraendurance sports continues to grow, and opportunities to push the physical and mental boundaries of human endurance are limitless. For our purposes, ultraendurance includes races that traditionally have served as the longest contests within a particular sport, such as the Ironman within the triathlon world, and endurance events and adventures lasting up to an entire day.

This chapter is for endurance athletes who choose to move up to ultralength challenges or for those striving to set a new PR in traditional ultraendurance events and races, such as the following:

Running: traditional and trail 50-mile, 100K, and 100-mile races and 24-hour runs; specialty road and off-road ultras like the Comrades Marathon (90 K), Sky Marathons, Death Valley Marathon (135 miles), and Pikes Peak Marathon (topping out at 14,110 feet, or 4,299 meters)

Duathlon, triathlon, or multisport races: traditional Ironman, double Ironman, or other daylong extreme multisport adventures, such as the Powerman Zofingen long-distance duathlon (10K run, 150K bike, and 30K run)

Cycling: organized rides (courses), brevets, and randonnees (e.g., 400 kilometers), especially if unsupported or ridden solo, as well as road races taking 10 to 24-plus hours, extreme off-road rides and races such as the Leadville Trail 100 Mountain Bike Race and the 24 Hours of Moab ridden solo

Adventure racing: 24- and 30-hour races (courses), one-day extremes

Hiking, trekking, winter sport adventures: sustained daylong (up to 24- to 30-hour) efforts and ascents, especially if fast-packing or self-sufficient, alpine-style climbing, or solo undertakings

What's the biggest difference as you move up from long distance to ultraendurance endeavors? Basically, you go slower and eat more, a lot more. If you don't, you won't finish or meet your time goal. For example, an Ironman is a swimming, cycling, running, eating, and drinking contest. No matter how much training you've put in or how accomplished you are in the first three, the last two can just as likely determine your success on race day. Former world champion and Hawaii Ironman winner Karen Smyers, for example, contends that her first Hawaii Ironman victory was half due to accomplishing the right training and half due to making the right nutritional decisions on race day. In the same vein, although her training during the following year indicated that she was in better physical condition to defend her title, she readily acknowledges that she was fortunate to rally and finish third after making one error in her drinking regimen during the bike segment.

Obviously, you can't complete an ultra without doing the proper training. You can't just show up and drink and eat your way to the finish. Nutrition, however, is often the area in which ultraendurance athletes can improve the most, especially if they are underprepared for the challenge ahead, approaching their limits, or are novice racers. As an ultraendurance athlete, you need to balance your nutritional awareness and knowledge against your training. Ignorance, laziness, or becoming too focused on your training will doom you on race or event day. Bending the basic rules of physiology and taking nutritional shortcuts has far greater potential to be disastrous (even fatal) during ultras than in other endurance-oriented events and races. Successfully completing and especially racing ultraendurance distances takes extreme willpower, a mastery of all disciplines involved—including drinking and eating while on the move—and a little luck.

Preevent Nutrition Game Plan

Your job as an ultraendurance athlete is to explore, practice, and hone your nutritional strategies, as much as is feasible, during training efforts and shorter events and races before you attempt an ultra. There is a reason why ultra-length competitions typically involve prequalifying or submitting a resume of prior ultraendurance experience. The dangers of kidney failure, hypoglycemia, heat exhaustion or heat stroke, hyponatremia, and hypothermia are very real. It's simple—you're not going to finish and may even end up in the hospital if you haven't learned to respect the nutritional aspect of endurance challenges.

All ultraendurance athletes face, to some degree or another, a myriad of nutrition-related challenges that affect their ability to be successful during ultras events and races:

- Managing precompetition stress and anxiety, the most likely cause of nausea, vomiting, and diarrhea before the start, to prevent underfueling caused by limiting or avoiding preevent meals.
- Handling the logistics of hydrating, refueling, and meeting electrolyte needs when on the move. What is available? How can I supply, carry, or access it? What goes down and stays down at race-day (or event-day) pace?
- Minimizing GI distress such as nausea, bloating, cramps, vomiting, and diarrhea during the event or race.
- Meeting the mental challenge of continuing to eat and drink when appetite is lacking, when feeling poorly, and during the latter stages of ultraendurance exercise.
- Coping with flavor fatigue.
- Dealing with personality changes and "brain fog" (loss of good judgment).
- Managing increased risk of kidney failure, hypoglycemia, and hyponatremia.
- Dealing with varied, changing, and often extreme environmental conditions, which increase the risk for heat illness, altitude sickness, or hypothermia.
- Contending with the effects of increasing fatigue, little or no sleep, or exercising through the night.
- Solving problems on the go or in a constantly shifting situation (for example, what worked last time may not work this time); determining when to try something new and what to try.
- Experiencing situations for the first time during the actual event or race (because, for example, replicating the last 30 miles of a 100-mile ultrarun in training isn't possible).
- Relying on and effectively dealing with others, such as volunteers, teammates, support crews, and pacers.

For ultraendurance athletes, practice does not make perfect, but it is the only road to follow to make progress. Practice during training and in shorter efforts should include preparing your gastrointestinal tract to handle and process fluids and foods during exercise; building a repertoire of acceptable drinks and foods to rely on to meet fluid, energy, and electrolyte needs; and experimenting with techniques (carbohydrate loading and prerace meals), supplements, and gear to find what best suits your individual needs. Essentially, practice hinges on building the mental discipline to do what you have to do when it doesn't seem necessary (when things are going well) and when you don't feel like doing it (when things are going poorly).

Learning more about what nutrition-related situations to anticipate or what to experiment with can come from reading about ultras and from talking with more experienced ultraendurance athletes. If you haven't already, read chapter 10, "Long-Distance Events." That information serves as a foundation or jumping-off point before moving on to the heightened nutritional concerns covered in this chapter. You will also learn a great deal from watching longer races, serving as a pacer, or being part of a support crew before you attempt an ultrarace. Watch races and visit specialty sport shops and Web sites to learn about the array of available gear options.

Every ultra athlete has different needs that he or she should determine well before the day of the race. At a minimum these include determining personal fluid requirements; choosing how to preload glycogen stores, meet energy needs, and prevent hyponatremia; and testing the effects of salt tablets, glycerol, caffeine, or other supplements when used before or during prolonged exercise. For example, based on science alone, hyperhydrating with glycerol would appear to be beneficial. The incidence of GI complaints is so high among ultraendurance athletes (particularly runners and triathletes), however, that the potential bloating, nausea, and abdominal distress associated with glycerol use may only further complicate the situation. The same goes for ingesting caffeine or using salt tablets—how much, when, in what form? What are the potential drawbacks and risks? (See chapter 5 for a review of supplements.) Your job is to use training bouts and other prolonged efforts, preferably in conditions similar to what you expect on race day, as dress rehearsals.

Being successful in ultra adventures and races will inevitably involve a lot of trial and error. Remember the caveat that every athlete, in the end, is an experiment of one. Also, despite the science, some things simply cannot be replicated in a lab or, for that matter, in training or during shorter efforts. For example, simulating the last third of a 100-mile ultrarun just can't be done. In the end, you just have to jump in and try it. Experience plays a large role in being successful. Knowing your body—what works, what doesn't, and what to try next—is truly what builds the self-confidence and mental discipline needed to be successful at ultralength challenges.

During the Event

Your job, from a nutritional standpoint, is to hydrate and refuel in a manner that is smart and safe, and if you're racing, helps you maintain your desired pace as long as possible. A mantra worth remembering is "Eat before you're hungry, drink before you're thirsty." Keep in mind that meeting your fluid, electrolyte, and energy needs during prolonged exercise is a twofold process—digestion and absorption. Particularly if you are an ultraracer, you must be prepared to slow down immediately when your digestive system isn't cooperating, regardless of your time or pacing goals. Trying to push through GI problems increases the likelihood that you won't finish.

Most ultraendurance athletes recognize the need to figure out what they can eat or digest while on the move, that is, what will go down and stay down.

This factor is essential because digestion, or the breakdown of food, begins to a small degree in the stomach. More important, however, is that ingested fluids and foods must empty from the stomach into the small intestine, where digestion of the three energy-giving nutrients (carbohydrate, fat, and protein) really gets going. The small intestine is also where these nutrients are absorbed, with water being reabsorbed or conserved by the colon or large intestine. Eventually, all absorbed nutrients end up in the blood, where they pass through the liver en route to being transported elsewhere in the body.

Finding beverages and foods that you can drink and eat during prolonged exercise simply isn't enough, and consuming them only when it's convenient or when you feel like it won't work. The total time that it takes for any given drink or food that you consume during exercise to be available as fuel to muscle and brain cells is really the critical factor. For example, your blood sugar can bottom out during prolonged exercise if you exceed the capacity of your stomach to absorb fluids that are providing supplemental carbohydrate. A sports drink that remains sloshing around in your stomach for a half hour doesn't help supply glucose to brain cells that are running on fumes.

In other words, to effectively supplement your body's limited internal glycogen stores during prolonged exercise, you must take into account the rate of digestion and absorption of what you consume. For example, some elite male endurance athletes purportedly have trained their bodies to be able to process as much as 400 to 500 carbohydrate calories per hour. Sports scientists, however, theorize that 280 carbohydrate calories (about 70 grams of carbohydrate) is the maximum amount that the body can successfully process in an hour. Thus, the general guideline to aim for is 25 to 60 grams of ingested carbohydrate per hour of prolonged exercise. To maximize your performance in ultras, carbohydrate supplementation needs to begin right from the start and occur at regular intervals (to maximize absorption), not after you have depleted your internal glycogen stores. Otherwise, you create a deficit that you can never overcome.

Athletes can burn 400 to 500 calories or more each hour during an ultra adventure or race. Even lean athletes have enough energy stored as fat to sustain days of exercise, albeit conducted at a much reduced intensity (50 percent of $\dot{V}O_2$max or less). Due to the constraints of digestion and absorption rates, however, our bodies are limited at fulfilling the hour-to-hour demand for carbohydrate, especially at the rate needed to sustain the faster paces and harder efforts associated with ultraracing. On top of that, the specific sport also has an effect. For example, athletes can generally consume more calories per hour cycling (as much as 400 to 500 calories per hour) than they can running (perhaps 200 calories per hour). Hence, the pace on race day is crucial to preserving internal muscle glycogen stores, as is the need to maximize these stores before you begin (through adequate training and carbohydrate loading—see chapters 2 and 4 for a review).

To delay the onset of fatigue during ultraendurance exercise, you must be committed right from the start to ingesting supplemental carbohydrate at regular intervals. Nevertheless, your body will rely increasingly on outside sources of glucose, and delivery will have to occur at a much faster rate to meet carbohydrate needs in the latter stages because internal glycogen stores will be depleted. The bottom line: if you don't drink and eat early on, you won't be around later on. And if you are around later on, you'll need to pay even closer attention to how often you eat and drink.

Fight Off Flavor Fatigue

The phenomenon of becoming turned off at the first taste (or even the mere thought or sight) of previously well-tolerated and liked beverages and foods is known as flavor fatigue. Consuming these items becomes increasingly difficult, and often impossible. The job of meeting fluid and fuel needs becomes even harder. To combat flavor fatigue, make certain that you have available various flavors of your preferred drinks, gels, and bars to choose from. Alternate flavors as much as possible. Don't be caught empty handed when an old standby loses its favored status (be on the move long enough and it will) and is no longer edible.

Most ultra athletes also complain of the increasing sweetness of what they consume (especially sports foods) as time passes, so prepare (as much as feasible) ahead of time. Include bland and especially salty-flavored options such as tomato juice, peanut butter or cheese and crackers, small potatoes and hard-boiled eggs eaten with salt, jerky, whatever—even if those foods don't typically appeal to you during shorter events or races. As the miles pile up or as time goes on, the goal is to hopefully find at least one item (in a drop bag, at an aid station, or in a turnaround or feed bag) that is appealing to you at that point. Although not always or entirely under your control, the more options that you have available, the better your chances are.

Eat Real Food

Some athletes can get the job done during ultras with rehydrating sports drinks (about 14 grams of carbohydrate and 50 calories per cup) and energy gels (20 to 25 grams of carbohydrate and 80 to 100 calories per packet) alone, along with perhaps an energy bar or two. Most athletes, however, will need more than just sports foods to meet their fluid and fuel goals as the hours pass, especially because they'll need to consume more carbohydrate at a faster rate during the latter stages as the body relies increasingly on outside fuel sources.

The easiest way to get in substantial calories is by drinking more concentrated (higher-calorie) carbohydrate or energy drinks, like Ultra Fuel and Carboplex, and using liquid meal replacement products, like Ensure or Boost. Every endurance athlete knows or soon figures out that drinking the calories that they need requires substantially less mental and physical energy than trying to eat them. (In training, practice under various conditions to find a drink that doesn't make you nauseous after just a few hours. See table 5.2 in chapter 5.) When blood flow to your digestive tract is low, which often occurs during running or intense cycling, lean toward liquid food.

As an ultra adventure or race progresses, however, especially beyond 10 hours, you will most likely find yourself increasingly challenged to meet your energy needs. At more moderate paces, such as during moderate-paced cycling, trekking, or walking during ultraruns, the blood flow to your digestive tract is greater (provided that you stay up with your fluid needs) and you should be able to tolerate easily digested carbohydrate-rich foods, like fruit, bagels, fig bars, and energy bars. Eating other solid foods, beyond just chocolate, cookies, and candy, can also be another real option. In fact, Pizza, potato chips, milk shakes, and even cheeseburgers may become your true lifesavers.

The protein-rich and higher-fat favorites just listed, or any others that you can tolerate during prolonged exercise, are digested more slowly than all-carbohydrate foods like energy gels and standard sports drinks used for rehydration. These solid foods empty from the stomach more slowly and take longer to be broken down (especially fat), so their absorption takes place over a longer period. You will feel full longer and experience less queasiness and hunger pangs. At the slower paces and lower intensity levels (50 to 60 percent of $\dot{V}O_2max$) necessitated by ultra distances, you also have enough time to actually use the calories or energy supplied by the fat that you consume during the race. (Keep in mind that the body resorts to using protein for fuel only when carbohydrate or overall calories are insufficient to meet energy needs.)

What may be most important of all, though, is that eating real food helps to combat the brain fog associated with prolonged exercise. Over the long haul, solid foods can be comforting and provide an invaluable morale boost. Remember, in the latter stages of an ultra, no calorie is a bad calorie!

Avoid Too Little and Too Much

Getting the drinking and eating parts of ultras just right on event or race day is part science and part art. Obviously, dehydration, depleted glycogen stores, or passing out from a precipitously low blood sugar level, all related to getting in too little fluid and fuel at the right time, do nothing to enhance your performance. Ingesting too much, however, can slow you down almost as fast and is just as likely to keep you from crossing the finish line.

Remember that your body can handle and process only a limited amount of calories (particularly from those all-important carbohydrate sources) each hour. Forcing down additional food in the hope of topping off or getting ahead of calorie needs, say in the early stages of an event to avoid having to eat later when it's less convenient or during the bike portion of an Ironman to try to prevent digestive problems during the run, typically backfires. Instead of having more calories available for fuel, you can turn your stomach into a whirling blender, especially if you will be running. Ingesting too much, most of which then sits in your stomach, will at the very least cause bloating, perhaps even nausea, and slow the emptying and absorption rate of everything else that you consume. It also greatly increases your chance of vomiting, which means that you don't get any benefit from what you ingested.

Hypertonic, or highly concentrated, carbohydrate-based drinks (above the 5 to 10 percent carbohydrate concentration of standard rehydration sports drinks), like juice, soda, and most caffeinated energy drinks, are more likely to cause trouble, but many athletes report no problems. These beverages take longer to empty the stomach, a scenario for potential digestive problems, and fructose (in the amounts found in juice) is known to be less well tolerated during exercise than are other sugars. (Diluting by at least half with water may be helpful if you want to keep these drinks as options.) Sports drinks with more complex carbohydrates like maltodextrins (long chains of carbohydrate that take longer to be broken down into individual glucose molecules) boost the calorie content of sports drinks and are generally very well tolerated.

Getting behind on fluid (water) can make whatever you ingest seem like too much because dehydration slows gastric emptying and absorption rates. Athletes then falsely blame nausea, vomiting, and other digestive problems on what they previously ate or drank. Other ways in which ultraendurance athletes may feel that they get too much and subsequently develop problems include washing down energy gels with a sports drink rather than diluting by drinking water; consuming too much of a concentrated (higher-calorie) liquid food (for example, drinks with sugar content above 10 percent or containing carbohydrate and protein) and too little actual water; or trying to do too much at once, such as consuming energy gels, a concentrated higher-energy drink, and energy bars or other solid food in a short time. Because eating on a bike is relatively easier, road cyclists and Ironman triathletes during the bike leg need to be particularly aware of overdoing it.

In terms of fluid, endurance athletes vary widely in how much they need to drink during ultraendurance events and races. You may have far different requirements from year to year at the same event or race, depending on the weather. Having said that, most athletes will need between one and two 20-oz bottles per hour. This is a lot of fluid for your body to process, especially because you want to avoid feeling queasy or nauseous.

Dehydration and heat illness are typically the most common reason that athletes do not finish ultraevents and races. The risk of kidney failure or renal shutdown is also far greater if you fall behind in meeting your fluid needs. Myoglobin, a protein material released into the bloodstream from injured muscle tissue, is normally cleared by the kidneys (looking brownish colored in the urine). Without adequate hydration, myoglobin accumulates and clogs the filtering system of the kidneys, leading to partial or total shutdown. The participant guide for the Western States Endurance Run (100 miles), for example, cautions that two Western States runners have required a series of dialysis treatments and that others have been hospitalized for several days with IV fluids to correct partial renal shutdown. If not treated, renal shutdown can permanently damage the kidneys.

Again, an important and limiting factor on performance is how much fluid the stomach can comfortably handle and how quickly it empties, with the consensus being a norm of one quart (one liter) per hour. Your body will not be able to keep up if you haven't practiced drinking this much (or more to meet your personal needs) during training. Remember that the oft-given guideline of drinking 20 to 40 ounces an hour or 5 to 8 ounces every 15 minutes, right from the start, is simply a general recommendation or starting place. At this point you should be very knowledgeable about your personal fluid needs.

Constantly monitor your body (your ability to urinate and sweat, signs of hyponatremia such as fluid retention). Drink at a reasonable pace to match your sweat losses as closely as possible. Staying hydrated can be particularly challenging in certain situations. Due to limited resources and extreme conditions, daylong self-supported adventure racers or climbers, for example, may need to focus on drinking the largest quantity of fluid that they can comfortably handle on every available occasion, and this approach will only minimize their fluid losses.

Two indicators will tell you how well you are hydrating during prolonged exercise: your weight and the color and frequency of your urine. A drop in weight from your preevent or race weight is a clear sign that you are dehydrated. Some competitions, ultraruns in particular, require athletes to be weighed before the race. Weight and other vital signs are monitored throughout the race, and medical personnel use this information to decide whether to allow an athlete to continue. The goal is to stay within two to three pounds (one kilogram or a little more) of your preevent or race weight during the entire time that you're on the move. In terms of urinating, you should feel the need to go at least once every two hours, and your urine should be very light or pale in color.

Gaining significant weight during prolonged exercise (more than 3 percent of preexercise weight) is just as dangerous. This circumstance indicates that your system is not processing fluids as fast as you are taking them in, increasing your risk for hyponatremia. Keeping the proper balance between fluid and electrolytes, particularly sodium, is crucial to maintaining proper weight, avoiding cramps, and most important, getting safely home or to the finish line. The only way to determine what amount of fluid and salt is right for you is to experiment in training. In general, most ultra athletes need 200 to 500 milligrams of sodium per hour (and for comparison, probably 20 to 50 milligrams of potassium). Every athlete is different, and your needs will even vary depending on how well heat trained you are on the day of the event or race.

Mind Your Sodium

If you're going to be an ultraendurance athlete, you must take seriously the increased risk of hyponatremia, particularly during ultras undertaken in the heat. (See chapters 4 and 14 for a review.) Again, the best way to prevent this potentially fatal fluid–electrolyte imbalance during prolonged exercise is to use a two-pronged approach. First, constantly monitor your body and adjust your fluid intake to your losses (sweat and urine) on that day. Second, don't restrict your fluid intake during the race but do increase your sodium intake before and during prolonged exercise with salty foods and sports drinks that contain sodium. (If you are gaining weight or are plagued by a sloshing stomach, you will need to stop drinking temporarily and slow down or stop to allow your body to adjust its fluid status. You accomplish this by getting rid of the excess fluid through urination. After that, you need to consume fluids with electrolytes or high-sodium foods.)

Recognize that juice and cola drinks supply fluid but little or no sodium, thereby increasing your risk of hyponatremia. Some popular sports drinks made specifically for endurance athletes also contain little or no sodium, because you are expected to customize your sodium intake by ingesting salt through foods or by taking electrolyte or salt tablets. Know beforehand the sodium content of the drinks, gels, bars, and other foods that you rely heavily on.

No clear-cut guidelines exist for ingesting sodium during prolonged exercise—200 to 500 milligrams an hour is only a general recommendation. Don't overdo it. Salt tablets can irritate the lining of the stomach and induce vomiting, so take them with at least 6 ounces of water. (If you have a health problem, check with your doctor beforehand about using salt tablets during prolonged exercise.) Some athletes do better with ingesting salt directly (with water, of course), such as provided by the small salt packets typically found at fast-food restaurants or in salty foods.

The bottom line: when it comes to replacing fluids and electrolytes and keeping up with the fuel needs of the body during ultras, you must develop and follow a plan. You cannot rely solely on thirst or hunger, and especially during ultras, your memory, or good judgment. Many interrelated factors conspire to make it extra challenging to get the nutritional aspect of ultra training just right:

- All exercise reduces blood flow to the digestive system to some degree, especially vigorous exercise (starting around 70 to 75 percent $\dot{V}O_2max$), and this reduced flow delays the rate at which the stomach empties.

  What you need to do is train adequately and intelligently to maximize your fitness level and adhere to a proper pace on event or race day, especially during the early stages.

- Dehydration also delays the rate at which the stomach empties, setting the stage for bloating, nausea, and vomiting. Dehydration further compromises the body's fluid and energy balance because it slows the rate of digestion and absorption of all drinks and foods consumed. (Whenever your overall blood volume falls, less blood is available to flow to your digestive system.)

  What you need to do right from the start (as much as humanly possible) is match your fluid and electrolyte needs with losses on an hour-to-hour basis.

- Activities like running that involve physical jostling (mechanical trauma) of the stomach and other abdominal organs interfere the most with stomach emptying and the rate of digestion and absorption.

  Right from the start of any ultra, regularly take in small amounts of carbohydrate-rich drinks and foods. Lean toward semiliquid or liquid calorie sources because liquids empty more quickly than solids do.

- Abdominal cramps and diarrhea arise during ultras due to overactivity, including the physical jostling, of the lower digestive system (small intestines and the colon). Reduced blood flow to the digestive system makes matters worse.

You need to have an hourly hydrating and refueling plan that aims to keep up with fluid, electrolyte, and energy needs without overloading the system at any one time.

Protect Your Brain

Usually the first thing to go for an ultraendurance athlete is good judgment. Although persistence is required during ultras, zoning out and operating on autopilot is not an indefinitely sustainable state. Stopping to rest and to feed your brain is sometimes what you need to do to get to the finish line faster, or even to continue, for that matter. Dips in your blood sugar level can leave you feeling overwhelmed, convinced that you aren't making any forward progress and questioning your ability to continue.

If your blood sugar bottoms out, reach for readily absorbable quick-energy carbohydrate sources such as energy gels, soda, juice, sports drinks, glucose tablets, or sugary candy. Slow your pace, walk, or stop altogether to give your body a chance to absorb the necessary carbohydrate. Your blood sugar level will usually stabilize within 15 minutes unless you're severely depleted. Seek or ask for medical attention if necessary. Heed slurred speech, blurred vision, excessive confusion, crying, or irritability as serious warning signs that you need to do a much better job at keeping up with your energy needs.

Remember, the first half of an ultra is mostly physical. The second half is mostly mental. When you hit a tough patch, rely on strategies that have worked in the past, but at the same time be willing to try something new. Successfully finishing an ultra challenge or race hinges on your ability to solve problems and keep yourself moving. Trust your training and give it a chance to come through. When you least feel like eating or drinking is when you most likely need to do so. The bottom line is that before you make any drastic decisions, such as whether to continue or not, feed your brain.

Finally, if you choose to use nonsteroidal anti-inflammatory drugs (NSAIDs, for example, Advil, Nuprin, Aleve, and Actron) during an ultrarace, be aware of the risks. Although acute kidney failure is rare, be extremely cautious. Taking NSAIDs during prolonged exercise when dealing with severe heat or dehydration magnifies the potential for kidney problems and may contribute to the development of hyponatremia. Pay particular attention to your fluid needs before and during the event to minimize these risks. Taking NSAIDs may also upset your stomach.

Ultraendurance athletes often take Tums, Rolaids, or Imodium before or throughout prolonged exercise to prevent or minimize GI problems. Again, no formal guidelines exist. Just remember that more is not necessarily better.

Sport-Specific Tips

Focusing only on running, cycling, or putting one foot in front of the other during ultralength challenges is simply not enough. Being competitive, achieving a personal best, or just making it across the finish line requires that you master the nutritional challenges inherent in ultras.

Ultrarunners

A 100-mile race is a running, drinking, and eating contest. You can't leave your nutrition game plan up to chance.

1. Know the location and timing of aid stations and drop points so that you can prepare what to have available and what to carry. This is why it's vital to write down or record your thoughts in some manner following training runs and shorter races and compile a database of what works for you and what doesn't.

2. Ultrarunners make three classic mistakes. Read on to learn what they are and how to avoid them.

   • Not drinking enough early in the race. Don't just tote fluid around with you; concentrate on drinking it. Most runners carry two sources of fluid—plain water and a rehydrating sports drink (which contains carbohydrate and electrolytes). Most bottles hold 20 ounces (600 milliliters), the minimum amount of fluid needed per hour. If you often arrive at aid stations with your bottles still full, consider adding handles to your bottles and carrying them as a reminder to drink more often (try this on training runs first). You should be urinating frequently (at least once every two hours), and it should be light in color.

   • Not taking in enough calories early. The crucial time to pay attention to your nutritional needs is the first 70 percent of the race. You must make smart decisions about your fuel needs (as well as fluid and sodium) during the first 70 miles, or you won't be around to finish the last 30. Forgetting to eat is easy when things are going well or seem under control early. If you dig yourself into a hole, however, you probably won't be able to recover enough to continue, even if you desperately shovel in calories during the latter stages of the race. All your training will be for naught if you aren't smart about eating early in the race.

   • Not paying enough attention to the need for salt. There are no clear-cut guidelines or recommendations because the need for sodium varies because of individual sweat rates and the weather. In hot and humid conditions, some runners may need as much as 800 to 1,000 milligrams of sodium per hour. Know beforehand the sodium content of the products that you intend to use (check the labels of energy gels, drinks, and so on) and determine how much you will be getting in the amounts of the foods that you intend to consume. During the race, at aid stations choose salty foods such as soup or broth, pretzels, chips, boiled potatoes sprinkled with salt, and so forth. If you plan to carry salt tablets with you, keep in mind that they disintegrate quickly if they contact moisture (sweat, for example) so place them in small plastic bags or other waterproof carriers. Take salt tablets with 6 to 8 ounces of water and don't overdo it. Salty foods tend to stimulate thirst, but salt tablets don't, so it is possible to ingest too much.

As an ultrarunner, you must definitely learn to drink your calories. Few athletes can go the distance on energy gels and water alone. Although gels supply quick energy that goes down easily, they provide only 80 to 100 calories per packet, and most ultrarunners need to consume roughly 250 to 500 calories per hour during a 100-mile race. The easiest way to get in substantial calories is by drinking highly concentrated energy drinks and using liquid meal replacement products like Ensure or Boost. Save caffeinated beverages such as cola and Mountain Dew for when you really need a quick pick-me-up, such as in the later stages of the race.

Supplement with solid foods as tolerated. Realize that nothing will taste good or sound appealing as time passes, so nibble on a variety of foods as you pass through aid stations or meet up with your crew. Foods that you are likely to find include salt replacement foods such as pretzels, soda crackers, chips and soup, fruit, energy bars, cookies, candy, boiled potatoes, and possibly sandwiches. Have your crew stock other foods that you've experimented with on training runs.

Time your eating and drinking so that you can do most of it when you're walking. In ultraruns, this typically means that you'll eat and drink when you're heading uphill. In the same vein, if your crew is meeting you somewhere other than an established aid station, have them meet you at the foot of a hill or mountain rather than at the top.

Your blood sugar can bottom out if you exceed the capacity of your stomach to absorb fluids. This may be the case if you feel uncomfortably full or bloated in your lower abdomen (as if you have two stomachs) or if the fluids that you've been ingesting seem just to sit in your belly and slosh around. In extreme cases, veteran ultrarunners report relief by vomiting, by wiping the slate clean and starting over. If you try this remedy, immediately begin your recovery by sipping on a properly formulated sports drink or broth made from bouillon cubes, not plain water. Remember, you will need fluid, carbohydrate, and sodium to be able to continue—the sooner, the better.

Periodic weigh-ins are a common practice at most 100-mile races. Be prepared to be detained (to drink and eat) or pulled from the race if you can't maintain your weight within an acceptable range (generally within 3 to 5 percent of your starting weight). As you attempt to rehydrate, consume sodium-containing sports drinks, soup or broth, and salty foods. The sodium in these items will help you retain the fluid that you consume.

Ironman Triathletes

During the race, aim to replace 30 to 50 percent of the calories that you expend, which translates into approximately 2,500 to 5,000 calories for most Ironman triathletes. To maintain hydration and a stable blood sugar level, most triathletes need roughly 250 to 400 calories per hour. Most of these calories (70 to 75 percent) should come from carbohydrate—sports drinks, energy gels and bars, and other solid foods that are well tolerated. Consuming a small amount of protein and fat will also help you over the long haul.

The goal is to enter the running leg in an energy-neutral state or slightly ahead, certainly not digging out from a calorie deficit that occurred from swimming and biking. Increasing fatigue and dehydration, dwindling glycogen stores, and the likelihood of digestive problems when running all combine to make eating and drinking extremely challenging during the final leg of an Ironman. Ingesting adequate calories just to stay up with the energy needs of running 26.2 miles is daunting enough. At this stage in the race, being behind and having to dig yourself out of a hole spells disaster.

Swim   Eating while swimming is obviously impossible. Due to the nonjostling nature of swimming, however, most athletes can comfortably tolerate eating and drinking fairly close to the onset of swimming. Preload with a final carbohydrate boost (energy gel or sports drink) about 30 to 60 minutes beforehand. You're trying to keep up with or "replace" at least some of the calories that you will be expending during the swim. Figure about 8 to 10 calories per minute.

Bike   Saltwater swallowed during ocean swims will cause a burning sensation in your throat. If you swallow enough, your tongue will swell and you may begin the bike ride feeling sick to your stomach. If necessary, let your stomach calm down a little. Start drinking about 10 minutes out on the bike and take your first substantial carbohydrate infusion (gel or higher-energy carbohydrate drink) within 20 minutes of starting the bike leg. But be aware that many triathletes get in trouble by drinking or eating too much, too soon during the bike leg. Blood redirected to the stomach for digestion can interfere with reestablishing blood flow to hardworking leg muscles. Concentrate initially on sipping drinks and hold off on eating anything for the first 20 minutes.

Triathletes spend the largest portion of time in a race cycling, so you absolutely must be proficient at eating and drinking on your bike. During the race, control or slow your pace (or stop entirely if need be) when it's time to rehydrate and refuel. If the race features individual feed bags at the turnaround and it contains something essential to your race plan, be prepared to stop for it (on the run too). Pack your turnaround bag full of many different foods to increase the chance that at least one item will seem appealing at that point in the race. Try including a treat that you can't get at aid stations on the course.

To stay up with the calories that you're expending and to overcome any calorie deficit that may have occurred during the swim, you must drink and snack in appropriate amounts at regular intervals (starting early) during the bike segment of an Ironman. Be mindful, however, to avoid overdoing it. Athletes who fear or who have previously experienced significant digestive problems while running will try to get ahead during the bike segment only to sabotage themselves later. Many triathletes find that they do better by getting fuel in at the start of the run (for example, by drinking a sports drink) than by cramming food down during the latter stages of the bike portion. If need be, try backing off the last 20 to 30 minutes on the bike to give the fluids and foods that you've ingested time to empty from your stomach before you begin the run.

Several hydration systems are options when you're on the bike, such as traditional mounted water bottles (on the down tube and seat tube), aerobar-mounted drinking systems, seat-mounted bottle carriers, and bladder hydration systems. Choose the one that works best for you. If you go with a bladder, choose an aerodynamic model made specifically for cyclists. Insulated water bottles that help keep liquids cold may help you consume more fluid while on the bike. Be careful of diluting your sports drink too much because doing so also dilutes the amount of sodium that you get. Some triathletes carry bottles of double-strength sports drink and dilute it by alternating with gulps from a water bottle picked up at an aid station. A safe system for novice racers is to start with two bottles—one of your preferred liquid food and one containing a sports drink. You can pick up water and additional sports drink from aid stations along the course.

Run Now begins the real challenge of meeting fluid and fuel needs while on the move. Gastrointestinal distress, such as nausea and bloating, is common during the running segment. The jostling nature of running and the progressive dehydration associated with several hours of continuous exercise slow the absorption of fluid and nutrients from the stomach. (Some fluid sloshing around in your stomach is to be expected.) At this point, stick to sports drinks, water, and energy gels or chews (and possibly soda) to minimize digestive problems. Take small amounts at regular intervals. Recognize that an inability to urinate during the run is a red flag that you've become too dehydrated. Slow or stop when you approach aid stations to ensure that you consume some fluid and aren't just pouring it on yourself or the ground.

If vomiting ensues during the run, think of it as wiping the slate clean. Slow or stop, regroup, and start over with your rehydrating and refueling efforts. Vomiting is definitely a setback, but you can rebound once your body starts to absorb the fluid and calories that it requires. Remind yourself that the only way to finish is by replacing, mile by mile, the fluid, calories, and carbohydrate that you need. Chewing solid food, such as an energy bar or a banana, can sometimes help settle a queasy stomach and provide a much-needed mental lift. Some athletes find that chewing on a Tums tablet also helps.

Transitions Relax and take your time as you execute the transition both onto the bike and into the run. Set up your transition area in a logical, organized manner so that you can't possibly exit the transition area without your essentials. Obviously, you should pack gel flasks, bento boxes, and bike jerseys beforehand. Always keep an extra water bottle handy in the transition area to drink from as you head out on the run. Again, rather than overdoing it during the last part of the bike segment, take advantage of your slower pace as you make the transition into running by using it as an opportunity to refuel.

Monitor your hydration efforts by keeping tabs on your ability to urinate; at least once every two hours (every 30 to 50 miles on the bike) throughout the race is a rough guideline. If you choose to drink soda (for example, Coca-Cola), consume water with it. You'll dilute the carbohydrate concentration of the soda into a more optimal range that favors absorption. Keep in mind that soft drinks also contain minimal amounts of sodium compared with a typical sports drink, increasing the risk of hyponatremia, especially in susceptible individuals. Some seasoned Ironman triathletes drink Coke from the outset of the run (at every aid station). Others prefer to hold off as long as possible. Reaching for Coke can provide an almost immediate psychological boost, but realize that in most cases the lift is only temporary. Be prepared to continue with Coke after you've started drinking it.

After the Event

Enhance your recovery by making smart nutritional choices following the race. Granted, you'll be sore and exhausted following an ultra adventure or race no matter what you eat or drink afterward. But you can lessen somewhat your discomfort and the extent of muscle damage (and rejoin the living sooner) by paying attention to your nutritional needs following prolonged, exhaustive exercise.

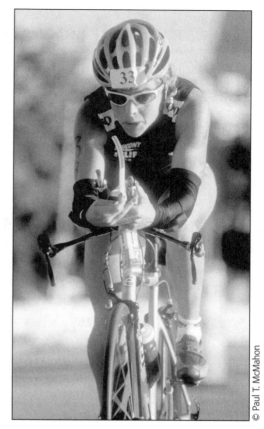

© Paul T. McMahon

Like many triathletes, three-time Ironman winner Heather Gollnick favors a hands-free aerodynamic hydration system.

Rehydrate with something other than plain water or alcohol. Drinking only plain water, especially if you're not able to get or keep any food down, can induce hyponatremia in the hours and first few days following prolonged exercise. It's crucial to consume electrolyte-containing fluids after ultras for the first few to several days, until your digestive system is fully functioning and your urine is clear and of normal frequency. This means drinking sports drinks, broth, soup, and tomato juice. Eating salty foods, as much as tolerated, will also help your body reestablish its normal fluid–electrolyte balance.

Drinking alcohol following all-out efforts may impede your recovery by hampering your efforts to rehydrate (alcohol is a diuretic) and refill your glycogen stores. Beyond that, realize that following an exhaustive physical effort, your body may not be able to tolerate or process alcohol as well as it normally does, so indulge in moderation, if at all.

Do the best that you can to ease nutritious foods in as soon as possible. Liquid calories provided by milk, low-fat milk shakes, fruit smoothies, and

Stop Reaching for the Water Bottle

Triathletes are needy people. Traditional bike shorts, running attire, and water bottles just don't work for them—especially over the long haul. The logistics of swimming, cycling, and running all in the same event have led to the development of a whole range of specialized equipment and clothing. Aerodynamic hydration systems, in particular, have evolved to meet the needs of the triathlete during a triathlon's cycling leg. Front-mounted to the handlebars or an aerobar, an aerodynamic hydration system offers many benefits during a race:

- Hands can always remain on the handlebars and eyes can remain on the road.
- Enables the rider to take frequent sips instead of big gulps.
- Front-mounted design means no more dropped water bottles from reaching down and behind while riding.
- Translucent container allows fluid levels to be seen at all times, eliminating the guesswork for a refill when approaching an aid station.
- Splash guard prevents spills.
- Bottles/reservoirs are easily refillable while riding.
- Eliminates the extra weight and hassle of carrying and reconstituting a sports drink powder (if using something other than course-supplied drink).
- Cool water (course supplied) added periodically makes the drink more palatable, which encourages more fluid to be consumed.
- Aerodynamic design reduces wind drag.
- Some designs have two separate liquid compartments (each with its own straw), allowing two different fluids to be carried in a single bottle.

Before using a new hydration system in an event, it's a good idea to practice with it first. The following tips will help you get the most out of a new system:

- Know the fluid volume of your system and the nutrient data of your sports drink (when reconstituted) in order to mix your drink at the proper carbohydrate concentration. For example, a 28-ounce drinking system can hold four ounces of a typical concentrated sports drink and 24 ounces of water. Eight ounces of this mixture will provide about 60 calories and 15 grams of carbohydrate—well within the 6 to 8 percent concentrated carbohydrate range that is recommended during moderate to vigorous exercise.
- Determine beforehand your sweat rate, calorie requirements, and carbohydrate needs while biking (ideally in conditions similar to what is expected on race day). These calculations will help you determine how many times you will need to refill the contents of your bottle during competition.

(continued)

(continued)

- Prior to the race, fill one regular water bottle with enough concentrated drink mix for the entire race. Mark the outside of the bottle at four-ounce increments (or some other predetermined amount).
- Upon approaching an aid station in a race, add four ounces of concentrate to the hydration system. Grab a bottle of water at the station (most races supply the 24-ounce size) and empty it into the hydration system as you ride—you're all set! Additional electrolytes can be added at any time as suits your need. Also, be sure to grab extra bottles of water throughout the race to take with energy gels or solid foods, as necessary.

canned meal replacement products are often the easiest place to start. (Many ultra athletes anecdotally report being able to tolerate dairy foods, such as milk and ice cream, well after ultras.) Focus on including quality protein sources with carbohydrate-rich foods at all meals for the next several days to help with glycogen resynthesis, as well as to hasten the repair of damaged skeletal muscle. Of course, don't ignore your cravings—you've earned the right to celebrate.

Some degree of muscle necrosis or muscle cell death occurs from participating in ultralength exercise, especially in the leg muscles of runners. This condition is further pronounced in athletes who became significantly dehydrated or overexerted themselves. Complete recovery can take months. Eating a well-balanced, nutrient-rich diet supports the recovery process, but simply eating right is not enough to fix this underlying damage. Don't resume serious training until you have fully recovered on all levels.

To improve your odds of being successful in the future, record your thoughts and observations about your nutritional strategies as soon as possible following ultra adventures and races. What worked? What didn't work? What do you want to try or remember for next time? Karen Smyers, International Triathlon Union World and Hawaii Ironman champion, recounted to me nutritional game plans of past Hawaii Ironman races simply by looking the details up in training logbooks that she always kept.

If you were foiled or slowed by your digestive system, particularly intestinal cramps and diarrhea, spend some time to think objectively about your training and physical preparation. Problems with your stomach are not only about what you did (or didn't) eat and drink before and during the event or race. The fitter that you are overall, the greater the blood flow is to your stomach and intestines at any given pace or level of exertion. This translates into being better able to handle and process the fluids and foods that you need to consume along the way.

Learning From the Best: Tips for Support Crews

Like all good ultrarunners, ultrarace champions Ann Trason (holder of multiple ultra world records and 14-time women's winner of Western States) and Tim Tweitmeyer (5-time winner of the Western States 100) often crewed for other ultrarunners when not racing themselves. Here's some advice they have for you when it's your turn to crew at an ultrarun. I put all these tips to good use when I crewed for my husband at the Leadville Trail 100 race in Colorado.

As a support-crew member, make sure that you have your own food and drinks. The event usually involves an extremely long day, and you don't want to become hungry. You are the brains behind the operation, so you need to be alert. You want to have fun too, and that's a lot easier to do when you have plenty on hand to eat and drink.

Have the runner write out a plan for you. If the runner won't do that, at least talk to him or her about the race as much as you can before the event. Do this a few days before the event, not the day before. A good ultrarunner will want to make your life easy. For example, you need to know anything unique the runner might need or crave along the way as well as what he or she must absolutely carry when departing the various aid stations.

Don't bombard your runner with questions as he or she arrives at an aid station. Before the race, have the runner give you a short list of questions that you should always ask. Trason, for example, would have her crew ask whether she wanted more ice in her bottles and whether she thought that she was getting enough salt. Make sure that your runner is eating and drinking. For example, make sure that you check the runner's bottles when he or she arrives at the aid station.

Because your runner might not even remember his or her name after 70 miles, Tweitmeyer suggests asking a basic set of questions to draw out important information that the runner might otherwise forget. As a support-crew member, take care of the details as well as the big things. Even simple stuff can bog down a runner late in the race.

Have available as much information as you can about the various drops and aid stations. Write it down so that there is no confusion. Most important is knowing what time to expect your runner to arrive so that you can be there! Be ready to share information with your runner, such as how far the person has run and the distance to the next aid station. Split times from previous years can be useful to have on hand. If you keep split times of other runners, you can share with your runner how the race is going.

Expect your runner to go through emotional difficulties. Stay positive, be flexible, and work at solving problems as they arise. Always think of yourself as the brains of the operation. Playing games with your runner to keep him or her going is OK. If the runner wants to drop out, for example, tell him or her that dropping is not an option at this point. Reassure the runner that if he or she makes it to the next scheduled place and still wants to drop, you will talk about it then.

Multiday and Multileg Endurance Events

12

"Make sure you eat well but don't overeat the night before a race. Meal planning for the morning of race day is also important as it is the last chance you will have to eat and hydrate without physical stress on your body."

—Ian Adamson, six-time adventure race world champion, including three-time Eco-Challenge champion, and winner of the Adventure Race World Championships, Primal Quest, Raid Gauloises, and Raid World Cup

Is one day of exertion simply not enough for you? More and more endurance athletes are asking their bodies to perform beyond 24 hours. Others expect their bodies to deliver shorter but higher-intensity performances over several days. Sixty to 80 hours of continuous adventure racing is a very long day. Taking part in a weeklong trail-running camp or a cross-state ride, which should include enjoying yourself and not getting injured, hinges on your being ready day after day. So, too, you must be ready to go again and again if others are counting on you to hold up for multiple legs of relay-type races and events.

These types of endurance endeavors are a real test of your nutritional strengths and weaknesses, as well as your mental discipline. Poor planning and lack of attention to detail, especially on how best to recover from day to day (or leg to leg), quickly become apparent. An otherwise challenging and fun endurance endeavor can dissolve into a slog fest or worse, a never-ending nightmare. Being smart about what and how you eat and drink during multiday adventures and races is a key component of the ultimate outcome—and it's one of the few factors under your control.

This chapter is for endurance athletes participating in multiday events and races, such as the following:

Running: road relay races such as Hood to Coast (12-person teams covering 197 miles, or 317 kilometers, from Mount Hood, Oregon, to the Pacific Ocean), cross-state and cross-country runs

Cycling: organized cross-state and cross-country rides, randonnees (400 to 1,200 kilometers), cycling classics, Race Across America (solo, tandem, and teams) and qualifiers

Adventure racing: expedition-length races (a few to 10 days) like the Raid, solo adventure race (250 kilometers)

Trekking and skiing: climbing trips and expeditions, through-hiking, back-country trips, and winter hut-to-hut trips

All-endurance sports: organized tours or personal adventures, sports camps, multisport relay-type races (for example, each person required to perform two or more legs)

The scope of multiday endurance events and races is enormous, including everything from a two-day organized ride with supported rest stops to months of being self-sufficient while through-hiking the Appalachian Trail. In this chapter I attempt to provide an overview of the most important nutrition-related principles that come into play. These basic recommendations work well with specific tips and strategies provided elsewhere throughout the book (see chapters 9 through 11 and 13 through 16).

One of the greatest challenges facing participants of multiday endurance endeavors is knowing when to eat. Many things get in the way—the actual activity (running, cycling, climbing, and so on), maintaining gear and clothing, personal hygiene and tending to injuries (blisters, saddle sores, and so forth), the need to rest or sleep, and, if racing, competitive strategy. Throw into the mix getting lost, spending time connecting with support crews, lost drop bags, misplaced supplies, weather delays, extreme heat or cold, altitude, fickle stomachs, loss of appetite, extreme fatigue, mental apathy, and a host of other unexpected surprises, and you can see how something as basic as eating and drinking can slip off the radar screen. You can't neglect eating and drinking during multiday endeavors, however, or you will pay the price. Although mental toughness, patience, and first-rate problem-solving skills are prerequisites, your body always has final veto power.

Energy Needs

Before multiday and multileg events and races, your job is fourfold:

1. Start out well hydrated by drinking adequate amounts of appropriate fluids during the two or three days before the event.

2. Start out with a healthy fluid–electrolyte balance by normal use of salt-containing foods and salting to taste, and increasing salt intake for three to five days beforehand if extreme heat, high humidity, or conditions warmer than what you trained in are expected.

3. Start out well fueled by carbohydrate loading (begin at least three days before the event) to ensure that muscle glycogen stores are at their fullest.

4. Eat a substantial carbohydrate-rich breakfast one to four hours beforehand (depending on how important it is for you to start with an empty stomach).

From then on, your job is to take advantage of every opportunity that you have to rehydrate, refuel, and recover. In other words, make smart use of the time, any time, that you have.

Multiple Shorter, Higher-Intensity Efforts

To maintain the faster paces and higher-intensity efforts required in relay races and events during which you alternate being on and off (for example, cycling pulls or running legs), you burn carbohydrate as fuel almost exclusively. Hence, carbohydrate loading is appropriate before these types of events. If your on time is 30 to 60 minutes or less, you are unlikely to need or benefit from eating during your pull or leg because you'll likely be working hard and near your anaerobic threshold. Drink once more before you go. For example, drink 5 to 10 ounces 10 to 20 minutes beforehand or take an energy gel with water 5 to 10 minutes before you go. Consider carrying fluid with you (water or a sports drink, especially during all-out efforts of 45 to 60 minutes) to help with cooling and sensations of dry mouth.

What you do nutrition-wise during your breaks is much more critical. During short "off" breaks, like 30 to 60 minutes, you must refuel to cover the carbohydrate that you'll burn during the break and the carbohydrate that your body will use during your next "on" effort. As a rule, consume 60 grams of carbohydrate per break or during down time lasting 30 to 60 minutes to keep pace with the ability of your body to process or oxidize up to one gram per minute of carbohydrate ingested during exercise. Obviously, a 30- to 60-minute break doesn't give you a lot of time for digestion. Liquids and gels are most efficient at this point—four cups of a sports drink or two gel packages and water will supply 60 grams of carbohydrate.

During longer breaks of up to two hours, be prepared to consume a liquid-food drink or small amount of well-tolerated carbohydrate-rich foods such as a banana, breakfast bar, or energy bar in addition to water or a sports drink. You can use real food if desired and available during longer blocks of time off, such as when you have three hours or more (runners may need at least four hours off). The key is to eat at the start of your break period (and definitely before you collapse and go to sleep), not to do a hundred other things or wait until you feel hungry.

Multiday Events

The biggest danger with multiday rides, runs, treks and tours, cycling classics, sports camps, and climbing expeditions is incomplete recovery—you slowly become glycogen depleted as each day passes and thus become increasingly fatigued. You find yourself less and less able to respond quickly or maintain your desired pace, and mentally you find that your commitment and enthusiasm start to wane. (Of course, chronic fatigue can set in as early as day 2 or 3 if you haven't trained adequately with long back-to-back efforts, but you can't do anything about that now.)

When it comes to eating and drinking, think before, during, and after. Fuel up every day before you start with a carbohydrate-rich breakfast to maximize your glycogen stores. If you'll be pushing the pace or racing (working at moderate to high intensity, above 60 percent of $\dot{V}O_2$max) you'll need to eat and drink at the earlier end of your acceptable breakfast window to start out on an empty stomach and minimize digestive problems. Drink again as near the start time as you can or top off with an energy gel taken with water. If the day is going to be more of a long, slow effort, then it's generally OK to eat closer to the start (say, two to three hours beforehand) and to include fattier foods that take longer to empty from your stomach and be digested.

During the event or race, you'll need to drink regularly (every 15 to 20 minutes) and refuel (every 30 to 60 minutes) from the onset so that you consume at least 30 to 60 grams of carbohydrate per hour. Sports drinks are the rehydrating beverage of choice to replace fluid and electrolytes. Along with sports drinks, a safe approach is to rely on energy gels and well-tolerated carbohydrate snacks during faster-paced efforts. Be prepared with salty foods or electrolyte tablets to help keep pace with your sodium needs. On long, slow days, incorporate real food, especially for the mental boost that it provides.

The key is to drink and snack regularly as you go, keeping pace with the calories that you're expending. Unless you have a four-hour or longer break planned, eating a large amount at any one time, such as a lunchtime meal or a meal during a rest stop, will divert blood away from working muscles when you resume exercising. You will feel lethargic and unresponsive and end the day lamenting how much harder the second half was.

When you've stopped moving for the day, your job is not done. You must consciously take advantage of the carbohydrate window, particularly the first 15 minutes, to maximize the glycogen replenishment process (see chapter 4 for a review). Ingest a substantial amount of carbohydrate calories immediately—at least .5 grams of carbohydrate per pound (~1.0 grams per kilogram) of body weight. (Even better, take in .75 grams per pound.) Remember, these are carbohydrate calories, not just calories from anything, like beer, nacho chips, or a candy bar. A recovery drink or meal replacement beverage can make the job easier (see the chart in chapter 5), and a small amount of protein may help reduce muscle soreness.

Each evening eat a high-carbohydrate meal that includes a good source of quality protein (for example, 20 to 30 grams as supplied by 3 to 4 ounces, or 85 to 112 grams, of meat). If need be, eat another carbohydrate-rich snack before bedtime.

Weighing yourself (if feasible) before you begin and right afterward can be very useful because you can quickly ascertain how well you are doing at meeting your fluid needs during the event or race. Over the next few hours, drink at least 2.5 cups of fluid for every pound (or 1.3 liters for every kilogram) that you are down. If you're down more than a few pounds, adjust your drinking plan for subsequent efforts and pay attention to your sodium intake too. Losing weight from day to day (especially in events and races lasting longer than three to five days) and having sore or "dead" legs that are struggling to respond are prime signs of chronic glycogen depletion. Your job is to stop the damage from occurring before it becomes too much to reverse by eating more (especially carbohydrate calories), taking more time to recover, or most likely some of both.

Continuous Events

Endurance endeavors such as multiday adventure races or continuous cycling races in which the goal is to keep moving no matter what (especially if you must meet timed cutoff points) present the most complex and challenging nutritional scenarios. How do you consume massive amounts of calories to keep your muscles fueled and working while at the same time making sure that this high caloric infusion doesn't hinder your performance? A few themes become clear.

First, you must refuel on the go at every opportunity and rely on liquid calories as much as possible (and feasible) to get the job done. Liquids are more efficient because they are absorbed more easily and quickly than solids are and thus lessen the risk of digestive problems. Second, successful multiday endurance athletes report using training sessions to develop both smart eating habits and the ability to eat constantly. In other words, eating while continuously on the move is a learned skill that requires a lot of mindful practice. Given the wide variation in individual tastes and preferences, the only way to determine what types of food you best tolerate is to experiment. You'll need to try various foods under different conditions, such as heat, cold, and at altitude, and determine how much you can tolerate. Being confident in your ability to cope with the mind-boggling variety of conditions and circumstances that you will inevitably confront during a multiday event or race won't come from a book, a Web site, or a friend. You develop confidence in your ability only through detailed trial-and-error experimentation.

Third, you must be able to keep separate your nutrition (calorie) and hydration (fluid) needs. Your body requires adequate water and fuel to keep moving continuously. Staying adequately hydrated (with water or a rehydrating sports drink), however, is the key to everything else you need to have happen (and keep happening) while on the move. Dehydration disrupts everything: Less blood flows to working muscles and your brain; your ability to tolerate heat decreases because you are less able to dissipate heat from working muscles;

less blood flows to the gastrointestinal tract, creating a greater risk of digestive problems; digestion and absorption is less efficient, resulting in slower conversion of food into usable energy; and the mechanisms that your body uses to regulate or restore normal fluid balance are further compromised.

Meeting your body's need for fluid during continuous endurance exercise is a whole separate ballgame from meeting energy or caloric needs. Relying on a concentrated liquid-food beverage to meet the fluid needs of your body or drinking more of it in an attempt to rehydrate spells disaster. As with fuel needs, however, the only way to get a handle on what and how much you need to drink to be optimally hydrated is to experiment during training under various conditions.

Salt and Fluid Balance

Sensitive internal balancing mechanisms constantly regulate the total amount of fluid in the body. Your mouth (by sensing thirst), brain (by stimulating you to drink when your blood is too concentrated), and stomach govern your fluid intake, and your brain (by antidiuretic or vasopressin hormone from the pituitary gland) and kidneys are involved in how much fluid is excreted (urinated). Imbalances, such as dehydration and water intoxication (excessive body water) can occur, but your body works hard to restore them to normal as promptly as it can. During long-distance, ultra, and multiday events and races (continuous or day after day), however, your body can find that maintaining this delicate balance is much more complicated. What you do or don't do further complicates the picture.

Endurance athletes have been told repeatedly over the years about the importance of drinking during prolonged exercise to avoid dehydration. Obviously, this is true and a critical piece of the puzzle if you want to perform at your best. But having too much water on board, or exercise-associated hyponatremia, is just as dangerous and can be life threatening for endurance athletes.

Hyponatremia doesn't occur just in athletes who substantially overdrink or overhydrate, especially with plain water, although this is one route. It also occurs in endurance athletes who are drinking modestly more than they need but whose kidneys can't keep up by excreting (urinating) the excess, as normally occurs at rest. The retained water dilutes the sodium in the blood. As a defense mechanism, water moves into cells (including brain cells), causing them to swell. This circumstance is particularly problematic in your brain because little room is available to accommodate extra fluid. Thus, changes in mental status, loss of coordination, bizarre behaviors, seizures, and coma are indicative of advanced hyponatremia.

Gaining weight during prolonged exercise is a definite sign of too much water. Using a scale to monitor body weight during multiday events and races is recommended but obviously not always feasible. Drinking a properly formulated sports drink that contains electrolytes (sodium and potassium) is beneficial. But sports drinks alone, even in combination with salty foods, are not enough to prevent hyponatremia if you overdrink or exceed the ability of your kidneys to excrete excess fluid. In other words, taking in sodium during exercise does not make it OK to overdrink.

Following a reasonable eating and drinking plan, even sticking to a tried-and true schedule, isn't foolproof either. In fact, doing so can be downright dangerous. Water retention can set in at any time, and you may not be able to determine why it happens. Besides weight gain, you (and a crew in supported races) must look for and be immediately aware of other signs of water overload, such as bloating, puffiness at sock or short lines, tightening rings and watchbands, tight or shiny skin, nausea and vomiting, and feeling a prominent forehead headache when descending or traveling over bumpy surfaces.

If you associate bloating with getting too much sodium, you're not alone. This is what we've always been told. But the universal finding is that the more weight an athlete gains during prolonged exercise compared with his or her starting weight, the lower the athlete's blood sodium level is likely to be. Bloated athletes are also much more likely to be hyponatremic.

To complicate the picture further, you can't simply go by your ability to urinate or lack thereof, especially during prolonged continuous exercise. This information isn't always reliable in regard to your hydration status. You can be not urinating and thus be relatively overdrinking if you continue to consume fluids over this same period. For example, urinary shutdown can occur because of a jammed urinary overflow valve (why this occurs in some people during exercise is not clear) or an inappropriate release of the antidiuretic hormone vasopressin, which stimulates the kidneys to reabsorb or hold on to water. In other words, we all know that we stop urinating if we're dehydrated. But you also may stop urinating when you are suffering from fluid overload!

Bloated athletes, and often those who are vomiting, who are not urinating but have been drinking are fluid overloaded, not dehydrated. These athletes are on the way to being hyponatremic, if they're not already there. In this situation, concluding that they need to hydrate more until their urine runs clear is incorrect and will only lead to more problems. The bottom line is always the same: Listen to your body. Bloating is the opposite of dehydration—you have too much water on board. The treatment is to stop drinking (even rehydrating sports drinks) and ingest sodium. Do not resume drinking (unless the fluid is a vehicle to deliver sodium, such as a salty broth) until you have urinated the excess fluid. Obviously, to give your body the best chance to accomplish this, you will most likely need to slow your pace dramatically or even stop completely.

Although electrolytes haven't gotten nearly the attention that they deserve, sodium is the other half of the fluid–salt equation. Keeping body fluids (water) and electrolytes (primarily sodium) in balance, especially during prolonged exercise, is what it's really all about. During exercise, water is lost in many ways—through sweat, expired air, urine, diarrhea, vomiting, and bleeding wounds. Electrolytes are also lost by all these routes with the exception of expired air. Sodium is the chief extracellular (outside cells) electrolyte of the body. The amount of sodium that you lose through sweat and urine depends on how fit you are, the preexercise electrolyte stores in your body, and how acclimated you are to the heat.

Sweat is the major route for the loss of sodium. You also lose some potassium through sweat. Potassium, however, is the principal intracellular electrolyte of the body (90 percent of the potassium in the body is stored inside cells). The body actively works to keep potassium within cells, so you don't lose potassium at a rate anywhere near the high rates that you lose sodium. Normal sweat rates for endurance athletes can range from .75 to 2 liters per

Pass the Salt!

Endurance athletes need to consume supplemental salt during prolonged exercise, such as long-distance endeavors, ultras, and events and races lasting longer than a day. Fortunately, sodium comes in many different forms. Your job is threefold: Know the sodium content of the items that you intend to use, realistically estimate the amount that you will need to consume to meet your personal electrolyte needs, and practice your electrolyte replacement in training under various conditions. (Smart athletes also get heat acclimated and continually work at staying cool during prolonged exercise to reduce their sweat losses.)

Item	Amount	Sodium content
Sport Beans	1 oz (28 g)	60 mg
Clif Shot Bloks	1 oz (approx. 3 pieces)	70 mg
Sharkies Organic Energy Fruit Chews	1.58 oz package (45 g)	105 mg
Energy gel	1 packet	40 mg–55 mg
Typical sports drink	8 oz (250 ml)	70 mg–110 mg
Endurance-type sports drink	8 oz	200 mg
Meal replacement beverage	8 oz	130 mg
V8 tomato juice	6 oz (175 ml)	420 mg–550 mg
Potato chips	1 oz	170 mg
Pretzels	1 oz	490 mg
Keebler Toast & Peanut Butter Sandwich Crackers	1 package	410 mg
Table salt	1 pinch (1/8 tsp)	300 mg
Broth	1 cup (one bouillion cube)	900 mg
Hammer Endurolytes	1 capsule	40 mg
Hammer Endurolytes Powder	1 scoop	40 mg
Electrolyte Stamina Tablets	1 tablet	45 mg
Thermotabs	1 tablet	180 mg
Succeed! Caps	1 capsule	341 mg

hour, with a rate of 1 liter an hour being common for an acclimated athlete. This rate of sweating means that the athlete is also losing on average 800 to 1,300 milligrams of sodium per hour.

Our bodies are extremely sensitive to the sodium concentration in the blood and in the fluids outside cells. Compensatory mechanisms help the body retain sodium when faced with sodium losses (such as the hormone aldosterone produced by the adrenal glands), but your body can only do so much. If you keep sweating heavily or long enough without replacing the sodium that you're losing, you will end up with an electrolyte imbalance, such as hyponatremia.

Keep in mind that your sodium needs during exercise are not based on the length of time that you are exercising. Rather, how much sodium you need depends proportionately on how much fluid you need to consume (ingest per hour) to maintain an adequately hydrated weight. Obviously, your fluid needs vary depending on the weather and your acclimatization to the heat. During exercise, you lose sodium primarily through sweat and urine. The sodium concentration in sweat varies considerably among individuals, and during exercise the sodium concentration of urine is about the same as that of sweat. A loss of 1,000 milligrams of sodium per liter of sweat is a reasonable average to assume. One liter equals approximately four cups, so every pound lost during exercise due to body-water loss is equivalent to about .5 liters or two cups.

Before the Event

Give the same time and attention to what, when, and how you're going to eat and drink as you do to your clothing, gear, navigation needs, and other logistical concerns. Remember, a chain is only as strong as its weakest link. If your nutrition game plan falls apart during multiday endurance adventures, so will you.

Knowledge is power: Know what you are getting into. First, is the event or race supported or unsupported? If supported, what fluids and foods are provided, how often, and in what amounts? What will you need to carry or take with you between aid stations or provided meals? During unsupported ventures, such as randonneuring and backcountry adventures, you are responsible for supplying, carrying, or buying what you need along the way. How will you get the job done? What gear do you need? Will you be relying on others?

Gather as much information as you can beforehand regarding the logistics of hydration and fueling along the way so that you know what to expect and plan for. Read books, visit official Web sites, and carefully review participant manuals and nutrition-related recommendations given by credible race directors and event promoters. Talk to other endurance athletes to gain insight and practical advice. Refer to notes that you've kept regarding what has and hasn't worked for you personally during past endurance endeavors.

Have a flexible game plan. You must have a personal nutrition game plan built on basic principles that addresses all your needs: fluid, energy (calories), and electrolytes. You can't just duplicate someone else's plan because what works for a teammate, friend, or highly conditioned elite athlete may not work for you. Practice and become proficient at eating, drinking, and problem solving in shorter events and races before tackling a multiday epic.

That said, what works on one occasion may simply, even mysteriously, stop working or not be tolerated on another day. An upset stomach, for example, is one of the most common problems that an endurance athlete faces. This condition can result from a multitude of factors, however, including unforeseen circumstances. You can often remedy the situation if you stay calm, slow down, and patiently experiment. Your job is to keep trying.

Real problems can arise during a multiday event or race when a strong-willed and uncompromising endurance athlete continues to stick with a game plan that is clearly not working. For example, you may continue to force down a set number of calories, despite evidence that your stomach (through bloating and nausea, for example) isn't able to keep pace. The mistaken belief is that deviating will be worse than making a change on the fly. In reality, every day (or leg of a relay race) is a balancing act between following your preplanned drinking and eating schedule and listening to your body. You'll need to monitor, interpret, and make adjustments depending on the feedback that your body gives. The bottom line: approach hydrating and refueling on the move as a flexible work in progress, not as a rigid schedule.

Choose teammates and support people with care. When you must trust and rely on others, give some serious thought to whom you form partnerships with. Things go much smoother when everyone involved exhibits the same level of commitment, which includes meeting personal fluid and fuel needs from day to day (or leg to leg). Take into account the personalities of all those involved—especially when they are fatigued, sleep deprived, and underfueled. Personality issues can make or break your experience. At the very least, they can make the adventure or race less enjoyable. At worst, not respecting the nutritional component of multiday endurance endeavors can prevent you from finishing or endanger someone's life.

If your race or event takes you outside your country, prepare by researching local resources. Take with you any foodstuffs that you can't do without. If gastrointestinal risks are associated with eating the local cuisine or drinking the water, be cautious leading up to a race or important adventure. Drink only bottled water, pasteurized juice, and soda (without ice). Consider taking extra supplies for the days before you start. Powdered meal replacement products and dehydrated camping fare come in handy before, as well as during, longer events and races. You can prepare all these items with bottled or purified water.

Protein-rich foods are particularly challenging to locate in some countries. Besides protein powders and energy bars, be creative and try jerky, pop-top cans of tuna or chicken, string cheese, individually wrapped rounds of hard cheese, peanut butter, and nuts. These foods provide substantial calories and are appealing complements to the array of sweet-tasting sports foods that you will typically be eating.

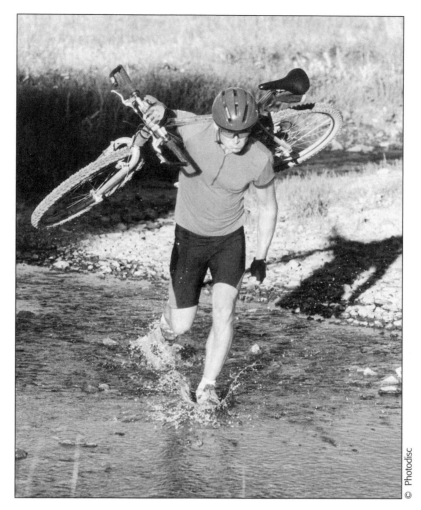

Competing over several days requires drinking and eating continually—no matter what the conditions.

During the Event

Start from the start. Stay on top of your fluid, electrolyte, and fuel needs right from the outset. Your best defense against dehydration, glycogen depletion, hyponatremia, and hypoglycemia is prevention: Never allow yourself to become too depleted of anything. If you go too low, you won't come back. Snack at regular intervals and eat at the start of breaks. This approach allows you to ingest as much as you can reasonably tolerate and have the maximal time to digest and absorb it, thus reducing the risk of digestive system problems.

Divide and conquer. Address hydration, energy, and electrolyte (sodium) needs individually. In other words, don't tie replacing your electrolyte losses with meeting your calorie needs. If you can't eat for a while, for whatever reason, you won't get the electrolytes that you counted on either. Constantly monitor your body. Don't ignore signs such as bloating, mental confusion, or the inability to sweat. For example, you can't become fluid overloaded unless the amount of fluid that you consume exceeds the amount that you lose (through sweat and urine). Drink to thirst and to match your fluid losses, which can vary tremendously depending on your fitness level, sweat rate, and weather conditions.

Stop the bloat. Don't ignore bloating or other signs of having too much water on board. Stop drinking immediately to avoid making the fluid overload worse (unless the fluid is a means to consume salt, such as a salty broth). Ingest salt. Medical experts familiar with endurance exercise suggest using the standard emergency room treatment of 300 to 500 milligrams of sodium, followed by the same amount 10 to 15 minutes later. Athletes typically report feeling better fairly quickly, within 5 to 20 minutes, if the hyponatremia is mild and caught early enough. As soon as your symptoms abate, slow down on ingesting sodium. But you may not be out of the woods. Don't resume drinking until you've urinated the excess fluid. From here on, be extra vigilant at meeting both your fluid needs and your electrolyte needs.

Keep an eye on friends and teammates. Obviously, everyone needs to be responsible for staying on top of personal fluid and fuel needs, but at the same time you must look out for all group members. In adventure races, for example, the first team to cross the finish line together wins. Teams that lose a member because of illness, fatigue, injury, or a team disagreement are disqualified. Relay races and even personal adventures can also end prematurely if someone is unable to continue or needs medical treatment.

Be sure that everyone is eating and drinking. Share fluids and food as needed. Dehydration, depletion of muscle glycogen stores, or a low blood sugar level makes whatever you're doing seem even harder than it is. Be particularly sensitive to mood swings; a friend or teammate in trouble may become extremely quiet or irritable and argumentative.

After the Event

Just do it. Accept the fact that you aren't going to feel hungry or want to eat after exhaustive exercise, especially in warm weather or other extreme conditions. Rely on liquid food. Find a carbohydrate-rich recovery drink and have it ready to go. Start drinking it within the first 15 minutes (no later than 30 minutes after you've stopped for the day) to maximize glycogen replenishment. Include some high-quality protein if feasible (in a meal replacement beverage, for example). At the very least, consume some protein within one to two hours at your next meal.

Replace all three. After long bouts of exercise, especially day after day, you will be deficient in water, calories, and sodium. Don't just consume large amounts of fluid (water or a sports drink), especially if you can't get or keep other items down, or if you're bloated or have gained weight from your starting weight. The smoothest and most complete recovery requires replacing all three components promptly and consistently—water; sodium in a salty beverage, food, or electrolyte supplement; and at least 200 to 300 carbohydrate calories.

Strategies for Team Efforts

Teamwork, efficiency, and constant communication are crucial to the success of a team. During multiday efforts, you, your partner or teammates, or your fellow adventurers, must apply the same skills to hydrating and refueling. Serious adventure racers, in particular, need to learn to travel light and fast.

Determine the food preferences of your teammates or companions beforehand (as well as any food allergies), so that you don't end up carrying food that someone doesn't like or can't eat. Assemble food items in one place, check labels, and together make up food bags containing predetermined amounts of calories.

Keep food and fluids near at hand. Easy access is the name of the game. Wear a bladder system or attach water bottles to the outside of your pack for easy access. Carry your own small stash of quick energy such as dried fruit, fruit-to-go strips, energy bars and gels, trail mix, hard candy, or chocolate in easy-to-reach pockets. In races, don't waste time taking your own pack off and repacking its contents every time you need to eat. Put your stash into the outer pocket of one of your teammates' packs.

Coordinate your refueling efforts with the inevitable stops that you'll be making. Serious adventure racing, for example, requires a considerable amount of stopping for navigational purposes. Plan to access more substantial pre-assembled team food (packaged in large zip-lock bags) at that time (as well as make adjustments in clothing and attend to foot problems). Keep it simple. If racing, place the food in one person's pack so that accessing it doesn't require a lot of effort or thought when you're in a hurry or feeling the effects of sleep deprivation. Remember, if one person needs to eat to continue, then everybody in the group should refuel.

If you're going to race, learn to eat on the run. Experienced adventure racers often combine cold water and dehydrated fare in a resealable container (to avoid spending time heating the water) and throw it into someone's pack. After 20 minutes the concoction is ready to eat. Share with teammates. Take turns passing the container around and squeezing the contents out of one corner—all while on the move, of course.

Make room for extra powdered sports drink (containing sodium) and electrolyte (salt) tablets. These items are worth their weight in gold during multiday races and events. For example, adventure racers competing in weeklong races are required to carry electrolyte tablets because the possibility of consuming only plain water for long periods increases the risk of hyponatremia.

Learning From the Best: Crew-Supported Bike Races and Events

Kerry Ryan, bicycle shop owner and RAAM winner (team division), and Cindy Staiger, a two-time solo finisher and highly sought-after RAAM crew chief who now works as an official for the race, offer their expertise on crew-supported cycling races.

For the Rider

1. Be selective about who makes your crew team. Choose at least one person you respect more than yourself. Otherwise, you won't have anyone to answer to when the going gets tough. In multiday races, in which you increasingly rely on your crew as time passes, be certain that at least one crew person has considerable nutrition knowledge.

2. Be aware of your needs—your typical eating and drinking habits on the bike, what usually works well, what doesn't work—and share this information freely with your crew.

3. Be mentally prepared to drink and eat the calories that you need. If you can't successfully meet your estimated calorie needs in shorter events (for example, a century ride), don't fool yourself into thinking that you can do it for a daylong relay race or multiday race. Establish good habits in shorter rides or races before stepping up to more challenging events.

4. Eat before you get hungry. Devise an hourly refueling schedule and stick to it, whether you feel hungry or not. A stable blood sugar level allows you to think better and stay awake longer. Consume liquid calories and small snacks on the bike. Solid foods tend to promote sleepiness, so supplement with solid foods only when you're not riding. Avoid eating large quantities of food at any one time unless you have a substantial rest break or are going to sleep.

5. Drink plenty of water. Stay on top of your hydration status by monitoring your urine output. If you have difficulty urinating or if your urine is dark yellow, you're dehydrated. Urine that is too clear (like water) indicates that you're overhydrated. Staiger figures that solo riders need to drink at least one full bottle (12 to 16 ounces, or 350 to 500 milliliters) of plain water per hour, besides the high-energy beverages that they are consuming. A rule of thumb is that a rider should be able to urinate a minimum of once every four to six hours.

6. Don't rely on supplements or drugs to improve your performance. The keys to success are training, pacing, eating, and drinking.

7. Go easy on caffeine. Caffeine provides a mental boost and helps you stay awake, but don't underestimate its dehydrating effects during multiday rides and races. Limit your intake, especially during hot weather.

8. To avoid mouth sores, which can make eating unbearable, routinely rinse your mouth with a dilute, tepid solution of 1 tablespoon of antiseptic mouthwash stirred into 8 ounces of water.

9. Settle an upset stomach by consuming saltine crackers or drinking a can of ginger ale, bottled seltzer water, or plain water with a small amount of baking soda stirred in.

For the Crew Team

1. Keep a detailed log. A little planning can go a long way, especially if you're in charge of more than one rider. Make extensive notes on each rider as the race unfolds—weather and terrain; speed and distance covered; estimates of calories required and consumed hourly or per leg; fluids and sodium needed and consumed; pit stops; presence or absence of gastrointestinal distress, muscle cramps, cravings, and low blood sugar; and any other information that you find useful. Keeping a log helps you anticipate and ward off problems before they become insurmountable.

2. Monitor your rider's calorie intake closely. Aim for your rider to stay ahead of, or at least match, estimated calorie needs; otherwise, the body begins to break down its muscles to use as fuel. Individual needs vary, but Staiger figures that riders generally need at least 400 to 600 calories per hour. Don't focus on overloading your rider with protein. Consuming enough overall calories (from whatever source) is what counts.

3. Think of endurance cycling as cycling with scheduled breaks. Plan breaks carefully to incorporate as much as possible into each stop, especially when crewing for solo endurance cyclists. Establish from the start that the rider is required to eat whenever possible, including while standing up during a rest break.

4. Babysit your rider or riders. A rider's success depends on the ability of his or her crew to take care of the smallest details. For example, keep fluids cold to encourage consumption, be certain that riders start each leg with clean water bottles, and keep plenty of salty foods and electrolyte replacement beverages on hand during hot-weather rides. In multiday events, recognize that two to three days of around-the-clock cycling may pass before a rider gives up total decision-making control to his or her crew. When the time comes, be prepared to do everything but push the pedals for your rider.

5. Keep your rider or riders happy about their food. Solid normal food helps riders stay properly fueled and mentally satisfied. Expect the unexpected. As the day or days progress, riders will crave weird foods. Be prepared to get them a small amount of it or a close substitute. If the food they desire goes against your better judgment, convince them to wait until a slightly better time (before going to sleep, for example).

6. Recognize the symptoms of bonking and intervene immediately. Warning signs include lethargy, decreased pedaling cadence or speed, inconsistent thought patterns, shakiness, glazed eyes, and acting spaced out. Treat a low blood sugar level immediately with liquid foods, such as juice, soda, and energy gels (taken with water). In severe cases, the rider may need 60 minutes or longer to revive sufficiently. Monitor your rider's calorie intake more closely after a bonk.

7. Feed yourself. Your rider's safety and success hinge on your ability to carry out your duties. You may not be able to do anything about getting more sleep, but frequent snacking will help you stay awake and be more alert.

13

Rowing and Long-Distance Swimming

"Rhythm and consistency are as important to nutrition as they are to your stroke technique and race strategy. No matter what may be going on during the race, never miss a scheduled feeding."

—Tobie Smith,
Open-Water 25K World Champion
(Perth, Australia, 5:31:20.1)

You may not think that long-distance swimmers and rowers have much in common. After all, long-distance swimmers succeed only by getting in the water, whereas rowers accomplish their goals only by staying out of the water. You may wonder why advice for oarsmen and women is even included in a sports nutrition book for endurance athletes. Rowers classically take part in races lasting less than eight minutes. They don't eat and drink during these races!

From a physiological standpoint, however, rowing is considered a power–endurance sport. To excel as a rower, you must improve your endurance capacity or the ability to perform (produce energy and endure physical demands placed on the body) at a given load over a period of time. The energy systems used during traditional sprint rowing races (as well as the long hours of training required for these intense efforts) mimic those in play during other shorter-range endurance activities, such as running a 5K or 10K road race or competing in a 30K cycling time trial.

A 2,000-meter rowing race can be broken down into three parts: the start phase; the middle, or distance, phase; and the finish, or sprint, phase. Sandwiched between a fast start and, ideally, a fast finish (both fueled by anaerobic metabolism) is the middle, or distance, phase. The longest phase of the race, lasting four to six minutes, this middle phase is fueled by energy produced by the body's aerobic energy system. In fact, the aerobic energy system produces 75 to 80 percent of the metabolic energy used during a rowing race. So, just as foods are grouped with similar items according to their nutrition profiles (eggs are in the meat group not the milk group, because despite being in the dairy case, eggs provide virtually no calcium), rowing is categorized as an endurance sport despite the concurrent emphasis on power and technique.

Today, those who enjoy competing in long-distance swimming and rowing have many opportunities. You may be swimming in a pool or in open water, rowing outside (sprints or longer head races or even marathons), or on an indoor ergometer. Rowathlons, similar to triathlons except that indoor rowing replaces the swimming leg, are also growing in popularity. Like all other endurance athletes, active people and athletes involved in long-distance swimming and rowing require a well-thought-out nutrition game plan on race day.

Rowing

Despite being engaged in one of the most physically demanding endurance sports, competitive rowers as a group are often hampered by nutrition misinformation, dehydration, the risk of chronic glycogen depletion due to high-volume training, difficulty maintaining weight as the season progresses (among male heavyweights, for example), and unhealthy practices to manage or lose weight (especially among lightweight rowers). Chapters 1 through 8 on eating smart every day while training are definitely appropriate and essential for all rowers to read and put into practice.

2,000-Meter Race

In collegiate and international rowing, the standard racing course is a distance of 2,000 meters (2K), requiring an all-out effort lasting approximately six to eight minutes. Rowers, depending on their individual size and fitness level, will burn approximately 25 to 35 calories per minute during this intense effort. If a rower goes into the race having followed a smart sports diet during the training period, he or she should have more than adequate glycogen stored in the muscles (up to 300 to 400 grams of glycogen or 1,200 to 1,600 calories) and liver (100 grams or 400 calories) to fuel the anaerobic and aerobic demands placed on working muscles during the race. In other words, rowers do not have to carbohydrate-load or superload the muscles with glycogen as a marathoner or cyclist attempting a century ride (100 miles) would benefit from doing.

Regattas typically last from two days to a week, with competitors progressing through heats and semifinals (and possibly repecharges) to earn a berth in the finals. Outside the top echelons of the sport, rowers typically compete in more than one race per day. As a rower, your goal on race day, with regard to nutrition, is to show up at each race with enough glycogen stored in your working muscles to fuel about eight minutes or less of intense exercise. Remember, carbohydrate is the only fuel that you can burn during flat-out exercise because of the limited availability of oxygen.

The primary issue, however, is not so much what you eat prerace (for example, what you eat for dinner the night before) but how good a job you do at maintaining glycogen levels in your muscles from day to day. Rowers, especially those overly concerned about or struggling to maintain a desired weight, run the greatest risk of gradually depleting glycogen stores while preparing for competitions and never allowing their muscles to regain their full potential supply. A rower may then enter a competition with glycogen stores that are unable to sustain an all-out competitive effort. During competitions, with much of the race day tied up in prerace preparations and the race itself, rowers also need to make recovery nutrition a priority. Keep appropriate carbohydrate-rich snacks at your fingertips at all times and commit to consuming those items as soon as possible after each race.

Dehydration is a common and often underappreciated foe of competitive rowers because of sweat losses incurred during rowing (even in cold weather), making-weight practices, or simply from being outdoors in the sun watching the competition. Dehydration is particularly detrimental to rowers who engage in drastic regimes to make weight, such as severely restricting fluids, reducing food intake, and continuing to exercise strenuously in the days leading up to the race. Despite what you tell yourself, it's simply not possible after the weigh-in to normalize your physiology and restore your blood volume to its full capacity. A study published in the *Journal of Medicine and Science in Sports and Exercise* ("Rowing Performance, Fluid Balance and Metabolic Function Following Dehydration and Rehydration") simulating these very conditions found that rowers were able to restore only half of the lost blood plasma by drinking fluids following their weigh-in. In terms of performance over a 2,000-meter course, rowers who had dehydrated and attempted to rehydrate were 15 meters behind. To top off stores of fluid, carbohydrate, and electrolytes, sports drinks are the drink of choice for all rowers, prerace and afterward, especially those who are rehydrating after weigh-ins.

Due to the limited weight classifications in the sport of rowing, many rowers find themselves struggling to reach or maintain a weight required for lightweight classification. Internationally, the maximum race weight for lightweight men is 72.5 kilograms (159.84 pounds). At the elite level, the boat (crew) average must not exceed 70 kilograms (154.32 pounds). For lightweight women, the maximum race weight is generally 59.0 kilograms (130 pounds). At the women's elite level, the boat average must not exceed 57 kilograms (125 pounds).

Further complicating the rower's preparation is that lightweight rowers must weigh in before each race, resulting in less than ideal race preparations. As with all athletes in weight-making sports, lightweight rowers will benefit from partnering with qualified medical professionals, such as sports medicine physicians and sports dietitians, to receive expert individualized advice about establishing an optimal weight with minimal consequences to health and performance. As the previously mentioned study reveals, a long-term plan to manage body weight that allows the rower to start the race fully hydrated is the best approach.

Head Races, Marathon Rows, and Other Rowing Events

Rowers may compete in venues other than 2,000-meter races, from head races (time trials of five to seven kilometers, or three to more than four miles, in length) to marathon rows. Extreme endurance athletes may tackle ultra ocean rowing challenges, such as rowing across the Atlantic! As for endurance sports in general, as the duration of the rowing event increases, prerace fueling and what and how you drink and eat during the race become more and more critical to your success.

Carbohydrate loading is necessary, for example, if you'll be rowing continuously for 90 to 120 minutes or more at race pace or if you will be rowing several times over a period of several hours or longer (see chapter 4). Rowers, like mountain bikers and Nordic skiers, literally have their hands full during a race, so marathon rowers and ultrarowers can experiment with wearing a hip belt or backpack-style reservoir hydration pack that holds a considerable volume of fluid that is delivered through a flexible drinking tube. Sports drinks, supplying needed fluid, carbohydrate, and electrolytes, are the drink of choice during these prolonged races.

All calories are good calories during prolonged exercise, so keep sports foods like energy gels and bars (in various flavors to combat flavor fatigue) and other tolerated solid foods readily accessible. As the distance (or time rowing) increases, food plays an increasingly significant role in maintaining a positive frame of mind, so have a variety of your favorites available. Athletes involved in extreme rowing challenges, such as the Woodvale Atlantic Rowing Race (more than 2,500 nautical miles) will benefit greatly from seeking personalized nutritional advice, including preplanned high-calorie meal plans, from a qualified sports nutrition expert.

Learning From the Best:
Nutrition Race-Day Tips for Competitive Rowers

As a rower involved in sprint events and head races, your nutrition goals for race day are simple. You want to top off your fluid and fuel (glycogen) stores and correctly time your last meal so that you feel comfortable rowing during the race. Stacey Borgman, half of the winning duo in the B Final of the Olympic women's lightweight double sculls (7:23:40) held in Athens, shares tips on how to get the job done. Borgman currently coaches a junior recreational rowing program in Lake Oswego, Oregon.

(continued)

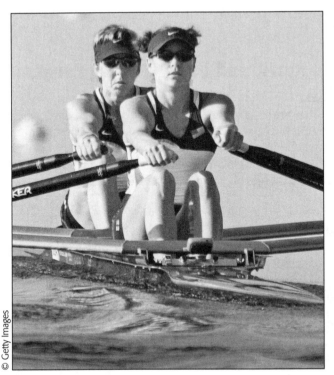

© Getty Images

Stacey Borgman (at stern) relies on high-performance eating habits, not diets, to make weight and preserve muscle mass.

Get Ready Before the Race

No matter how early in the day your race is scheduled, have something for breakfast! If the race is later in the day, Borgman recommends eating a normal breakfast and to avoid trying to row on a full stomach, eating a light lunch slightly earlier than you normally would. From there, if you get hungry, eat small snacks like fruit, granola bars, or a few nuts, or sip on a sports drink. Energy bars are also good to eat between races or if you're hungry right before a race and want to avoid that full or sluggish feeling.

Establish a Routine After the Race

Get off the water, put your boat up, and get a drink. Borgman made it a habit to carry a sports drink and snacks in her gear bag so that she could get started right away, especially if she was racing again that day.

Nutrition Recommendations for Head Races

Head races can be brutal because of the cold and wind. Keep in mind that you'll be on the water twice as long as the time that you spend actually racing, rowing to the starting line or back from the finish line, so you'll be rowing for an hour or more. Expect that you'll also be rowing into the wind in at least one direction! You'll get thirsty and hungry, so plan for it. Borgman requires all her athletes to carry at least a water bottle filled with a sports drink in their boat, as well as an energy gel or bar to have after crossing the finish line.

Avoid the Most Common Nutrition Mistakes

From her perspective as a lightweight, Borgman routinely sees rowers who believe that they can stop eating entire food groups and still keep rowing to make weight. Unhealthy and unsuccessful approaches typically include cutting out all foods with fat or attempting to avoid carbohydrates and eat just protein. Borgman stresses balance—carbohydrate, protein, and fat and the need to eat meals that include all three. Eliminating one or two of these elements for any length of time is senseless. Your body isn't going to last. Borgman always relied on real food, not bars and sports drinks, to keep her system going from day to day.

Advice for Lightweight and Other Weight-Conscious Rowers

To keep your metabolism going, you have to eat! I never was dieting. What I was doing was for my sport, not for the way I looked. I spent three months getting down to weight so I could go to the championships! I would always relax in the winter and let my body go back to its natural weight. I've watched a lot of rowers with potential who never make it because they get caught up in the weight stuff versus the sport itself. Don't do something to look good, like trying to keep at your racing weight year round. Do what is best for your performance.

How to Maintain Weight as the Season Progresses

The number-one priority is to keep eating, but not by filling up on junk to keep weight on. Make sure that you eat three to four real meals and eat snacks between them. Take in lots of protein and carbohydrate from real food. Always carry healthy snacks with you. Protein shakes or fruit smoothies and sports drinks really help.

Indoor Rowing

The sport of indoor rowing was born in 1981 after the advent of the rowing machine. Today it attracts millions of competitors throughout the world. The blue-ribbon championship race distance is 2,000 meters, with recognized age-group records for this distance as well as a range of other distances. Every winter, national championships take place in the United States, almost every European country, and many other countries throughout the world. A world indoor rowing championship is held every February in Boston (United States).

For those with hardy seats and hands, indoor marathon and ultrarowing races are also available. The individual marathon distance is 42,195 meters, and the half-marathon distance is 21,097 meters. Other events include group or individual 100,000-meter rows, group or individual million-meter rows, group or individual 24-hour rows, and group or individual longest continuous time rows. For individual efforts in the standard distances, records are kept for lightweight (165 pounds, or 75 kilograms, and under for men; 135 pounds, or 61.4 kilograms, and under for women) and heavyweight categories. The weight is taken at the beginning of the row.

Outdoors or inside—it doesn't matter. The longer the rowing challenge, the more you enhance your odds of being successful by embracing an endurance athlete's nutrition weapons. This means drinking fluids with all your meals and snacks and including some salty foods (or adding extra salt to the foods that you eat) in the days leading up to the race, carbohydrate loading, topping off your liver glycogen stores by eating breakfast, and managing your energy and carbohydrate needs (at least 30 to 60 grams per hour) throughout the event by consistently consuming sports drinks, sports foods, and as many other solid foods as you can tolerate.

Long-Distance Swimming

As defined by United States Master Swimming, a long-distance pool event is any distance-based swimming event over 1,650 yards (1508.8 meters) or a time-based event equal to or greater than one hour. The event may occur in any body of water, either natural or manmade. A long-distance open-water event is a swimming event of any distance conducted in an open body of water, either natural or manmade. Open-water championship races are held at various distances (from 1 mile to 6 or more miles), and a myriad of other open-water swimming events and challenges exist today for adventuresome ultraswimmers. A 10K open-water race is now part of the Olympics (as of 2008).

Open-water swimmers face particular challenges on race day—not only swimming the required distance and maintaining a good pace throughout the swim but also withstanding the cold for the requisite time and appreciating the general weather conditions (particularly the wind). If refueling (30 to 60 grams of carbohydrate per hour) during a long-distance open-water race is not possible, preloading is the next best option. This is best accomplished by eating small meals frequently (for example, three meals and three snacks, including one at bedtime, followed by breakfast) rather than stuffing yourself the night before or the morning of the swim.

Learning From the Best: Tips for Open-Water Swimmers

With help from competitive open-water swimmer Karen Burton, a two-time U.S. marathon swim champion and long-time national open-water team coordinator, and Tobie Smith, a former open-water 25K world champion, I put together these nutrition pointers:

1. **Prerace: Start the race well hydrated and well fueled.** Increase your glycogen stores by preloading with carbohydrate-rich foods and supplemental high-carbohydrate drinks (50 to 70 grams per 8 ounces) for at least three days before the race. You may experience some lethargy and feel sleepier than normal, so you may need to nap more than usual. Drink plenty of fluid leading up to the race. Smith advises choosing bland foods that go down easily and settle well the night before. And she reminds swimmers that going to bed hungry the night before a long race is foolish! Plan to eat the morning of the race too.

2. **During the race: Feed on a regular, consistent schedule.** The standard feeding schedule is 8 ounces of an electrolyte and fluid-recovery drink every 15 minutes. Aim for 20 grams of carbohydrate per feed, or 70 to 80 grams per hour. In warm-water races, try to keep drinks slightly chilled on the boat,

but not freezing cold. Smith made her drinks at a slightly stronger concentration so that she could really taste them. A flavored drink is particularly refreshing when swimming in saltwater, because your mouth and tongue start to swell and your throat burns from the saltwater. In cold-water races, warm drinks can help you insulate from the inside out.

Avoid drinking only water if you will be swimming for more than 90 minutes, because you need the carbohydrate and electrolytes provided by a sports drink. In five seconds or less you should be able to grab a cup held out on a feeding stick or by hand, roll on your back, drink, dump the cup, and return to swimming.

Don't skip feeds, especially if you're feeling good and everything is going to plan. Be sure to experiment in training with the drink that you plan to use during the race. Plan to drink most of the calories that you need. Urinating every 30 minutes or so is a good sign that you're drinking enough, although this interval varies depending on the water temperature. You may urinate more frequently when swimming in cold water, and you will likely urinate less frequently while swimming in warm-water races.

3. **Bring solid foods as backup energy.** Cookies, energy bars (precut into small pieces), canned fruit, bananas, and candy are some options. You need something on the boat to give yourself a lift during low points in the middle of the race. The calories that these foods supply should supplement the calories provided by your drink. Be sure to drop your feeds to every 10 to 12 minutes, or even less, if you are feeling poorly. A low blood sugar level can manifest as weakness and loss of power. If your crew hasn't caught on, yell, "Feed!" if you want quicker feeds.

4. **Postrace: Replenish glycogen stores soon after the race.** Expect to be tired, achy, and uncomfortable afterward. Speed your recovery time by immediately drinking 32 ounces (1 liter) of a high-carbohydrate beverage. Eat a meal within two hours of completing the race. The race isn't over when you stop swimming. During the open-water swimming season, you may swim three or four weekends in a row, so recovery is paramount. Expect your appetite to increase during the few days following a race. You may become hungry quickly, so eat often and be prepared by keeping essential foods on hand.

5. **Be sensitive to air and water temperatures.** Open-water swims can take place in conditions ranging from 60°F (16°C) water with 50°F (10°C) air temperatures all the way up to 83°F (28°C) water with 90°F (32°C) air temperatures.

In general, you'll need extra fluids and feeds for both extremes. In hot-weather races especially, you run the risk of dehydration. In cold-water races, you burn fuel much more quickly trying to keep up your core body temperature. In warm-weather races, increase your feeds to as often as every six to eight minutes or double your feeds by drinking one cup of water along with a

(continued)

cup of a fluid and electrolyte-replacement drink. Pack a cooler of ice to keep drinks cool during warm-weather races. For cold-water races, bring hot water to make feeds.

6. **Be aware of the symptoms of hypothermia, which can occur in warm water as well as cold water.** Remember, if you've been swimming in a pool with water temperatures above 80°F (27°C), competing in 70°F (21°C) water can feel cold. Becoming dehydrated also predisposes you to hypothermia. Early signs include feeling cold (especially along the back), being unable to hold your fingers together while swimming, and shivering.

   The trainer or coach on the boat makes the call of when to pull a swimmer from the water. Don't leave this decision up to the swimmer. A swimmer in trouble will be unable to swim in a straight line, appear blue, have difficulty speaking, and may be disoriented. If in doubt, the coach should ask the swimmer some thought-provoking questions, such as the name of a family member, or ask the swimmer to count backward from 20.

7. **Feed the crew.** Be sure that the boat crew has enough food and beverages. An open-water swim means a long day on the water for the crew, and you depend on them always to be alert.

8. **Develop a healthy relationship about your body weight and body-fat percentage.** A couple of extra pounds and a higher body-fat percentage can be advantageous for open-water swimmers, providing buoyancy and improving tolerance for cold water. Follow a sensible diet of mostly carbohydrate and adequate protein and fat, and let your weight fall where it will.

9. **Be prepared for the challenges associated with international races.** Bring with you any drink mixes or foods that you plan to use during the race. Prepare your own bottles using powdered mixes and bottled water. Because you may be without your usual support crew, be sure to discuss your feeding schedule with whoever will be in charge on your boat. If necessary, set a watch alarm to beep every 15 minutes to remind yourself of your feeds.

   To avoid becoming sick before the race, follow the standard precautions for eating and drinking in a foreign country. If you have concerns about the quality of the water that you'll be swimming in, don't wait until you arrive and are ready to dive in. Contact your physician or local health department and obtain a gamma globulin injection, as well as a tetanus booster if necessary (once every 10 years), before you depart.

Extreme Heat

14

"In the heat, I especially don't overdo things early in the race (like energy gels) that I know I'm going to rely on late in the race."

—Scott Jurek, the course-record holder and seven-time defending champion of the Western States 100-Mile Endurance Run and the course-record holder and defending champion of the Badwater Ultramarathon

You've probably heard the saying "When the going gets tough, the tough get going." Obviously, this adage refers to endurance athletes. Who else would be dedicated (or crazy) enough to push their bodies to the limit for a T-shirt or a belt buckle? And I mean push—through snowdrifts, haze shimmering off sun-baked asphalt roads, and thin air found on high mountain ridges.

Often held under mind-boggling conditions, endurance events ultimately come down to a battle with Mother Nature. She sets the rules, and anything goes. Be prepared to broil, pant, and freeze, sometimes all in one day. To persevere (or just plain survive) you must be able to handle challenging conditions. Heat, humidity, cold, and high altitude challenge the best of athletes. Whether you want to compete in endurance sports or you simply enjoy hiking, mountaineering, or skiing, reading the next three chapters will help you learn about nutritional strategies for dealing with extreme environmental conditions. First, let's look at how to beat the heat!

Temperature Regulation

How is it possible to go from freezing temperatures to 90°F (32°C) without breaking a stride? Thank your body's thermostat—the hypothalamus. Located at the base of the brain, the hypothalamus receives signals from two sets of thermoreceptors. Central receptors sense changes in the temperature of your blood as it circulates through the hypothalamus; peripheral receptors monitor the temperature of your skin and the environment around you. Because your hypothalamus has a predetermined temperature, or set point, that it seeks to maintain, your body must deal quickly with fluctuations in body temperature.

When your body temperature rises, your hypothalamus signals into action the sweat glands and blood vessels in your skin. Your blood vessels dilate, or open wider, bringing more blood and the heat that it carries to your skin, where the heat can escape to the environment. At the same time, your sweat glands produce more sweat. As this moisture evaporates, it pulls heat from the skin. If your body temperature falls, your blood vessels constrict, so you lose less heat across the skin. You also begin to shiver, which raises your metabolism and generates heat. Several hormones, such as thyroxine (from your thyroid gland) and epinephrine and norepinephrine (from your adrenal glands) can also increase your metabolic rate, thereby increasing the amount of heat that you produce internally.

Extreme cold and heat limit your ability to exercise, particularly if you're trying to compete. For example, in hot weather your working muscles and skin compete for a limited supply of blood. Your muscles need blood and the oxygen that it carries to keep working. Your body, however, must divert blood to the skin to take the heat generated by working muscles to the surface to keep you cool. At some point, neither your muscles nor your skin receive enough blood flow to function optimally. In cold environments, trouble sets in when you dissipate heat faster than you produce it. In either case, you can exacerbate the situation by not paying close attention to your fuel and fluid needs.

Performing in Extreme Heat

From a physiological standpoint, you encounter the most severe stress when you exercise in the heat. You must deal with the heat gained from the combination of physical exertion and the hot environment. Nevertheless, you still rely primarily on the evaporation of sweat to shed excess heat and remain (relatively) cool. Although sweating is a vital thermoregulatory mechanism for removing heat, it comes at a price. Dehydration results if you don't take in enough fluids to keep pace with your sweat loss. An average-size person (110 to 165 pounds, or 50 to 75 kilograms) might lose 1.5 to 2.5 quarts (liters) of sweat, or 2 to 4 percent of his or her body weight, each hour during an intense effort on a hot, humid day. Fluid losses of as little as 2 percent of body weight (for example, a weight loss of three pounds for a 150-pound athlete, or 1.4 kilograms for a 68-kilogram athlete) can impair performance (see table 14.1).

To provide a cooling effect, sweat must evaporate, not just drip off your skin. That's why humid conditions hinder your athletic performance—less sweat evaporates off your skin because the air is already saturated with water. Consequently, you dramatically increase your risk of heat illness when you face the dual challenge of exercising in heat and high humidity. For example, exercise physiologists estimate that a marathoner who typically runs a mara-

Table 14.1 Effects of Dehydration

Body weight lost from sweating	Physiological effect
1%–2%	Thirst, some fatigue, minor loss of strength
3%–4%	Reduced maximal aerobic power and endurance, compromised ability to regulate body temperature, increased chance of overheating
5%–6%	Headache, decreased concentration, decreased cardiac output, chills, nausea, faster breathing, rapid pulse
7%–10%	Dizziness, muscle spasms, poor balance, exhaustion, collapse, potential cardiogenic shock, coma

thon in two and a half hours will be almost five minutes slower over the same distance when the thermometer hits 80 degrees.

Exercising in hot weather decreases your economy, or efficiency. In other words, you use more fuel to perform at a particular pace or intensity compared with exercising under cooler conditions. As you become progressively dehydrated from failing to take in enough fluids to match your sweat losses, your blood volume falls and your heart compensates by beating faster. Working muscles receive less blood flow and less oxygen in the heat (as blood is rerouted to the skin for cooling purposes), so they use more muscle glycogen and produce more lactic acid. This adjustment helps explain why a given effort in the heat leaves you feeling more fatigued and exhausted than undertaking the same effort in cooler weather.

Heat Acclimatization

The body acclimatizes to heat after approximately 7 to 14 days of training in warm conditions, although how quickly you adapt and to what extent is highly individual. The physiological adaptations that occur better prepare you for future exercise bouts in the heat. Within the first few days, you begin to sweat earlier and at an increased rate. (Remember, sweating allows you to eliminate excess heat and hold down your internal body temperature, so more blood flows to your working muscles.) Various hormonal messages will signal your sweat glands to reabsorb valuable electrolytes such as sodium and chloride. Sweating triggers the release of other hormones, which stimulate your kidneys to excrete less sodium and reabsorb more water. Thus, your body attempts to compensate for fluid and minerals lost through heavy sweating by reducing their losses in urine. After you are acclimated to the heat, you reduce the rate at which your muscles use glycogen during exercise in the heat by as much as 50 to 60 percent.

Don't underestimate the importance of making small adjustments when training in the heat, such as wearing light-colored, loose-fitting clothing, seeking out shady training routes, and taking longer rest breaks. While training in the swamplike conditions of Washington, D.C. (often 80 degrees and 85 percent humidity at 6:30 a.m. during the summer), I managed with early morning runs or headed to the pool for water-running sessions instead. When weather patterns change abruptly or you travel to a warmer climate, reduce your pace and training volume for at least the first few days. If you're competing, lower your expectations of what you can reasonably and safely accomplish.

Dehydration, Hyponatremia, and Heat Illnesses

The dangers of exercising in the heat include severe dehydration, heat cramps, and potentially more serious conditions such as heat exhaustion, heat stroke, and hyponatremia (blood sodium depletion).

Dehydration

Dehydration, or the loss of body fluid, is the most common problem that plagues athletes of all ages and abilities who undertake endurance events or races in the heat. Besides throwing off track your ability to regulate your body temperature, dehydration reduces your strength, power, endurance, and aerobic capacity. Many endurance athletes I meet believe that they need to be less careful about replacing fluids as they become acclimated to the heat. In fact, you need to drink more to offset your enhanced sweating response. As you become progressively dehydrated, you negate your improved ability to tolerate heat. Dehydration may also be behind the gastrointestinal woes that many marathoners and ultrarunners suffer from.

Think of dehydration as a fierce competitor that won't let go. When you become dehydrated beyond 2 percent of your body weight during exercise, your heart rate and body temperature rise and your performance really begins to suffer. Fluid losses of 3 to 5 percent of your body weight can significantly impair your performance, and losses of more than 5 percent of your body weight are dangerous. There is no way to adapt to dehydration, so don't even try.

Hyponatremia

Athletes (especially women) competing in endurance and ultraendurance events in the heat and humidity are at particular risk of developing hyponatremia, or a blood sodium level below the normal range of 136 to 143 millimoles per liter. Research done in the 1990s on triathletes who were competing in the Hawaii Ironman triathlon, for example, found that almost 30 percent of the finishers were hyponatremic. Hyponatremia can result from losing large amounts of sodium (for example, through prolonged sweating), but the more likely cause is drinking too much fluid (especially plain water) beyond what you need, either before, during, or following prolonged exercise. Your blood sodium level drops as you replace the fluid, but not the sodium, lost through sweating by drinking large amounts of sodium-free (plain water) or low-sodium fluid. Essentially, the sodium concentration in your body becomes diluted.

Meltdown Man

Although many anecdotes relate the travails suffered by those who become dehydrated when exercising in the heat, one of the most highly publicized and horrifying encounters befell Australian Mark Dorrity, often referred to as the Meltdown Man. In the Australian summer of 1988, Mark and a few friends began an 8K run at 2:30 in the afternoon when the ambient temperature was in excess of 100°F (38°C). In fact, the fun run in which the men were supposed to take part had been postponed from 2:30 until 5:30 in the hope that temperatures would be cooler. Well in the lead near the end of the run, Mr. Dorrity, 28 years old and in good physical condition, suddenly collapsed and was in such obvious trouble that he was transported directly to a hospital.

Upon admission, his body temperature was 107.6°F (42°C). A tracheotomy was immediately performed to support the pulmonary ventilation that his impaired respiratory system could not maintain. Because his immune system was subdued and his blood-clotting mechanisms were impaired by his high body temperature, an opportunistic infection set in, a result of a scrape sustained on his left leg when he initially collapsed. Over the next few days, the muscles of his left leg turned a khaki color and had the stringy texture of overcooked meat. This accelerated rhabdomyolosis (degeneration of skeletal muscle tissue)—overenthusiastically and inaccurately referred to as meltdown in the Australian press—caused acute renal failure, requiring months of dialysis. Twenty-seven days after admission, the leg was amputated at the hip. Mark remained comatose for 132 days before regaining consciousness and beginning years of convalescence.

Reprinted, by permission, from R. Murray, 1995, "Fluid needs in hot and cold environments," *International Journal of Sport Nutrition* 5: S62–73.

Although consuming a sports drink rather than just plain water during exercise isn't a definitive cure-all, it's a must for those athletes at the highest risk for hyponatremia, such as slower-pace marathoners (those who run or walk for more than four hours) and triathletes on the move for longer than 9 to 13 hours. Female athletes in general tend to be at higher risk for hyponatremia because of their comparatively smaller starting blood volume. Women are also more apt to heed published guidelines about drinking during exercise!

If you develop a headache while exercising and become nauseous, lethargic, confused, or disoriented, seek medical attention immediately. In severe cases of hyponatremia, athletes lapse into unconsciousness, develop epileptic-like seizures, and may stop breathing or suffer cardiac arrest (see table 14.2.). Just one example is a woman who died because of hyponatremia after having collapsed at mile 24 of the 1998 LaSalle Bank Chicago Marathon. Despite the fact that an international panel of hydration experts declared that exertional hyponatremia during exercise was relatively rare (evidence-based studies

Table 14.2 Warning Signs of Dehydration and Hyponatremia

Dehydration	Hyponatremia
Early: headache, fatigue, dizziness, nausea, vomiting, dry mouth and eyes, loss of appetite, flushed skin, heat intolerance or exhaustion, dark-colored urine with a strong odor, irritability, muscle cramps, weight loss	**Early:** feeling bloated, nausea and vomiting, visible bloating (swollen hands and feet, watch or rings feel tight, bloated stomach), dizziness, throbbing headache, rapid weight gain, pale-colored urine (looks like water), cramping
More advanced: difficulty swallowing, clumsiness, abnormal chills, shriveled skin, sunken eyes and dim vision, inability to urinate, delirium, heat stroke	**More advanced:** restlessness, malaise, apathy, confusion, disorientation, severe fatigue or weakness, respiratory distress, seizure, coma

predict that probably less than 1 in 1,000 finishers of endurance events such as a marathon or triathlon will be affected), the American College of Sports Medicine released updated guidelines on hydration and physical activity in 2005 to educate the public on both dehydration and hyponatremia.

If the ultraendurance event that you compete in features weigh-ins, be aware that gaining weight while exercising is a red flag that you are overhydrated and at increased risk for developing hyponatremia. Eating salty foods in the days before the event and consuming beverages containing sodium before, during, and after prolonged exercise, such as sports drinks and soup or broth, is usually sufficient to ward off or slow the progression of hyponatremia.

Heat Cramps

If you've ever suffered from heat cramps or watched someone else do so, you won't soon forget the experience. Severe cramps hit the skeletal muscles most heavily used during exercise. For endurance athletes, that means abdomen, calf (lower leg), quadriceps (front of the thigh), and hamstring (back of the thigh) muscles. During my first adventure race, our three-person team had to kayak, mountain bike, trail run, and conquer various obstacles together along the course. We encountered a hot (over 90°F, or 32°C), sunny day in Portland, Oregon. Unfortunately, our star athlete, although blessed with a competitive spirit, was low on physical conditioning and had just stepped off a plane from England, where he had been working for the previous year. An hour in the kayak and two more on the bike didn't seem to faze him, until he hopped off the bike. He collapsed to the ground with severe cramps in both quadriceps. Having survived two hours of single-track mountain biking, I was not about to miss the chance to put my running background to good use. With the help of a sports drink and electrolyte tablets, we got him up and running.

You don't necessarily have to be dehydrated to experience heat cramps. Low levels of minerals involved in muscle contraction such as sodium and chloride, are most likely the major cause of heat cramps. You put yourself at risk if you sweat heavily for several hours and rehydrate only with plain water. To prevent heat cramps, acclimate to hot and humid conditions as much as possible, be liberal with the saltshaker in your daily diet, and rely on sports drinks rather than plain water for prolonged, strenuous exercise in the heat.

Heat Exhaustion

Heat exhaustion, or the inability to continue exercising in the heat, results from dehydration. You might recall photographs of then-President Jimmy Carter attempting to race the hilly Catoctin Mountain Park 10K run on a hot, humid September morning. Ashen-faced, staggering, and dazed, he was forced to drop out slightly past the halfway mark even though he had trained for the race. When you suffer from heat exhaustion, your cardiovascular system simply can't meet the simultaneous demands of sending blood to your active muscles and your skin. This situation occurs as your blood volume drops because of the excessive loss of fluid or minerals from sweating. Your thermoregulatory mechanisms are still working, but you can't dissipate heat quickly enough because too little blood (and the heat it carries) goes to your skin.

Signs of heat exhaustion to watch for during exercise include extreme thirst, headache, weakness, dizziness, heat sensations on the head or neck, abdominal cramps, chills, goose bumps, nausea, and vomiting. You may also hyperventilate (breathe rapidly and deeply), act confused, and possibly even faint. The risk of suffering heat exhaustion increases if you're exercising at or near your maximum capacity, are dehydrated, aren't physically fit, or are not yet acclimated to the heat. Athletes suffering from heat exhaustion should stop all activity immediately and seek a cooler environment (get in the shade or an air-conditioned area if available). If you're coherent and conscious, consume fluids, preferably beverages that contain sodium such as sports drinks, tomato juice, or soup. Force yourself to drink, even if you're feeling nauseous.

Heat Stroke

If left untreated, heat exhaustion can deteriorate to a potentially life-threatening disorder called heat stroke. Characterized by severe hyperthermia, when the body temperature rises to dangerously high levels (exceeding 104°F, or 40°C), heat stroke can permanently damage the central nervous system or even kill the person. During heat stroke, the thermoregulatory mechanisms of the body fail because of excessive heat buildup and excessive dehydration. Symptoms include vomiting, diarrhea, disorientation, convulsions, and unconsciousness. The person may stop sweating altogether, and the skin will feel hot and dry. Rapid cooling of the entire body is crucial.

Don't be lulled into thinking that heat stroke is a possibility only on the hottest day of the year. Incidents of heat stroke have been reported in cool to moderate environments (55°F to 82°F, or 13°C to 28°C). Several factors that may increase your risk of heat stroke include being overweight or in poor physical condition, advanced age, lack of sleep, alcohol or drug use, having a sunburn, not being acclimated to the heat, and having previously suffered a heat injury.

Nutritional Strategies for Beating the Heat

Let's assume that you are physically fit, heat acclimated, well rested, and well fueled for whatever endeavor you choose to undertake in the heat. What else can you do to maximize your chances of performing well? You can work to minimize the risk of both dehydration and hyponatremia in several ways.

Before the Event

- **Know your hourly sweat rate.** Fluid and electrolyte needs of fitness and sports-minded people are widely variable depending on a person's genetics and the specific environmental conditions under which the endurance exercise takes place. Cyclists, for example, may not appreciate how much they sweat because of how quickly it evaporates. Aim to determine your hourly sweat rate while training under the same or similar heat and humidity conditions that you expect to encounter during the event or on race day. You can estimate your average hourly sweat rate by this formula (see page 80 for more examples):

  Preexercise weight (convert to ounces) – postexercise weight (ounces) + fluid intake during exercise (ounces) = individual hourly sweat rate

  Notes: Pre- and postexercise weights refer to nude body weight.
  Duration of exercise is one hour.
  Every pound lost = 16 ounces of fluid.
  This formula assumes no urine output during this period.

- **Practice drinking while on the move during longer training or preevent efforts.** Your main job before you undertake or compete in an endurance event, especially one that takes place in the heat, is to practice how to replace or match as closely as possible during exercise the total amount of fluid and electrolytes that you lose through sweating (your hourly sweat rate). Now is the time to develop a fluid plan and to experiment with bladders and other hydration systems to determine which is best for your particular sport or situation. If you're responsible for meeting your own fluid needs (no aid stations), figure out how you are going to carry the fluid that you need or how you will resupply along the way. If the race organizers will be supplying the sports drink, find out in advance what brand will be offered on the course so that you can experiment with it during your longer training efforts.

- **Pass the saltshaker.** If you're a normal healthy adult, your body has several sophisticated mechanisms for regulating how much sodium you take in and retain, so you don't have to make a conscious effort to restrict your intake. When faced with hot weather, especially seasonal changes or an event in a hotter region that you will travel to, add salt to the foods that you eat or consume sodium-rich foods such as bouillon, canned soup or beans, cheese, tomato or vegetable juice, pretzels, salted crackers, and other low-fat snack foods. The sodium in these foods (and in the sports beverages that you drink before and during exercise) will help you retain water and avoid a sodium deficit, as well as boost your drive to drink.

Even if you're fit and well acclimated to the heat, you can lose large amounts of sodium and chloride through extensive and repetitive sweating (115 to 700 milligrams of sodium or more per liter of sweat), along with the sodium typically excreted in urine. For some endurance athletes during prolonged exercise, such as those with high sweat rates of 2.5 liters per hour, this could translate into a substantial loss of sodium exceeding 1,500 milligrams per hour. You can exacerbate this sodium deficit if you consciously follow a low-salt diet (as in the 2,400 milligram a day recommended limit for inactive people) and incur persistent sodium losses from prolonged training and competitions.

- **Experiment with electrolytes (salt) tablets and other salty foods.** For those who undertake prolonged efforts or have previously suffered a heat illness, ingesting salt or electrolyte tablets (which contain primarily sodium) during prolonged endurance exercise may be necessary if sports drinks and salty foods (if available) don't get the job done. You may experience nausea, vomiting, or diarrhea when taking electrolyte tablets, so don't wait until an important race or event to figure out what works for you. Be sure to carry tablets in a plastic bag or waterproof case because they will disintegrate if they come into contact with any moisture, such as sweat.

- **Experiment with glycerol.** Glycerol, a hyperhydrating agent, acts like a sponge in the body, soaking up and holding on to extra water. Now available as a sports supplement, glycerol is to be ingested with water or sports drinks before exercise to help reduce or delay dehydration (see chapter 5, "Using Supplements Effectively"). If you're considering giving glycerol a try, experiment with it before using it in an important event or competition because it can cause nausea or vomiting, as well as leave you initially feeling heavy and bloated.

- **Start out with a full tank.** Common sense should tell you that if you set out to exercise without being adequately hydrated, things will only get worse, especially in the heat. Consciously remind yourself to drink during the day by carrying a water bottle with you (especially during air travel) or leaving one in plain view, such as on your desk. Every time you eat a meal or a snack, make sure that you also drink a healthy beverage (see page 25). Drinking at regular intervals throughout the day is better than downing a large volume of fluid at any one time—which is only going to send you running to the bathroom.

Don't become anxious and overhydrate (especially by drinking excessive amounts of plain water) the day or two before your event or race. If you're running to the bathroom every hour or if your urine is very pale (if it looks like water), you're exceeding the fluid needs of your body and setting yourself up for more troubles when you finally begin to exercise.

If practical, freeze bottles beforehand or buy an insulated bottle to help keep liquids cool and refreshing. Young athletes dehydrate quickly, especially on warm days, so if you are with kids or teenagers make sure that each child has his or her own water bottle or bladder. If you're venturing into the backcountry, pack a water filtration device or iodine tablets and be certain that you know how to use them.

During the Event

- **Stick to a predetermined drinking schedule.** Remember, the goal is to minimize both dehydration and hyponatremia. Dehydration is far more common, however, so plan to drink early and often, about every 15 to 20 minutes. Our thirst mechanism fails to keep up with the actual fluid needs of our bodies, especially during exercise, so set your watch alarm as a reminder if need be. Generally, water is adequate for events lasting an hour or less (like a 10K road race) although a sports drink shouldn't do you any harm and is likely to provide an extra boost for a finishing kick.

  If you'll be on the move for more than 60 minutes at a moderate pace, drink a sports drink to meet your fluid, carbohydrate, and sodium needs. (Ideally, it's the same one that you've been training with.) Research has shown that athletes who are exercising in the heat and have free access to water replace only one-half to two-thirds of their fluid losses. Sports drinks can help you drink more because they contain electrolytes that boost your drive to drink.

  Drinking on a predetermined schedule is mandatory on warm, windy days or hot days with low humidity when you may not be as aware that you're sweating. Any time that you're with kids and teens, you'll also need to schedule and take mandatory fluid breaks, because young athletes can quickly become dehydrated. Young athletes typically do a much better job of rehydrating if a flavored beverage, such as a sports drink, is readily available.

- **Drink to match your fluid losses.** You can't simply wing it during endurance events and races or try to drink as much as you can—you need to drink intelligently. Both severe underdrinking and severe overdrinking are dangerous! For example, consuming fluid beyond what you're losing as sweat increases your risk of developing hyponatremia, but simply not drinking at all is not a safe option to prevent hyponatremia. You have to know your body and constantly monitor the signals that it sends.

  Because endurance athletes can't rely on the perception of thirst alone, you will need to monitor your body weight and the rate at which you are sweating. If you're gaining weight (in events with mandatory weight checks), if you are noticeably bloated or feel puffy, or if your rings, watch, or belt become tight, be alert to the fact that you may be overhydrating. This scenario is a real risk if you've chosen to drink mostly plain water or have been reduced to doing so in an attempt to deal with gastro-

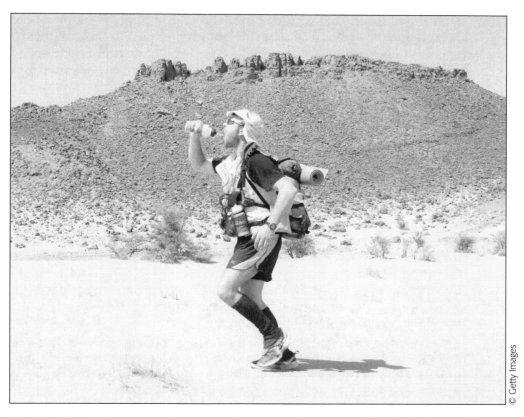

© Getty Images

Drink intelligently in extreme heat: every 15 to 20 minutes to avoid dehydration and hyponatremia.

intestinal woes. If you're not sweating heavily (as may occur if you are running slowly) and aren't thirsty, then you need to replace your fluid losses at only a modest rate. Obviously, you can also find relief from the heat by pouring cool fluid over your body, using sponges, or passing through sprinklers, but none of these practices can substitute for ingesting fluids.

- **Be prepared to carry what you need.** In many endurance events and races, you will be responsible for meeting your own fluid needs most of the time. Don't let the concern of carrying extra weight prevent you from wearing a bladder or a waist belt that holds a water bottle or two. The benefit of having fluid readily accessible, especially during prolonged events, far exceeds any negative consequence of carrying additional weight in the form of water or powdered sports drink. For example, drinking at regular intervals promotes sweating—your primary avenue to heat loss. If you can't cool off adequately, trust me—your brain will find a way to slow (or even completely shut down) your body.

Even in situations in which fluids are provided, such as organized rides, triathlons, and marathons, you may still benefit (or even find it necessary) to carry some of your own. For example, planned aid stations or rest stops with food and drinks may not be frequent enough for marathoners and others who sweat heavily or larger athletes with high fluid needs. Be honest with yourself. You will lose far more time if you're reduced to a crawl or if you have to stop and deal with muscle cramps than you ever will because of being weighed down by a pound of extra fluid or sports drink powder.

- **Consume salty foods and beverages (and possibly electrolyte tablets).** In most cases, consuming a sports drink during exercise, along with getting enough salt on a daily basis, will be enough for most endurance athletes. Look for salty foods at organized events (soup, cheese, pretzels, pickles, tomato juice) or foods that you can add salt to, such as potatoes or sandwiches. If you're participating in prolonged events and plan to be on the move for four hours or more and you choose to supplement with electrolyte tablets, don't overdo it. Keep in mind that no definitive guidelines exist. Generally, don't take more than one tablet (200 to 350 milligrams of sodium) per hour of exercise and take it with plenty (6 to 8 ounces) of water. Some athletes may need two tablets per hour during long, hot races, as may athletes participating in multiday events who have access only to plain water.

- **If need be, force yourself to eat.** Be aware that hot conditions and intense or prolonged exercise can doubly suppress your appetite. If you're in for a long day of exercise, such as all-day hike or an adventure race that may even stretch past a day, you will have to force yourself to eat. Eating anything is better than eating nothing, so don't be worried if you survive on the same few foods. Carbohydrate-rich foods, either sports foods like energy bars and gels or real food like fig bars and gumdrops, will work. Basically, anything that goes down and stays down is a winner.

After the Event

- **Rehydrate to match your fluid losses.** For one-day events, aim to drink at least 2.5 cups of fluid for every pound (~1.5 liters for every kilogram) of body weight that you're down. Don't consume only plain water—athletes have been known to induce hyponatremia in the hours following prolonged exercise when they avoid or are unable to eat solid food and they rehydrate by drinking only plain water or other low-sodium beverages, like beer. Monitor your ability to urinate and its color—you want it to be pale yellow.

- **Refuel promptly.** Anticipate a decrease in appetite. Drinking the calories (and carbohydrate) that you need for refueling purposes is usually easier at this time. Lemonade, fruit juices, milk shakes, yogurt, instant breakfast drinks, fruit smoothies, and complete meal replacement products go down fairly easily. Ease in other high-carbohydrate foods, such as bagels, cereal, and energy bars, as soon as you can tolerate them.

  Resist the urge to wait until your appetite returns because you'll miss the valuable window of opportunity (the first 30 to 60 minutes) immediately

The Beauty of a Bladder Hydration System

Whether you're traveling by foot, bike, ski, snowshoe, or kayak, you need to hydrate or you'll die—figuratively, if not literally. Many of the problems encountered during endurance activities, such as nausea, headaches, heat illness, and altitude sickness, often occur from not drinking enough. Bladder hydration systems encourage you to drink by making fluids readily accessible. You don't have to come to a stop, miss a step, or tie up your hands while reaching for a water bottle. Bladders also allow you to carry large quantities of fluid comfortably. A 50-ounce (1.5-liter) bladder is equal to two large water bottles, and a 70-ounce (2-liter) bladder equates to three large bottles. The granddaddy of all bladders can hold 100 ounces (3 liters), the equivalent of four large water bottles. Bladder hydration systems come in various styles and forms, designed specifically for different sports and activities. Worn alone or as part of a pack, sport vest, or hip-mounted belt, a bladder hydration system can efficiently distribute the weight of the fluid without interfering with normal movement. Bladders are available at outdoor and sporting goods stores or specialty shops that cater to cyclists, runners, and skiers.

Fully insulated bladders help liquids stay cool as temperatures rise, and you can add ice to some models. During winter, keep your hydration system bladder and hose from freezing by wearing a layer of clothing on top of it. Keep the drinking hose under cover until it's time to drink. Drinking small amounts at regular intervals will help keep the contents from freezing. In severe cold, blow air into the tube and force the liquid back into the bladder or experiment with winterizing adaptation kits available from some manufacturers.

Keep your bladder system clean and free from mold and bacteria by rinsing it with warm water following every use. For more thorough cleaning, use a biodegradable dishwashing detergent and a bottlebrush to clean the tube. You can buy bottlebrushes at a local hardware store or supermarket, or you can buy a cleaning kit from the manufacturer. To sanitize your bladder, add a teaspoon or two of household bleach to a full bladder. Shake vigorously, and then rinse the bladder and tube well with hot water. Don't overkill potential germs. You can make yourself sick from using too much bleach or not rinsing well enough with hot water. Use a paper towel to dry the inside of the bladder and then prop the sides open with a paper towel or similar item and hang to air dry. If residual tastes and odors bother you, fill the bladder with water, add two teaspoons of baking soda, and let it sit overnight. Rinse well and dry as explained earlier.

after exercise to jumpstart the process of replenishing muscle glycogen stores and promoting the repair of damaged muscle fibers. Refueling promptly is essential for any athlete! Eating solid foods will also help replace the other electrolytes that you lose through sweating (in much smaller amounts than sodium), such as potassium. Potassium-rich foods include juices, fruits, vegetables, milk, and yogurt.

Learn From the Best: Performing in the Heat

Ultrarunner Scott Jurek knows how to beat the heat. The course-record holder and seven-time defending champion of the Western States 100-Mile Endurance Run, Jurek decided to take on the Badwater Ultramarathon, a 135-mile (217-kilometer) nonstop run from Death Valley to Mount Whitney, California, in temperatures up to 130°F (55°C). He won that, too—on his first attempt, running to a new course record of 24 hours and 36 minutes. Jurek, who at age 25 became the youngest male runner to win Western States, has more than 12 years of racing ultras under his belt and a 2:38 marathon PR. Although you may never literally face the heat of Death Valley, here's his advice on how to do more than merely survive hot-weather endurance events and races.

Training Priorities for Racing Well in the Heat

You need to do two main things before the start of your event: Figure out your sweat rate (what you lose each hour) and train your digestive tract to handle drinking large volumes of fluid during exercise. For a sweat test, replicate as closely as possible the conditions that you expect and then see what you've lost after 60 to 90 minutes of exercise (see formula in chapter 4). Then factor in duration (how long you will be out there), the intensity at which you'll be working during the race, and any extenuating circumstances, such as being at altitude or in high humidity, that will further increase the amount of fluid that you'll be losing.

There are no shortcuts. You have to figure out what your body needs and then train your digestive tract, which means improving your gastric emptying rate. As Jurek emphasizes, you can't expect to be able to handle 60 to 70 ounces of fluid per hour on race day if you've been drinking only 30 ounces in training.

Day of the Race

On race day, concentrate on hydration and getting in adequate carbohydrate. Stay on top of it from the beginning. Know what you need to drink each hour and stick with it. Ultraendurance athletes, especially, can't make it up as they go along. Jurek reminds athletes that although they may be able to gut out a marathon in five or six hours, they have very little wiggle room in longer races. You can't make up for falling behind. You will require hours to get back because your body will need time to absorb and process what it needs. Slow down if necessary so that you can digest what you're taking in.

Some dehydration is going to happen. But Jurek agrees with most experts that a loss of 2 to 3 percent from preexercise weight is the defining edge. At Badwater, Jurek brought his own scale and monitored his weight throughout the race.

As for carbohydrate, make sure that you know what you need per hour based on your body weight and then stick to it. Jurek uses the following formula: .7 to 1.0 × body weight in kilograms = grams of carbohydrate per hour. (This equates to 30 to 60 grams per hour for most endurance athletes.) Look at the total time or number of hours that you will be competing. Although elite athletes seem not to eat or drink that much when racing marathons, realize that they're out there for little more than two hours! In addition, they are extremely fit and thus can burn more fat for fuel. Endurance athletes, especially ultra athletes, need a steady supply of carbohydrate, as much for brain power as for fueling muscles.

Diluting Sports Drinks During Hot Weather

Jurek doesn't believe in diluting sports drinks. He agrees with sports nutrition experts that it's too easy to get behind on carbohydrate and electrolytes as these components go too when a sports drink is diluted. Jurek makes sure that he has both plain water and a sports drink available. If he craves water, then he drinks water and gets his carbohydrate some other way (with energy gels, for example). Jurek always has some plain water available to help ensure that things don't become too concentrated in his stomach from, for example, mixing a concentrated sports drink and gels.

Meeting Electrolyte Needs

Jurek thinks that most serious ultra athletes appear to have learned how important sodium is during prolonged exercise, but he's concerned that less experienced or less competitive endurance athletes, or newcomers like marathon runners who are moving up in distance, may not have gotten the message. He stresses the fact that most sports drinks, even if consumed in appropriate quantities, aren't high enough in sodium to meet the needs of marathoners who are going to be out there for four to eight hours.

As the heat, humidity, or your intensity picks up, you sweat more, especially if you're not heat acclimated, and you can lose sodium at an extremely high rate. Depending on the event and conditions, Jurek advises the athletes he coaches to either mix their drinks very strongly or to keep it simple and use salt tablets.

Tried-and-True Strategies for Competing in the Heat

Jurek's first strategy is to keep his drinks as cold as possible. Second, for any sports drink or food that he plans to use, he always brings a variety of flavors. Third, because not eating is simply not an option, he doesn't overdo anything early in the race (for example, energy gels) that he knows he'll have to rely on late in the race. If you carry salt tablets, you need to keep them dry. Jurek uses a widget (a small squeezable pill purse), but baggies work as well. Be sure to reseal the baggie completely after each use.

Last, during hot-weather races Jurek advises athletes to keep it simple. He eats less fibrous solid foods and goes with sports foods like sports drinks and gels and simple foods like potatoes and bananas. The bottom line is that if you don't eat, you'll be forced to go very slowly because of insufficient fuel, and as Jurek says, that's not a fun way to do long races.

15

Extreme Cold

Thanks to year-round sporting activities and advances in performance clothing, you may find yourself out in the cold for long periods. Like those who deal with extreme heat and humidity, cold-weather athletes must learn to master the unique challenges of exercising in less than ideal conditions, especially if they want to compete. In cold environments, we must maintain our internal, or core, temperature. Our bodies rely on three main mechanisms to avoid excessive cooling: shivering (uncontrolled muscular contractions that can raise the body's resting rate of heat production four to five times), nonshivering thermogenesis (whereby the nervous system increases the metabolic rate to produce more internal heat), and the vasoconstriction of peripheral blood vessels to prevent unnecessary heat loss. Proper clothing and subcutaneous fat (found just below the skin's surface) are also necessary to help insulate deep body tissues from the cold.

Performing in Extreme Cold

During exercise in the cold, trouble sets in when you dissipate heat faster than you produce it. Although prolonged exercise increases the use of free fatty acids for fuel, this process is attenuated in the cold because vasoconstriction impairs blood flow to the subcutaneous fat, the major storage site for free fatty acids. As fatigue sets in, as may occur during prolonged running, swimming, or skiing, muscle activity slows and your body struggles to generate enough internal heat to maintain its temperature. Blood glucose plays an important role in how you tolerate the cold. Hypoglycemia, or low blood sugar, for example, suppresses shivering. Muscle glycogen also appears to be affected: for example, being used at a somewhat faster rate in cold water than it is in warmer conditions. No matter what activity or sport you're involved in, you'll be better prepared to withstand the rigors of exercising in a cold environment if you're well hydrated and well fueled.

Cold Acclimatization

Exercising in cold weather may be something that you grin and bear, or it may be an activity that you relish. Although acclimating to the cold is possible, the process is not well understood and it appears to be harder to accomplish than is warm-weather acclimatization. Generally, extremely fit athletes and those with slightly higher body-fat levels tolerate cold-weather exercise most comfortably.

As anyone who lives and trains in the cold can attest, adjusting psychologically to the cold may be what counts the most. Whether it was growing up running in the snowbelt of upstate New York, surviving ice and snowstorms while attending Georgetown University in Washington, D.C. (a city with few snowplows), or tolerating seven winters in Boston and two more in Colorado, I simply know that I can handle the cold.

Dehydration and Hypothermia

Performing in the cold brings its own set of challenges. Endurance athletes must be aware of two potential problems that can strike at any time: dehydration and hypothermia. To perform at your best, you'll need to be just as savvy about fluids and fuel while exercising in the cold as you are during warmer conditions.

Dehydration

Although you may not believe it, dehydration can hinder your ability to perform in cold weather just as it does when you exercise in the heat. Do you ever wonder how you could possibly have to make a pit stop in the middle of a snowstorm? Blame it on cold-induced diuresis. When you venture out into the cold, the peripheral blood vessels that carry blood to your skin and to regions of your body such as the ears, hands, and feet constrict to conserve heat and maintain your core temperature. This peripheral vasoconstriction causes your blood pressure to rise, including the blood pressure in your kidneys, which induces you to urinate and lose fluid.

You also lose a considerable amount of fluid when you exercise in the cold as your respiratory passages warm and humidify incoming cold, dry air (the air that you exhale is saturated with water). This process can lead to a loss of as much as one quart of fluid daily. Athletes often don't consume as much fluid during cold-weather exercise because suitable drinks aren't as readily available. On top of that, you may simply not feel as thirsty when you exercise in the cold, or you struggle with keeping drinks from freezing, or you consciously restrict your fluid intake to avoid the logistical problems or discomfort associated with making pit stops in the cold.

And although Jack Frost is nipping at your ears and toes, you don't stop sweating. Any time your body temperature rises sufficiently, you sweat. If you tend to overdress when you exercise in the cold, you can sweat profusely, especially during intense efforts. Researchers estimate that if you wear clothing with insulating properties equivalent to four business suits, your sweat losses could reach two quarts per hour during moderate to heavy exercise in freezing conditions. So it's easy to see why athletes become dehydrated during cold-weather exercise.

Hypothermia

Hypothermia, a decrease in core body temperature below 98.6°F (37°C), occurs when you lose more heat than you produce. Occurring in stages, warning signs of mild hypothermia include shivering, a red face, and increased respiration and heart rates. Often accompanied by dehydration and exhaustion, hypothermia can quickly progress to lethargy, weakness, slurred speech, disorientation, and combative behavior as the core temperature continues to fall. Left untreated, a hypothermic person may stop shivering, become progressively delirious, and lapse into a coma.

You don't have to scale the world's tallest mountain in the dead of winter to be at risk for hypothermia. Because it can develop in relatively mild temperatures (50°F to 65°F, or 10°C to 18°C), hypothermia is a real danger any time you exercise in cool or cold weather. Be alert for the signs of hypothermia in the following high-risk situations: whenever the weather changes quickly (for example, in spring and fall or at high altitudes), during windy days, in events that involve swimming or passing through water, and during the second half of long races, such as marathons and triathlons, when you may fail to generate enough heat because you are moving at a slower pace and may be losing heat through wet clothing (from sweat, rain, or snow).

You may be able to generate enough heat during exercise as long as you keep moving but face trouble when you stop. I encountered hypothermia while climbing Mont Blanc, the tallest of the Alps (15,771 feet, or 4,807 meters), on a sunny August morning in relatively light wind conditions. Unfortunately, I don't remember the spectacular views of Italy and France from the top because I was too busy shivering uncontrollably. Caught up in the moment (and not wishing to slow our French guide), I kept on record pace to the summit (5,000 vertical feet, or 1,500 meters, in four hours) without taking any major stops to adjust clothing or eat anything beyond the candy that we carried in our pockets. I was in trouble as soon as we reached the top when I stopped generating heat from kicking steps into the snow with heavy double boots. Luckily, I'm still around to tell you how to avoid this scenario!

Nutritional Strategies for Beating the Cold

Mom's advice to have a bowl of stick-to-your ribs oatmeal before you head out into the snow makes a lot of sense, not because the temperature has dropped (you can compensate by dressing appropriately) but because you're less efficient moving over slippery surfaces. In other words, you expend more energy (calories) performing most outdoor activities in cold conditions than you do in temperate conditions. For example, the simple act of walking on snow requires almost twice as much energy as traversing the same route on dry ground at the same speed. You also burn more calories because of the extra weight of heavy boots and winter clothing, which can increase your energy needs by 5 to 15 percent. No universally accepted standard exists for figuring your caloric needs in the cold, but the U.S. Army sets a goal of 4,500 calories a day (for the average male).

Your ability to think clearly and avoid injury and hypothermia decreases when you don't consume enough carbohydrate to replenish your glycogen stores and keep your blood sugar level steady. Look at the scientific basis behind the adage "Never ski tired." As you deplete the glycogen in your fast-twitch muscle fibers, you lose muscular strength and, consequently, power. You rely to a large degree on your fast-twitch muscle fibers to correct and control your movements while skiing (and during similar activities), so your ability to execute a series of perfect telemark turns late in the day may hinge on stopping to refuel with a midafternoon snack.

Along with your muscles' need for carbohydrate, your brain relies exclusively on glucose (a simple carbohydrate) for fuel. If your blood sugar falls below a critical level, your judgment and ability to perform skilled maneuvers will severely deteriorate, which could result in injury or death. (Skiers often lament ignoring their desire to call it a day and then being injured on their last trip down the mountain.) Shivering, the body's attempt to raise its core temperature, uses carbohydrate, and severe shivering can deplete glycogen stores. Exercising in cold water also uses muscle glycogen at a somewhat higher rate than does exercising in warm water.

When it comes time to consume the calories needed for cold-weather exercise, athletes and experts alike continue to debate the merits of a carbohydrate-rich diet versus a diet higher in fat. This debate likely endures because people who live in cold regions often appear to favor higher-fat (and higher-protein)

Hot Chocolate Smoothie

Here is a rich, thick beverage that you can eat or drink.

- 4 teaspoons of sugar
- 4 teaspoons of cocoa powder
- 4 tablespoons of powdered milk
- 4 teaspoons of potato starch (used as a thickener; available at your local supermarket or an Asian market)

At home: Combine all ingredients and place in a zip-lock bag.

On the trail: Place ingredients into an insulated mug, water bottle, or thermos. Add 1 cup of boiling water, stir well, cover, and let stand 5 minutes. Makes one 8-ounce serving.

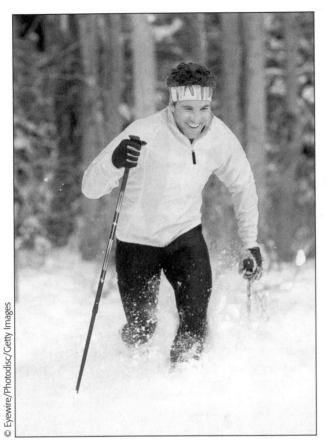

© Eyewire/Photodisc/Getty Images

Cold weather requires taking in extra calories to fend off hypothermia and boost energy.

foods. Keep in mind, however, that the relative use of carbohydrate and fat for energy varies widely among individuals. Your fitness level and degree of cold acclimatization, the intensity of the exercise, and the severity of the cold all factor in. For example, the more fit and acclimatized you are, the more fat you burn, which helps conserve your limited glycogen reserves. Studies on energy metabolism in prolonged cold are limited, but the findings suggest that we metabolize both fat and carbohydrate at a higher rate in the cold. The bulk of the calories that you consume during cold-weather exercise, however, should still come from carbohydrate-rich foods because the increase in carbohydrate metabolism is substantially larger than the increase in fat metabolism.

When it comes to improving your ability to tolerate the cold, look at both the source of your calories and the timing of your snacks and meals. Despite conventional wisdom, a high-carbohydrate diet has been found superior to a high-protein diet in improving cold tolerance, and a high-fat or a high-carbohydrate diet has essentially the same effect when meals and snacks are consumed every four hours. A high-fat diet may be superior, though, when snacks and meals are eaten more frequently, every two hours, for example. (Adequate amounts of carbohydrate must still be consumed, however, to replace muscle glycogen and prevent excess fatigue.) The best advice that I have for athletes looking to stay out in the cold (especially for prolonged adventures that involve overnight stays) is to be in good physical condition, wear proper clothing, and eat enough calories (regardless of the source) to maintain body temperature.

Assuming that you're properly clothed, venturing out into the cold doesn't increase your requirement for any specific nutrient per se. But negotiating difficult terrain and carrying the extra weight of a pack and heavy cold-weather clothing will increase your calorie needs. We tend to feel less thirsty in cold weather, so eating may be logistically difficult or uncomfortable. Without consciously and deliberately fulfilling your fluid and fuel needs, prolonged exercise in the cold can deplete carbohydrate reserves to the extent that hypoglycemia (low blood sugar) and hypothermia (low body temperature) occur. Here's how to give yourself the best chance to perform well in the cold.

Before the Event

Respect the added challenges of performing in the cold. As with clothing and gear, preparing nutritionally beforehand really pays off.

Mind your iron stores   You may be more susceptible to the cold if your iron levels are low. Researchers have found that iron-deficient women were able to produce heat but had difficulty retaining it to maintain their body temperature. Men who suffer from iron deficiency, although not studied, probably respond in a similar manner. Have your serum hemoglobin, hematocrit, and ferritin (stored iron) checked before you pop any iron supplements. There is no evidence that you can enhance your cold tolerance by taking excess iron if you're not deficient (see chapter 6, "Solving Peak Performance Challenges").

Find fluids and foods that work in the cold   Now is the time to discover that your favorite energy or candy bar turns into an inedible rock when the temperatures dip, not when you're clinging to the side of a cliff or halfway through a skiing adventure that you've been dreaming about for the last year. Before any cold-weather adventure or race, try all your favorite energy-boosting snacks to make sure that they pass the test. Do this during training efforts outdoors in cold conditions or put the item in the freezer for a few hours and see what happens. If you can't eat it, don't bother packing it.

If you rely on a bladder to carry fluid, choose an insulated one designed for cold-weather activities and choose clothing that allows you to wear it underneath, as close to your body as possible. Experiment with the bladder over a range of temperatures, because the hoses on even the best models can freeze up. If possible preheat drinks and pour the fluid into an insulated water bottle (even closed-cell foam secured by duct tape will help) or a sturdy thermos in the morning. Remove unnecessary wrappings and packages from food to save time and reduce the weight that you have to carry. To avoid having to remove your mittens or gloves, chop, slice, and dice foods such as energy bars and cheese before you leave home and repackage the bite-size pieces into plastic food storage bags.

Experiment with glycerol   You may have heard about ingesting glycerol, a hyperhydrating agent that helps the body hold on to water, as a strategy to use when exercising in hot weather. Researchers at the Thermal and Mountain Medicine Division, United States Army Research Institute of Environmental Medicine in Natick, Massachusetts, found that glycerol could also be useful for athletes in cold weather. In three separate double-blind trials, seven men ingested either water alone, water and glycerol, or no fluid 30 minutes before being exposed to four hours of cold air (57°F [15°C] and 30 percent relative humidity). When they ingested water and glycerol beforehand, the men urinated less and retained more fluid during the cold-air exposure than they did when they drank only water. In other words, they stayed better hydrated over time, which would probably improve their ability to perform physically. If you want to try glycerol, be sure to experiment in training efforts first (see chapter 5, "Using Supplements Effectively"). Incidentally, previous research on subjects actually immersed in cold water (versus exposed to cold air) has failed to find any hydration-boosting effect due to glycerol ingestion.

Rise and dine that morning   The mere act of eating revs up your metabolism and generates heat (although not nearly enough to warrant throwing away your long johns). At the very least, warm and nourishing foods provide a psychological boost. If rich in calories, they'll also help you meet your anticipated calorie needs. If you're heading out for a single, short bout of cold-weather exercise, you don't need to worry as much. But hours of continuous exercise can really boost your calorie needs. For example, depending on your body size, pace, pack weight, and terrain, you can expend 3,000 calories (or more) on top of your normal daily needs during a six-hour hike with a full backpack.

Unless you fuel up before you set out, you'll dig a big hole by lunchtime, even if you snack along the way. And I don't mean a Starbucks grande and biscotti. Carbohydrate-rich foods are the fuel of choice for hard-working muscles. Dress up oatmeal, a classic sendoff, by stirring in raisins or other dried fruit, brown sugar, honey, or a scoop of peanut butter. If oatmeal isn't high on your list of favorite foods (it's not on mine), opt for a peanut butter sandwich or just-add-water products that take only minutes to prepare, such as individual serving cups of chili, couscous with lentils, mashed potatoes, or grits. My breakfast of choice before a long hike, for example, includes a just-add-water cup of macaroni and cheese (230 calories—71 percent from carbohydrate, 14 percent from protein, and 14 percent from fat). If you're worried about gastrointestinal woes, try drinking your calories instead. An ultrarunner friend swears by a couple cans of Ensure before he hits the trail. Instant breakfast and meal replacement drinks are another option.

During the Event

As is true for exercising in any conditions, don't rely on thirst to trigger your need for fluids. To generate heat, you'll need to keep moving, and to keep moving, you need fuel. It's simple—drink and eat at regular intervals to improve your chances of performing well in the cold.

Plan to drink early and often   Dehydration is often coupled with hypoglycemia (low blood sugar level), and both compromise your ability to perform in the cold, as well as significantly increase your risk of becoming hypothermic. You must have access to a source of safe, drinkable water or other acceptable fluids. A good rule of thumb is that you need a minimum of two quarts (liters) per person for a daylong (six-hour) event. Drink small amounts at regular intervals (ideally a few gulps every 15 to 20 minutes) rather than a large amount at lunchtime and then again later in the day. Performing with dehydrated muscles will increase the risk that you'll injure yourself, and if you wait to consume a large amount in one sitting, you'll simply urinate out much of the fluid.

Keep fluids from freezing by stashing your container near your body, in a breast jacket pocket rather than in your backpack, for example, or strap on a bladder hydration system that you know performs well in the cold. Depending on your activity, instant fruit or fluid replacement drinks, herbal teas, apple cider, cocoa, and soup make good choices. (Be aware that tea or coffee provides no calories unless it's spiked with sugar or honey.) Stay away from alcohol because it causes you to urinate. Although you may feel warmer when you first drink alcohol, the core temperature of your body doesn't increase. In fact, drinking alcohol causes you to lose heat by opening the blood vessels to your skin.

Eating snow is a poor option too. The energy that you expend warming the snow can lower your core body temperature enough to induce hypothermia. If you're a winter camper and want to obtain water by melting snow, be prepared to spend two precious commodities—time and fuel. You will have to melt approximately five cups of snow to obtain one cup of water. Be sure to bring the water to a rolling boil (keep an eye on it; five minutes isn't necessary) to kill waterborne microorganisms. If you're on the move, speed up the process by packing snow into your water bottle while the bottle still has liquid in it. Filter or chemically disinfect any melted snow or water that you don't bring to a rolling boil. Despite your best intentions, eating snow or drinking untreated water may be your only option to ward off dehydration and enable you to keep moving in an emergency. Look for clean snow or running water free of contaminants from animals or other humans.

Feed the furnace   Shovel in the carbohydrate at regular intervals to keep your liver and muscle glycogen tanks full. The longer you'll be out in the cold, the more fat you'll need in order to meet your elevated calorie needs and improve your tolerance for the cold. Choose high-calorie foods that pack a lot of wallop, especially if you'll be spending prolonged periods in the cold (like overnight) or are limited in what you can carry. Keep prepared food items readily accessible and stored in inner pockets where they can soak up body heat.

Snack or break for minimeals on a regular schedule. Don't wait until you're too wet, tired, or cold to think about your next snack or meal. Make sure that you actually down the calories. Because I like to travel light and fast while hiking, I often found myself carrying the food that I intended to eat in my hands for a long time, rather than ingesting it. I now consciously make myself stop and eat. Plan ahead by anticipating the terrain, weather, and other elements that you will likely encounter.

On longer excursions, such as four- to nine-day cold-weather excursions, figure on at least two pounds of food (precooked weight) per person per day. Don't skimp on protein but don't overdo it. Carbohydrate and fat are superior to protein when it comes to providing fuel for muscles and improving your

Cold-Weather Adventure Foods

Whenever you push your limits, you need to eat high-quality foods to replace calories, carbohydrate, and other nutrients, especially if you're exercising in the cold. Although energy bars and gels can certainly fill the bill some of the time, you may want to consider the following list of foods on your next cold-weather adventure. The foods that you select, obviously, will depend on your activity, tastes, length of time outside, and other practical considerations, such as how much you can carry and how long it takes to prepare the food.

Milk
Powdered milk, cocoa mixes, powdered breakfast drinks

Grains
Instant whole-grain cereals (oatmeal, Wheatena), granola (eat hot or cold), instant grits, rice, mashed potatoes, couscous and bulgur, quick-cooking pasta and bean products, instant ramen noodles, bagels, pita bread, tortillas, crackers, cookies (especially fruit filled), rice pudding, breakfast bars

Fruit
Fresh fruit such as apples, oranges, grapes, and so on; dried fruit such as raisins, apricots, banana chips, apples, prunes, dates, pineapple, and cherries; fruit leathers; freeze-dried dessert products

Vegetables
Freshly cut and peeled (packaged and ready to go), dehydrated, or freeze dried

Protein
Peanut butter, nuts, seeds; cured meats such as ham, sausage, and so on; dried meat sticks and jerky; assorted cheese; powdered hummus; powdered eggs; no-cook refried beans; canned or foil packets of turkey, chicken, tuna, and shrimp; prepackaged, freeze-dried, or dehydrated entrees

Snacks
Chocolate, candy bars, cookies, gumdrops, hard candies, licorice, instant pudding, trail mixes

Beverages
Fruit juices and drinks, lemonade, apple cider, herbal teas, coffee, cocoa, fluid replacement drinks, powdered drink mixes, no-cook soups

Others
Margarine, butter powder, seasonings, condiments (honey, sugar cubes, and so on)

Adapted, by permission, from D. Benardot, 1993, *Sports nutrition: A guide for the professional working with active people*, 2nd ed. (Chicago, IL: American Dietetic Association).

cold tolerance. The chief concern when exercising in the cold is to maintain your body temperature by eating enough calories, regardless of the source. Bring a small reserve of extra food in case you get lost or your adventure takes longer than expected.

If you're out for hours at a time or temperatures are extreme, you may be able to improve your cold tolerance by snacking on high-fat foods every two hours while exercising. Aim for 500 calories per snack. For example, try a peanut butter and jelly sandwich made with two tablespoons of peanut butter or gorp with two to three ounces (about 60 to 90 grams) of peanuts mixed with the same amount of raisins. If you plan to sleep in the cold, try another 500-calorie snack immediately before retiring to your sleeping bag. You may sleep better, and your extremities, your fingers and toes, may stay warmer through the night.

After the Event

Rehydrate and refuel promptly after your adventure. Basic recovery rules apply following cold-weather exercise—start rehydrating and refueling by drinking carbohydrate-rich beverages (with a small amount of protein if you can tolerate it) within 30 minutes of finishing, and eat solid real food as soon as you can. This habit is particularly important if the next day will require another long, intense effort. Campers and mountain climbers who drink and down a quick snack first rather than waiting to attend to their nutritional needs after taking care of every other task fare much better over the long haul.

Learning From the Best: Performing in the Cold

Ultraracer Nikki Kimball covers a lot of ground in her trail shoes and on her skis. Growing up in Vermont and now based in Montana, Kimball is not afraid of cold weather. Initially an accomplished country-country ski racer, she has excelled at road cycling, the biathlon, mountain running (three-time member of the U.S. Mountain Running team), and ultrarunning (two top-10 finishes in the 100K World Cup Championships). Kimball, a two-time winner of the Western States 100, now focuses on trail ultras, her specialty, with ski racing thrown in for fun. Here, Kimball shares her experience of returning to ski racing after 12 years away from it to illustrate valuable strategies for thriving in the cold.

Common Nutrition-Related Experiences When Performing in the Cold

In her final race of the season, a 50K in the American ski marathon series (the Yellowstone Rendezvous), Kimball did not handle her nutrition well. The day was extremely cold—negative 26°F (−32°C) when she woke up and only 0°F (−18°C) at the start. The snow, therefore, was very slow. The consequences of cold temperatures in cross-country skiing are at least twofold as they relate to nutrition, especially in racing. First, more calories are needed just to stay warm. Kimball knows that she

(continued)

becomes more fatigued in the extreme cold from normal prerace activities such as walking around, waxing her skis, and warming up because her body must expend extra energy just to maintain its core temperature. Kimball also found herself working harder than normal in the beginning of the race because she wanted to get warm, so she cautions that pacing yourself can be more difficult when you feel driven to attain a more comfortable body temperature. The second factor of extreme cold is that the snow is much slower. Therefore, you will work harder and need more time to cover a given distance. In the Rendezvous, Kimball acknowledges that she did not drink and eat enough partly because she didn't account for the extra time and effort required to race in cold temperatures.

Consequences of Nutritional Choices

Fortunately for Kimball (who won in 2:53:26), many experienced marathon ski racers made the same mistakes that she did. Kimball bonked at 47 kilometers, but she had already passed the lead women who bonked at about 43 kilometers. Had the race been any longer Kimball says that she would have been passed by her former coach (age 48) who, despite having had a hip replacement 16 months previously, had been passing the leaders in the final 6 kilometers because she had handled her pacing and nutrition much better than the rest of the field did. The race was a great example of experience trumping youth and biomechanical health (those with naturally healthy joints) in a sport in which the stars are typically in their 20s and 30s.

Challenges to Fueling While Skiing

Another factor in taking in adequate fuel during the cold can be the logistics of feeding, especially when ski racing. An accomplished ultrarunner, Kimball finds it comparatively easy to feed in ultrarunning because both hands are free, and she's confident that she can eat without slowing her pace at all. In skiing, she admits that she hadn't practiced feeding. Thus during the Rendezvous she had difficulty drinking at feed stations with poles in her hands, as well as difficulty feeding from her bottle in her hip pack.

Be Committed to Drinking and Eating

Kimball has frequently heard runners use the excuse that they don't want to lose time in aid stations drinking, which she finds ridiculous because she knows firsthand that the gains made by proper hydration and feeding far exceed any time lost in taking in the required nutrition. Nevertheless, here she was underfeeding because she didn't want to take time to mess with drinking with poles in her hands! The lesson according to Kimball is that if you're concerned about the time that it takes to feed—in running, skiing, or any event—then practice feeding in training. The logic of passing up feeds to save time is completely flawed. You can accomplish sufficient fueling in seconds, whereas dehydration or bonking will cost minutes or even hours, and will increase your risk of dropping from the event.

Additional Tips for Excelling in the Cold

The urge to urinate always comes on earlier in the cold, whether you drink or not, so you won't escape making pit stops by not drinking. Kimball advises athletes to update their cold weather wardrobe if necessary, particularly women who ski race, to take advantage of technical clothing that is now designed to make taking a pit stop easier. She also always tries to take in fluids that are warm (at least room temperature) because they're easier to drink, thereby encouraging her to drink more. Kimball starts out by making her drinks (tea or sports drink) with hot water. She usually relies on an insulated hydration pack, especially during ski endeavors, because it doesn't bounce up and down with the smooth motion of skiing. At the end of any cold-weather endeavor, Kimball has a thermos waiting with a hot drink inside it. She immediately begins to replenish the calories that she needs, and she swears by the boost that a warm beverage gives in helping her to warm up more quickly.

16

High Altitude

"If you don't like a certain food at sea level, you will most likely really dislike it at altitude. Spend all year eating healthy. When on the climb, eat to obtain calories (fuel)."

—Susan Ershler, part of the first couple in history to climb the highest mountain on each of the seven continents together, including Mount Everest

If your favorite endurance activity or competitive event has lost its challenge, try doing it at altitude. Rapidly changing weather and less oxygen to draw on for physical efforts, coupled with having a headache, queasy stomach, and a lack of appetite, can make things far more interesting. Mother Nature may rule when it comes to the weather, but you can stay in the game by acclimatizing, drinking adequate fluids, and making wise food choices.

Altitude Acclimatization

If you travel too quickly to higher elevations you may develop a headache, experience difficulty breathing, suffer from general weakness and nausea (even vomiting), lose your appetite, and have trouble sleeping. Welcome to the world of acute altitude, or mountain, sickness (AMS). Experts estimate that 6.5 percent of men and 22 percent of women will suffer from this malady when traveling above 6,000 to 8,000 feet (~1,800 to 2,400 meters). The underlying mechanism remains unclear, but the accumulation of carbon dioxide in tissues and the seeping of fluid into the brain are likely culprits as your body adjusts to less oxygen than it is accustomed to. Why women tend to suffer more from AMS than men do remains unclear.

What else is happening as you gasp for air and your working muscles scream for oxygen? Initially, you breathe more rapidly in an attempt to extract more oxygen from the air. Your plasma (the watery portion of your blood) volume drops to increase the concentration of red blood cells (oxygen carriers) in your blood, and your heart kicks into overdrive to deliver more blood (and thus more oxygen) to active muscles. If you stay long enough, at least 10 to 14 days, your body begins to acclimate and make adjustments that are more permanent. Your plasma volume expands, and your muscles begin to extract more oxygen from the blood, thus reducing the workload on your heart. If you stay even longer (4 to 8 weeks), you'll end up with more red blood cells, which will really help you compensate for the thinner air. By the way, the percentage of oxygen in the air (20.93 percent) remains constant regardless of the altitude. What varies is the atmospheric (barometric) pressure—it decreases as you ascend, thus decreasing the partial pressure of oxygen in your bloodstream. A substantially reduced pressure gradient between the oxygen in your blood and the oxygen in your active tissues hinders the transfer of oxygen from the blood to the tissues. Less oxygen being delivered to working muscles translates into reduced performances for endurance athletes.

Dehydration and Glycogen Depletion

Dehydration and glycogen depletion remain your nemeses at high elevations. The air holds little water (especially if it's cold), which increases the amount of water that you lose through respiration and perspiration, although you may not be aware of it.

Exercising at altitude, particularly extended stays at high altitude (9,000 feet, or 2,700 meters, and above) also influences the metabolism of the body. Upon acute exposure to high altitude, the body's basal metabolic rate, or the energy that it needs to maintain the processes that support life, rises as much as 30 percent. You thus need more calories just to maintain your body weight (about 30 to 35 calories per pound, or 65 to 75 calories per kilogram, of body weight). You also require more energy to fuel your high-intensity exercise efforts, such as carrying a heavy pack up a steep grade, compared with the same work done at sea level. A shift takes place in your muscles too, as they begin to rely less on fat and more on carbohydrate (glucose) for fuel. Increased reliance on glucose while at altitude may be advantageous because exercising muscles use carbohydrate more efficiently (in other words, they require less oxygen) than they do fat. Fortunately, carbohydrate-rich foods seem more palatable at altitude than protein and high-fat foods do.

If you spend several days to a few months above 14,000 feet (4,300 meters), you can expect to lose weight. As you go higher and stay longer, you will find it more difficult to maintain a balance between the calories that you take in and those that you expend. Initially, you can drop a few pounds of water as you acclimate. Your appetite may lag behind as well, especially if you suffer with AMS, so your food intake may be low for several days. Of course, if your adventure involves a lot of physical activity at high altitude, you will be expending a substantial amount of calories that you need to replace daily. (Aim for 30 to 35 calories per pound of body weight.) Fortunately, you may be able to avoid losing significant weight (at least up to 16,500 feet, or 5,000 meters) by making sure that you have access to a variety of tasty foods. Researchers followed eight healthy male Caucasians at the Italian Research Laboratory in Nepal (16,650 feet, or 5,050 meters) to test this theory. After one month in comfortable surroundings with a wide choice of palatable foods available, the men did not experience significant change in weight, body-fat percentage, circumference of arms or legs (measures of muscle mass), or performance on strength and vertical-jumping tests.

Overall, digestibility and absorption of nutrients do not appear to contribute to weight loss unless you're at extreme altitude (above 23,000 feet, or 7,000 meters), in which case your digestive tract may lose some of its absorptive capacity. Of course, at that altitude, you may experience a few other problems too! Most of the weight that you lose after prolonged altitude exposure is simply loss of body fat and muscle mass. The cause is a combination of taking in too few calories—because of the lack of appetite and limited food choices—and expending more calories, in part because of an elevated resting metabolic rate.

A sizable portion of altitude-related weight loss, up to 70 percent, is loss of muscle mass. In elite mountain climbers, researchers have documented losses that decrease the thigh cross-sectional area by 15 percent over a two-month period at altitudes above 18,000 feet (5,500 meters). Detraining may be a partial cause of this muscle loss. If you arrive in top condition, you may lose muscle because of a relative lack of exercise while you acclimate or wait out weather delays. On the other hand, the lack of oxygen may directly affect protein metabolism by decreasing your ability to synthesize new protein.

Nutritional Strategies for Handling High Altitude

If possible, give yourself a chance to acclimatize when traveling to a higher altitude. Arrive at least two weeks before a competitive event. If that's not possible, compete within 24 hours of your arrival to minimize the effects of AMS. On hikes and expeditions during which you plan to spend the night, ascend slowly, in stages. A good rule to follow over 10,000 feet (3,000 meters) is to climb only 1,000 feet (300 meters) per day. To limit your weight loss, bring a variety of palatable food and limit the time spent at high altitude.

The bottom line is that those who do best at altitude are those who drink and eat the most, and doing that basically takes a lot of willpower. On my trip to Kilimanjaro, Africa's tallest peak (19,341 feet, or 5,895 meters), I could tell which group members were experiencing AMS just from their lack of mealtime conversation! Underfueling not only puts you at risk (especially during multiday events) but also, if you're with a group, threatens your companions' enjoyment and safety.

Before the Event

Undertaking endurance challenges at high elevations demands that you be mentally ready and physically prepared. Boost your confidence and give yourself that extra edge by eating smart in advance.

Eat iron-rich foods and supplement as necessary   If you live and train at moderate altitude (3,000 to 8,000 feet, or 900 to 2,400 meters) or you're planning an extended trip to high altitude, be sure to consume plenty of iron-rich foods on a regular basis. Meat (especially red meat), fortified breakfast cereals, dark leafy greens, dried beans and peas, dried fruit, and prune juice make good choices. You want to take advantage of your body's desire to build new red blood cells. Iron is a crucial component of hemoglobin (housed in red blood cells), the prime carrier of oxygen in blood. Female athletes must pay particular attention to their iron status while training at altitude. The need for supplementation can be easily determined though routine blood tests (see chapter 6).

Explore the merits of vitamin E   Vitamin E, a powerful antioxidant, helps keep cell membranes healthy. Without enough of it, your red blood and muscle cells are destroyed more rapidly by oxidative damage from free radical molecules. Exercise raises your need for vitamin E, and exercise at high altitude probably raises it even more. Eat a training diet rich in whole-grain products, wheat germ, vegetable oils, green leafy vegetables, nuts and seeds, and liver and eggs (yolks) to ensure an adequate intake of vitamin E. Supplementation may help protect against chronic oxidative damage to membranes during intense, prolonged exercise (for example, at high altitudes), although not all scientists agree and no firm recommendations exist. A suggested reasonable daily dose for endurance athletes is 100 to 200 IU per day. Vitamin E has low toxicity (the tolerable upper intake level is 1,500 IU daily), but some people report flulike symptoms when taking more than 400 IU daily for prolonged periods.

Plan ahead: bring what you need   Any time that you travel with others, especially as part of a prearranged or supported trekking trip, the time to speak up about nutritional concerns is before you go. You should inquire about the planned menus anyway, rather than complain about the food (or lack of it) after the trip is underway. Those who have additional concerns, such as food allergies or gluten intolerance (or if you're a vegetarian), must make requests and develop an alternative plan ahead of time.

Experiment and determine what works up high   Use short adventures and forays at altitude to become comfortable with a variety of foods and drinks that you will need for longer events. You can't go wrong with items that are premade, crushproof, and require no cooking. (For expeditions, never underestimate the importance of the cook.) Practice eating and drinking in high altitude conditions and line up a reliable hydration system. Anticipate that your tastes will change as you go higher. Talk to experienced old-timers and listen to their advice. They may suggest particular foods that you wouldn't normally choose or identify foods that you should leave behind. To enhance appetite and boost morale, a good idea is for all members of the group to bring (within reason) some of their favorite treats to enjoy, as well as share with friends and teammates.

Play it safe   For the few days or the week before your altitude adventure, play it safe and eat familiar foods that you like. Now is not the time to be adventurous because working hard at altitude quickly exacerbates dehydration or weakness (and increases AMS) because of having the runs or not being able to eat. Going to high altitude (for treks and adventure races, for example) often means traveling to a non-Westernized country. Staying healthy is particularly challenging. Do not sample the local street cuisine beforehand. No matter how good it looks, do not eat salads, fruit that you can't peel, or ice cream. Make sure that any drinks you order (request the can or bottle) do not contain ice. Stick to dining at the best hotels and restaurants that cater to tourists, or (if reasonable) bring your own prepackaged foods.

During the Event

Don't throw away your hard work and preevent planning by becoming lazy about your nutritional needs after you hit the trail. Food is what gets you to the top and, even more important, what gets you back down.

Drink on a schedule Exercising at altitude increases the rate at which you lose water, so your fluid intake must increase to match this loss. Based on my experience, don't be surprised if you require double the amount of fluid that you normally do. For example, by the time you reach 10,000 feet (3,000 meters) you might need four to five quarts (liters) or more per day. Set an alarm on your watch, if necessary, to remind yourself to drink. Alternatively, put a group member in charge of predetermined breaks.

Energy drinks provide both calories (in the form of carbohydrate) and fluid. Other good choices (besides plain water) include instant fruit drinks, reconstituted powdered milk or meal replacement drinks, hot chocolate, tea loaded with honey or sugar, and soup. Avoid alcohol completely because it contributes to both dehydration and nausea. The oft-repeated advice that urine runs clear (pale yellow) when you're well hydrated holds true at any elevation.

Ignore your lack of appetite Being nauseated or not feeling hungry doesn't get you off the hook. In fact, with less oxygen going to your brain and stomach, expect to lose your appetite, especially during the first few days as you acclimatize (or during extended stays at high altitude). Unfortunately, active muscles can't wait that long. Food is fuel, so the more you eat, the more you'll be able to do. Besides, you'll feel better and enjoy the experience more. It's your job to keep yourself adequately fueled. Eating during endurance events and races at altitude can require as much willpower as continuing to put one foot in front of the other.

Don't worry about chowing down on exactly the right thing. At high altitude, all calories are good calories! Just be sure to bring a variety of appetizing foods with you because your tastes will change as you go higher. At the very least, bring several flavors of energy bars and gels to ward off flavor fatigue. Foods that you love at home are typically the ones that you are most likely to eat when you're up high.

Keep in mind that sweet-tasting foods, in particular, can become overwhelming at altitude. I was caught off guard by the complete lack of appetite that can strike at higher elevations as I hiked up to 15,000 feet (4,500 meters) on Kilimanjaro. Partial to sweet-tasting, red-colored sports drinks at sea level, I couldn't even look at my favorite drink, never mind stomach it. Finding a canister of lemon-lime powered sports drink in the bottom of my pack saved the trip. (Butterfinger candy bars and potato chips helped me reach a new "high" too.) Eat small, frequent meals to keep your energy up and help combat nausea.

Load up on carbohydrate and keep the fat Fill up on carbohydrate (ideally at least 60 percent of your total calories) because they require significantly less oxygen for metabolism and are generally better tolerated than high-fat foods are at altitude. If you don't constantly replenish your liver and muscle glycogen stores by eating foods rich in simple and complex carbohydrates (for example, bread, cereal, rice, pasta, fruit, powdered milk, candy, and sugar), you'll end up exhausted and less able to tolerate the effects of being at altitude. On top of that, your body will use valuable protein stores as energy instead. In addition to sports drinks, energy bars, and gels, keep carbohydrate-rich portable items handy to snack on, such as bagels, pita bread, instant pudding, fresh and dried fruit, carrot sticks, pretzels, gorp, granola or breakfast bars, Pop-Tarts, fig bars, and candy.

That said, don't be surprised if you crave and can tolerate high-fat foods, such as nuts, cheese, pepperoni, sausage, chocolate, and peanut butter. These foods are the best way to consume calories quickly. Adding oil, margarine, or butter to foods is another efficient (and often necessary) way to boost calories. Relatively lightweight and easy to carry, high-carbohydrate or meal replacement drink powders (some provide as much as 200 calories and 15 to 30 grams of protein per cup) can be a real lifesaver.

Cook simple fare while on the trail Preparing even routine foods at altitude can be tedious, so get everyone to pitch in. Don't weigh yourself down with foods that take a long time to cook, such as beans, brown rice, and elbow or shell pasta. Concentrate on instant mashed potatoes, couscous, thin pastas, low-fat ramen noodles, quick-cooking rice, dehydrated foods, and freeze-dried foods. Be sure to estimate how many cups of hot water and fuel you'll need to prepare these items. To save time and energy, pack whole meals together ahead of time and label them with the dates that you will eat them. Soak dehydrated foods during the day in an extra water bottle to shorten their cooking time.

Don't worry about trying to prepare gourmet fare. That's not the goal. A simple spice kit can beef up ordinary fare. Of course, you could always carry a bigger pack and bring your whole kitchen. I observed a woman at base camp at 10,000 feet (3,000 meters) on Mount Rainier who brought a fresh lemon and a kitchen knife to slice it just so she could flavor her drinking water!

After the Event

Refuel promptly. As with all physically challenging and prolonged bouts of exercise, take advantage of the carbohydrate window and begin refueling as soon as possible. Anticipate a decrease in appetite by initially drinking the calories and carbohydrate that you need to replace. Refueling promptly after the day's endeavor is particularly essential for through-hikers, those on expeditions, and other athletes involved in multiday adventures and races at altitude. Those able to finish, and finish strongly, are almost always those who paid attention to their fluid and fuel needs from the very first day.

Learn From the Best: Performing at Altitude

Phil and Susan Ershler became the first couple in history to climb the highest mountain on each of the seven continents together, including Mount Everest. Phil is a world-renowned mountain-climbing guide and partner of International Mountain Guides. Susan, now a motivational speaker, was a 35-year-old corporate executive when she met Phil. Always athletic but never having climbed or even hiked, she conquered the Seven Summits by systematically mastering what was needed. Following is Susan's tried-and-true nutritional advice for performing your best at altitude.

Three nutritional strategies are particularly important for succeeding at altitude:

1. Prepare ahead of time by eating a healthy diet and limiting nonnutritious foods throughout the year—not just during the few days or weeks beforehand.
2. Eat something at every break, or approximately every 60 to 90 minutes minimum. While performing at altitude, we often break rule number one—in other words, we can't always eat the most nutritious foods. Healthy foods may not be available, or, like many trekkers and climbers, you may completely lose your appetite. In this case, the important thing is to ingest calories—candy bars, chocolate, anything that you can tolerate as long as you get in calories.
3. Drink fluids constantly.

Getting the Fueling Job Done in Less Than Ideal Conditions

When Susan sets out for a day hike, she likes to use a bladder hydration system. But she notes three potential problems with using this type of system at higher altitudes and on certain treks. First, in cold conditions the hose may freeze, even the insulated ones. Second, the common practice of sitting on your pack during breaks can cause the bag to break and end up soaking everything in your pack. Third, if the trail is dusty, the mouthpiece can pick up dirt constantly. For example, on the trek to Everest base camp, the trail is dusty and often littered with yak dung. The mouthpiece of a bladder system can quickly become dirty. Therefore, on climbs or long treks the Ershlers always carry 32-ounce (1-liter) neoprene water bottles.

As mentioned previously, be prepared to force yourself to eat. Susan, like most experienced climbers, finds that the higher she climbs, the less she wants to drink and eat. Therefore, carrying foods that you love is a must. Echoing her highly experienced husband, she stressed, "As Phil always says, 'If you don't like a certain food at sea level, you will most likely really dislike it at high altitude.' Spend all year eating healthy. When on the climb, we eat to obtain calories—*fuel*. As a rule, we take rest breaks approximately every hour. We need to eat every hour as well."

A Powerful Nutritional Learning Experience at Altitude

Phil constantly reminds his climbers to eat and drink something at every break. On one of Susan's first major climbs, Mount Elbrus in Russia (18,513 feet, or 5,643 meters), she felt physically spent coming into the high break just before the summit. What followed was a lesson learned the hard way: "I sat down on my pack and said to myself, 'The heck with eating and drinking.' The rest at the break felt good, but as we left that break, I felt completely spent. The last stretch I fully experienced 'hitting the wall.' I felt as if I could barely move my legs. Very slowly, with Phil's assistance, I did make the summit. As soon as we arrived, I ate a granola bar and snapped right out of my drained state. From that day forward I never stopped at a break without eating or drinking some calories." Another useful trick is to keep some candy or food in your pockets, not just in your pack. When exhausted, you need to make sure that food is easy to access.

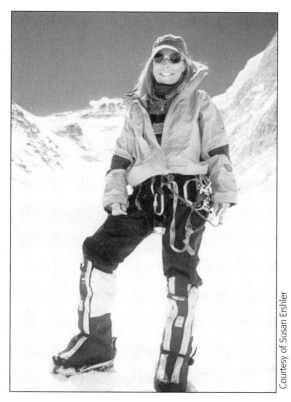

Climber Susan Ershler's nutrition secret is to never take a break without refueling.

Courtesy of Susan Ershler

Secret Nutrition Weapons for High Altitudes

Drink, drink, drink. At altitude, it's normal not to feel thirsty or not want to make the effort to drink. You need to force yourself to drink continuously. Susan reiterates that nothing will zap your energy and inhibit your performance faster than becoming dehydrated. Oftentimes (especially in the third world), the water is less tasty because you use iodine to treat it or because it tastes smoky from being heated over a fire. Susan always travels with Crystal Light powdered drink mix (and often powdered Gatorade as well). These products make the water appealing, which encourages drinking, especially when you don't feel thirsty. If you're using iodine, wait at least 30 minutes after treating the water to mix in a drink mix.

Bring a variety of your favorite foods. Tastes change quickly at altitude. For example, you may crave something salty at one moment and the next hour want something sweet. Then you may want something more nutritious (real food). Susan always packs for climbs and treks with that in mind. She always brings salty hard pretzels, dark chocolate, and some more nutritious foods like cheeses and beef jerky.

APPENDIX A
Measurement Conversion Charts

Energy in Foods

1 calorie (cal) = 4.18 kilojoules (kJ)

Converting information from food labels

Examples: 1/2 cup (120 ml) of orange juice = 60 calories
60 calories × 4.18 = 250 kilojoules

1/2 cup (120 ml) of orange juice = 250 kilojoules
250 kilojoules / 4.18 = 60 calories

Metric Conversion Made Easy

To change weight in	To	Multiply by
Ounces	Grams	28
Pounds	Kilograms	.45
To change volume in	**To**	**Multiply by**
Teaspoons	Milliliters	5
Tablespoons	Milliliters	15
Fluid ounces	Milliliters	30
Cups	Liters	.24
Pints	Liters	.47
Quarts	Liters	.95
Gallons	Liters	3.8

Copyright © 2006 Calorie Control Council
Available: http://www.caloriecontrol.org/metricconversion.html

Body Mass Index (BMI)

Imperial formula

$$BMI = [\text{weight in pounds} / (\text{height in inches})^2] \times 703$$

Metric formula

$$BMI = \text{weight in kilograms} / (\text{height in meters})^2$$

Temperature Measurement Equivalents

To convert Fahrenheit to Celsius: subtract 32 and multiply by .6.
To convert Celsius to Fahrenheit: multiply by 1.8 and add 32.

	Fahrenheit	Celsius
Boiling point of water	212°	100°
Freezing point of water	32°	0°
Normal body temperature	98.6°	37°

APPENDIX B

Facts About Vitamins and Minerals

Vitamins/ Minerals	Dietary reference intakes (DRIs) for ages 19 to 50	Best sources	Functions
Thiamin	1.1/1.2 mg/d	Wheat germ, whole-grain breads and cereals, organ meats, lean meats, legumes, fortified grains	Releases energy from carbohydrate; maintains healthy nervous system
Riboflavin	1.1/1.3 mg/d	Milk and dairy products, green leafy vegetables, lean meats, beans, fortified grains	Releases energy from protein, fat, and carbohydrate; promotes healthy skin
Niacin	14/16 mg/d	Lean meats, fish, poultry, legumes, whole grains, fortified grains	Releases energy from protein, fat, and carbohydrate; aids in synthesis of protein, fat, and DNA; promotes healthy skin and nervous system
Vitamin B_6	1.3 mg/d	Liver, lean meats, fish, poultry, legumes, whole grains	Aids in metabolism of protein; synthesis of essential fatty acids; forms hemoglobin and red blood cells
Vitamin B_{12}	2.4 µg/d	Lean meats, poultry, dairy products, eggs, fish	Aids in metabolism of carbohydrate, protein, fat; produces red blood cells; maintains nerve cells
Folate	400 µg/d	Green leafy vegetables, legumes	Aids growth of new cells; forms red blood cells
Biotin	30 µg/d	Meats, legumes, milk, egg yolk, whole grains	Aids in metabolism of carbohydrate, fat, protein

Vitamins/ Minerals	Dietary reference intakes (DRIs) for ages 19 to 50	Best sources	Functions
Pantothenic acid	5 mg/d	Found in variety of foods	Aids in metabolism of carbohydrate, fat, protein
Vitamin C	75/90 mg/d	Citrus fruits, green leafy vegetables, broccoli, peppers, potatoes, berries, kiwi, cantaloupe (rockmelon)	Maintains normal connective tissue; enhances iron absorption; serves as antioxidant; helps heal wounds
Vitamin A	700/900 µg/d	Liver, milk, cheese, fortified margarine, carotenoids in plant foods (orange, red, or deep green in color)	Maintains healthy skin, mucous membranes, vision, and immune system; serves as antioxidant
Vitamin D	200 IU pr 5 µg/d	Vitamin D fortified milk and margarine, fattier fish, fish oil, sunlight	Promotes normal bone growth; aids in calcium absorption
Vitamin E	15 mg/d	Vegetable oils, margarine, green leafy vegetables, wheat germ, eggs, whole grains	Serves as antioxidant; forms red blood cells
Vitamin K	90/120 µg/d	Liver, eggs, cauliflower, green leafy vegetables	Promotes normal blood clotting
Calcium	1,000 mg/d	Milk, cheese, yogurt, ice cream, legumes, dark green leafy vegetables	Helps in formation of bones and teeth; has role in muscle contractions, nerve impulse transmission, and blood clotting
Phosphorus	700 mg/d	Meat, poultry, fish, eggs, milk, cheese, legumes, whole grains	Aids in metabolism of protein, carbohydrate, and fat; repairs and maintains cells; helps in formation of teeth and bones
Magnesium	320/420 mg/d	Milk, yogurt, legumes, nuts, whole grains, tofu, green vegetables	Aids in metabolism of carbohydrate and protein; aids in neuromuscular contractions

Vitamins/ Minerals	Dietary reference intakes (DRIs) for ages 19 to 50	Best sources	Functions
Iron	18/8 mg/d	Organ meats, lean meats, poultry, shellfish, oysters, whole grains, legumes	Aids in formation of hemoglobin and transportation of oxygen in red blood cells
Zinc	8/11 mg/d	Lean meats, fish, poultry, shellfish, oysters, whole grains, legumes	Aids in energy metabolism; synthesizes protein; helps with immune function and wound healing
Copper	900 µg/d	Lean meats, poultry, shellfish, fish, eggs, nuts, beans, whole grains	Is necessary for iron absorption, manufacture of collagen; heals wounds
Fluoride	3/4 mg/d	Milk, egg yolks, water, seafood	Helps form teeth and bones
Selenium	55 µg/d	Meat, fish, poultry, organ meats, seafood, whole grains, and nuts from selenium-rich soil	Serves as component of antioxidant enzymes
Chromium	25/35 µg/d	Organ meats, meats, oysters, cheese, whole grains, beer	Regulates blood sugar; aids normal fat metabolism
Iodine	150 µg/d	Iodized salt, seafood, water	Serves as component of thyroid hormone that helps regulate growth and development rate
Manganese	1.8/2.3 mg/d	Green leafy vegetables, whole grains, nuts, legumes, egg yolks	Aids in synthesis of hemoglobin
Molybdenum	45 µg/d	Legumes, cereal grains, dark green leafy vegetables	Involved in carbohydrate and fat metabolism
Sodium	Based on sweat loss, at least 1,500 mg/d	Table salt; found in virtually all foods, especially processed items	Promotes acid–base balance, fluid balance, nerve impulses, muscle action
Potassium	4,700 mg/d; if high sweat rate may need more	Fruits and vegetables (bananas, orange juice, potatoes, tomatoes), milk, yogurt, legumes	Promotes fluid balance; acid–base balance, nerve impulses, muscle action, synthesis of protein and glycogen

Note: µg = microgram

APPENDIX C
High-Carbohydrate Foods

Food category	Calories	Carbohydrate (g)
Dairy		
Low-fat (1%) milk (1 cup, or 250 ml)	100	11
Skim milk (1 cup)	80	11
Low-fat chocolate milk (1 cup)	179	26
Pudding, any flavor (1/2 cup)	161	30
Frozen yogurt, low-fat (1 cup)	220	34
Fruit-flavored low-fat yogurt (1 cup)	225	42
Beans		
Black-eyed peas (1/2 cup)	134	22
Pinto beans (1 cup)	235	44
Navy beans (1 cup)	259	48
Refried beans (1/2 cup)	142	26
Garbanzo beans (chickpeas) (1 cup)	269	45
White beans (1 cup)	249	45
Fruits		
Apple (1 medium)	81	21
Apple juice (1 cup)	111	28
Applesauce (1 cup)	194	51
Banana (1)	105	27
Cantaloupe (rockmelon) (1 cup)	57	14
Dates, dried (10)	228	61
Fruit roll-ups (1 roll)	50	12
Grapes (1 cup)	114	28
Grape juice (1 cup)	96	23
Orange (1)	65	16
Orange juice (1 cup)	100	24
Pear (1)	98	25
Pineapple (1 cup)	77	19
Dried plums, (10)	201	53
Raisins (1/4 cup)	130	31
Raspberries (1 cup)	61	14
Strawberries (1 cup)	45	11
Watermelon (1 cup)	50	12

Food category	Calories	Carbohydrate (g)
Vegetables		
Three-bean salad (1/2 cup)	90	20
Carrots (1 medium, 3 oz or 85 g baby carrots)	31	8
Corn (1/2 cup)	89	21
Lima beans (1 cup)	217	40
Peas, green (1/2 cup)	63	12
Potato (1 large)	220	50
Sweet potato (1 large)	118	28
Bread and cereals		
Bagel (2.5 oz, or 70 g)	186	38
Biscuit (2 oz, or 56 g)	190	23
Breadsticks (2 sticks)	77	15
Cereal, ready-to-eat (1 cup)	110	24
Cream of rice (3/4 cup, cooked)	95	21
Cream of wheat (3/4 cup, cooked)	96	20
Cornbread (1 square)	178	28
English muffin	154	30
Fig bar (1)	50	10
Flavored oatmeal, instant (1 packet)	110	25
Flour tortilla (6.5 in., or 17 cm, diameter)	88	15
Graham crackers (2 full cracker sheets)	130	25
Granola bar (low fat, 1)	90	15
Hamburger bun (1)	123	22
Hot dog bun (1)	123	22
Noodles, spaghetti (1 cup, cooked)	197	40
Oatmeal (1 cup, cooked)	145	25
Oatmeal raisin cookie	62	9
Pancake (4 in., or 10 cm, diameter)	84	11
Pizza (cheese, 1 slice)	290	39
Popcorn, plain (1 cup, popped)	26	6
Pretzels (1 oz, or 28 g)	106	21
Rice (1 cup, cooked)	226	50
Rice, brown (1 cup, cooked)	226	45
Saltines (5 crackers)	60	10
Triscuit crackers (6 crackers)	120	20
Waffles (2, 3.5 by 5.5 in., or 9 by 14 cm)	230	30
White bread (1 slice)	80	15
Whole-wheat bread (1 slice)	80	14

Note: Equivalent units of volume: 1 cup (imperial) = .946 cup (metric) = 1.041 cup (Canada).

Adapted, by permission, from S. Nelson Steen, 1998, "Eating on the road: Where are the carbohydrates?," *Sports Science Exchange*, #71, 11(4):1–5.

APPENDIX D

Eating on the Run

Stocking Your Pantry

If you're like most athletes, you have the time to eat healthy meals and snacks. What you don't have time for is pedaling or hoofing it over to the nearest grocery store because you're missing some key ingredient or, worse, looking in the fridge and realizing that you forgot to go food shopping again. By keeping a stash of these nutritious staples on hand in your pantry, refrigerator, and freezer, grabbing healthy snacks and whipping up simple meals is easy.

Breads, Pasta, Rice, and Other Grains

Quick-cooking brown or white rice (cooking time: 10 minutes)

Pasta (cooking time: 10 minutes; fresh pasta: 3 to 5 minutes)

Other prepackaged quick-cooking pastas or grains: couscous (cooking time: 5 minutes), quinoa (cooking time: 10 to 15 minutes), cracked wheat bulgur, pasta and beans, wheat pilaf, tabouli (cooking time: 15 minutes)

Instant stuffing mixes (cooking time: 5 minutes)

Corn and flour tortillas

Whole-grain breads, bagels, rolls, pita bread, English muffins (store in the freezer)

Low-fat crackers (4 grams of fat or less per ounce, or per 28 grams)

Quick-cooking oatmeal, Farina, Wheatena (cooking time: 5 minutes)

Ready-to-eat whole-grain cereals, breakfast bars, granola bars

Pancake mix, toaster waffles

Fruits and Vegetables

Potatoes or sweet potatoes (store in a cool, dark area; bake in the microwave)

Instant mashed potato mixes (cooking time: 5 minutes)

Frozen or canned vegetables (rinse canned varieties to reduce sodium content)

Bags of prewashed salad greens

Bags of minicarrots

Prechopped vegetables or fruit from grocery store salad bars

Canned fruit such as mandarin oranges and pineapple chunks; frozen berries

Oranges, apples, bananas (store in the fridge to slow ripening)

Dates, raisins and other dried fruit

Frozen 100 percent juice concentrates and individual-serving juice boxes

Milk and Milk Products

Low-fat milk (regular or soy)

Low-fat yogurt

Low-fat cheese (including part-skim ricotta and mozzarella, and parmesan)

Low-fat cottage cheese

Meat and Meat Alternatives

Boneless, skinless chicken breasts (store in the freezer)

Lean ground meat (ground round, sirloin, turkey breast)

Cubed meat for kebabs or stir-fries

Cooked shrimp

Lean deli meats such as turkey, ham, or roast beef

Packets or cans of tuna (packed in water), chicken

Edamame (ready-to-eat or frozen), soynuts

Canned chili, baked beans, frozen burritos

Canned beans such as kidney, pinto, black, chickpeas, vegetarian or no-fat refried beans

Frozen veggie or garden burgers

Tofu

Eggs or egg substitutes (can be stored in the freezer)

Peanut or other nut butters

Healthy Oils and Fats

Soft (tub) or liquid margarine

Oil for cooking and baking—olive, canola, peanut

Low-fat salad dressing

Reduced-calorie mayonnaise

Nuts and seeds

Avocado

Olives

Extras

Condiments such as mustard, ketchup, salsa, cocktail sauce, soy sauce, vinegar, jelly or jam

Seasonings such as onion and garlic powders, dried herbs

Spaghetti sauce (4 grams of fat or less per 4 ounces, or per 125 grams)

Canned soup

Instant (just add boiling water) cups of polenta, lentils, beans

Sports bars

Pretzels, low-fat chips, low-fat popcorn

Lower fat "fun foods" (like cookies, fig bars, and angel food cake)

Tips: Perishables, such as milk and yogurt, fresh fruit and vegetables, fresh pasta, and deli meats, need to be replaced weekly. Other staples can be stored for longer periods, especially if unopened.

Dining Out

Dining away from home doesn't mean giving up on a well-balanced, healthy diet. Keep the food pyramid in mind and try to fill out the groups as you would at home. By choosing the restaurant or eatery carefully, you'll have plenty of options. Although some endurance athletes can afford to consume higher-fat items, this list emphasizes higher-carbohydrate, lower-fat selections for those who eat out regularly.

Fast Food

Pizza with vegetarian toppings

Broiled burgers or grilled chicken with lettuce and tomato on whole-wheat bun

Sandwich, sub, or wrap made with lean meat and vegetables

Chicken or grilled steak fajitas or soft tacos

Bean burrito

Salad bar, entrée salads with grilled chicken and low-calorie dressing

Soup

Baked potato with vegetables and low-fat toppings

Chili with crackers

Bagel or English muffin, lightly buttered or with jam

Waffle or pancakes with syrup

Ready-to-eat cereal (hot or cold) or oatmeal

Low-fat muffins or cookies

Regular or flavored nonfat or low-fat milk

Low-fat milk shake, yogurt, and fruit parfaits

Frozen yogurt or soft-serve ice cream

100 percent fruit juice, fruit cups, fruit salad, bags of sliced apples

Tips: Go easy on extra cheese or meat toppings on pizza, supersize burgers and fries, fried chicken and fish sandwiches, creamy soups, salad dressings, breakfast biscuits, sausage and bacon, tartar sauce, mayonnaise, special sauces, Danish pastries, and soft drinks.

Mexican Cuisine

Gazpacho or bean soup

Red or black beans

Refried beans (made without lard or fat)

Spanish rice

Marinated vegetables

Grilled shrimp and fish

Grilled chicken

Soft plain tortillas

Burritos (not deep fried)

Soft tacos

Fajitas

Enchiladas

Tamales

Pico de gallo

Salsa

Baked tortilla chips

Tips: Go easy on crispy fried tortillas (nachos) and taco shells, quesadillas, chile relleno, tostados, chimichangas, sour cream, cheese, and guacamole and always ask how the refried beans are prepared. Order a la carte if you can and choose your sides wisely.

Chinese Cuisine

Wonton or hot and sour soup

Steamed rice and vegetables

Steamed dumplings

Stir-fried dishes (chicken, beef, scallops, shrimp, or tofu) loaded with vegetables

Chow mein dishes

Moo goo gai pan

Chicken or beef chop suey

Fortune cookies

Tips: Go easy on fried rice, fried wontons, egg rolls, fried chow-mein noodles, spare ribs, sweet and sour dishes, crispy beef, Kung pao chicken, lemon chicken, General Tso's chicken, and Peking duck.

Italian Cuisine

Minestrone soup

Crudités (raw vegetables)

Bread sticks or plain bread

Pasta with lower-fat sauce (marinara, red clam, white clam)

Meat sauce (rather than meatballs)

Chicken cacciatore or primavera

Spinach or mushroom tortellini

Thick-crust plain or vegetable pizza

Salads with dressings on the side

Italian ice or fresh sorbet

Tips: Go easy on antipasto plates; butter, margarine, or olive oil served with bread; creamy salad dressings; extra cheese and meat toppings on pizza; alfredo or pesto sauce; Italian sausage, fried calamari, parmigiana dishes, manicotti, and lasagna.

Indian Cuisine

Dahl (bean soup)

Naan

Roti (breads)

Basmati rice

Shish kebab

Curries

Tips: Go easy on fried appetizers, samosas, and dishes that load up on cheese or sauces, such as Palak or Saag Paneer. Ask how sauces are made because many restaurants add cream besides the ghee (clarified butter) and coconut milk (Malai) normally used.

Classic Western Cuisine

Lentil or bean-based soups and side dishes

Plain bread

Salad with dressing on the side

Steamed vegetables

Baked or mashed potatoes

Brown or wild rice

Stir-fried dishes and kebabs made with lean meats and loaded with vegetables

Barbecued chicken

Pot roast

Turkey with stuffing

Hamburger or garden burger

Filet mignon or sirloin steak

Pork tenderloin

Grilled, broiled, or baked fish or skinless chicken

Fruit

Sorbet or frozen yogurt

Low-fat milk shakes

Tips: Go easy on salads already dressed (for example, Caesar salad); buffalo wings; stuffed potato skins; french fries; onion rings; fried items (chicken, steak, and shrimp); extra gravy; tartar sauce; creamy and buttery sauces; sour cream or butter on baked potatoes; pot pies; cheesy items like grilled cheese, cheese steak sandwich, and patty melts; and New York strip, T-bone, and porterhouse steaks. Watch out for excessively generous serving sizes—split with a friend or request a takeaway bag.

SELECTED RESOURCES

Sports Nutrition Information

Australian Institute of Sport, www.ais.org.au.

Gatorade Sports Science Institute (GSSI), www.gssiweb.com.

International Olympic Committee, www.olympic.org/uk/organisation/commissions/medical/index_uk.asp.

NCAA Nutrition and Performance, www.ncaa.org/nutritionandperformance.

Peak Performance, www.pponline.co.uk.

SCAN (Sports, Cardiovascular and Wellness Nutritionists), to locate a sports dietitian, www.scandpg.org.

USDA Nutrient Data Laboratory, www.ars.usda.gov/nutrientdata.

Hydration Systems and Gear

Camelbak Hydration Systems, 800-767-8725, www.camelbak.com.

Mountain Safety Research, 800-531-9531, www.msrcorp.com.

Nalgene Outdoor, 800-625-4327, www.nalgene-outdoor.com.

Bike Nashbar, 800-888-2710, www.nashbar.com.

Ultimate Direction, 800-426-7229, www.ultimatedirection.com.

Body Image and Disordered Eating

Anorexia Nervosa and Related Eating Disorders, www.anred.com.

National Eating Disorders Association (NEDA): Eating Disorders Information and Referral Line, 800-931-2237, www.nationaleatingdisorders.org.

Cookbooks, Dining Out, and Recipes

Eating on the Run, Evelyn Tribole, MS, RD, Human Kinetics, 2004.

What to Eat When You're Eating Out, Hope Warshaw, RD, CDE, American Diabetes Association, 2006.

The Volumetrics Eating Plan, Barbara Rolls, PhD, HarperCollins Publishers, 2005.

Meals for You, www.mealsforyou.com.

Supplement Information

ConsumerLab, www.consumerlab.com.

National Center for Drug Free Sport, 816-474-8655, www.drugfreesport.com.

Quackwatch, www.quackwatch.com.

Vegetarian Nutrition

Vegetarian Resource Group, www.vrg.org.

Vegetarian Resources, School of Public Health at Loma Linda University, www.llu.edu/llu/nutrition/veg.

Adventure Racing

Adventure Racing, www.adventureracing.net.

Checkpoint ZERO, www.checkpointzero.com.

Cycling

Cycling Research News, www.cyclingresearchnews.com.

Cycling Performance Tips, www.cptips.com.

RAAM: Race Across America, www.raceacrossamerica.org.

Randonneurs USA, www.rusa.org.

Ultra Marathon Cycling Association, www.ultracycling.com.

Endurance Adventures

Backpacker, www.backpacker.com.

Mountain Zone, www.mountainzone.com.

Rowing

Rowing News, www.rowingnews.com.

Running

Marathon & Beyond, www.marathonandbeyond.com.

Running Research News, www.runningresearchnews.com.

Ultrarunning Online, www.ultrarunning.com.

Skiing

American Birkebeiner, www.birkie.com.

Cross-Country Skiing, www.xcskiworld.com.

Swimming

Swimming Research News, www.swimmingresearchnews.com.

Triathlon and Duathlon

Inside Triathlon, www.insidetri.com.

Triathlete, www.triathletemag.com.

Note: The inclusion of a Web site does not constitute an endorsement of that site. At the time of publication, all phone numbers and URLs were correct.

BIBLIOGRAPHY

ACOG Committee. 2002. Opinion no. 267. Exercise during pregnancy and the post-partum period. *Obstetrics and Gynecology* 99(1):171–173.

American College of Sports Medicine, American Dietetic Association, Dietitians of Canada. 2000. Joint position stand on nutrition and athletic performance. *Journal of the American Dietetic Association* 100:1543–56.

Armstrong, L.E. et al. 1996. Heat and cold illnesses during distance running. American College of Sports Medicine position stand. *Medicine and Science in Sports and Exercise* 28:i–x.

Australian Institute of Sport. 2005. Sport nutrition: Sports supplement program fact sheets. www.ais.org.au.

Baker, J. et al. 2005. Effects of indomethacin and celecoxib on renal function in athletes. *Medicine and Science in Sports and Exercise* 37(5):712–7.

Beals, K.A. 2004. *Disordered eating among athletes: A comprehensive guide for health professionals.* Champaign, IL: Human Kinetics.

Benardot, D. et al. 2001. Can vitamin supplements improve sport performance? *Sports Science Exchange Roundtable* 12(3):1–4.

Bergeron, M. 2000. Sodium: The forgotten nutrient. *Sports Science Exchange* 13(3):1–4.

Borsheim, E. 2005. Enhancing muscle anabolism through nutrient composition and timing of intake. *SCAN's PULSE* 24(3):1–5.

Burke, L.M. 2001. Nutritional needs for exercise in the heat. *Comparative Biochemistry and Physiology—Part A: Molecular & Integrative Physiology* 128(4):735–48.

Burke, L.M., and V. Deakin, eds. 2006. *Clinical sports nutrition.* Sydney, Australia: McGraw-Hill.

Burke, L.M., B. Kiens, and J.L. Ivy. 2004. Carbohydrates and fat for training and recovery. *Journal of Sport Science* 22:15–30.

Burke, L.M. et al. 2001. Guidelines for daily carbohydrate intake: Do athletes achieve them? *Sports Medicine* 31(4):267–99.

Casa, D. et al. 2005. ACSM roundtable series on hydration and physical activity: Consensus statements. *Current Sports Medicine Reports* 4:115–127.

Chatard, J.C., I. Mujika, C. Guy, and J.R. Lacour. 1999. Anemia and iron deficiency in athletes—practical recommendations for treatment. *Sports Medicine* 27(4):229–40.

Clapp, J.F. 2002. *Exercising through your pregnancy.* Omaha, NE: Addicus.

Coleman, E. 2000. The glycemic index in sport. *SCAN's PULSE* 19(3):1–4.

Coleman, E. 2004. Does adding protein to a sports drink improve performance? *Sports Medicine Digest* 26(1):10–11.

Cox, G.R. et al. 2002. Effect of different protocols of caffeine intake on metabolism and endurance performance. *Journal of Applied Physiology* 93:990–99.

Doubt, T.J. 1991. Physiology of exercise in the cold. *Sports Medicine* 11:367–381.

Eberle, S.G. 2005. Disordered eating + runners: A troublesome combination. *Running Times*, September, 44–50.

Eichner, R.E. 2001. Anemia and blood boosting. *Sports Science Exchange* 14(2):1–4.

Eichner, R.E. 2002. Heat stroke in sports: Causes, prevention and treatment. *Sports Science Exchange* 15(3):1–4.

Farquhar, B., and W.L. Kennedy. 1997. Anti-inflammatory drugs, kidney function, and exercise. *Sports Science Exchange* 11(4):1–6.

Hargraves, M. 2005. Metabolic factors in fatigue. *Sports Science Exchange* 18(3):1–6.

Helge, J.W. 2000. Adaptation to a fat-rich diet: Effects on endurance performance in humans. *Sports Medicine* 30(5):347–57.

Hopkinson, R., and J. Lock. 2004. Athletics, perfectionism and disordered eating. *Eating and Weight Disorders* 9:99–106.

Hsieh M. 2004. Recommendations for treatment of hyponatremia at endurance events. *Sports Medicine* 34:231–238.

IOC Medical Committee Working Group Women in Sport. 2005. Position stand on the female athlete triad. http://multimedia.olympic.org/pdf/en_report_917.pdf.

Jeukendrup, A.E., W.H. Saris, and J.M. Wagenmakers. 1998. Fat metabolism during exercise: A review (part I). *International Journal of Sports Medicine* 19:231–244.

Jeukendrup, A.E., W.H. Saris, and J.M. Wagenmakers. 1998. Fat metabolism during exercise: A review (part II). *International Journal of Sports Medicine* 19:293–302.

Jeukendrup, A.E., and M. Gleeson. 2004. *Sport nutrition: An introduction to energy production and performance*. Champaign, IL: Human Kinetics.

Kayser, B. 1994. Nutrition and energetics of exercise at altitude. *Sports Medicine* 17:309–323.

Kayser, B. 1992. Nutrition and high altitude exposure. *International Journal of Sports Medicine* 13:S129–32.

Kayser, B. 1994. Nutrition and energetics of exercise at altitude. *Sports Medicine* 17:309–23.

Lambert, E.V. et al. 2001. High-fat diet versus habitual diet prior to carbohydrate loading: Effects of exercise metabolism and cycling performance. *International Journal of Sport Nutrition and Exercise Metabolism* 11(2):209–25.

Lambert, E.V., and J.H. Goedecke. 2003. The role of dietary macronutrients in optimizing endurance performance. *Current Sport Medicine Reports* 2(4):194–201.

Levey, J.M. 2000. Runner's diarrhea: An overview. *AMAA Quarterly* 14:6–7.

Littlefied, K. et al. 2006. Athletes with eating disorders. *The Remuda Review* 5(1):2–11.

Loosli, A.R., and J.S. Rudd. 1998. Meatless diets in female athletes: A red flag. *The Physician and Sportsmedicine* 26:45–48.

Lowery, L.M. 2004. Dietary fat and sports nutrition: a primer. *Journal of Sport Science* 3:106–17.

Manore, M., and J. Thompson. 2000. *Sport nutrition for health and performance*. Champaign, IL: Human Kinetics.

McArdle, W., F.I. Katch, and V.L. Katch. 2005. *Sports & exercise nutrition*. 2nd ed. United States: Lippincott Williams & Wilkins.

Messina, V., R. Mangels, and M. Messina. 2004. *The dietitian's guide to vegetarian diets*. 2nd ed. Jones & Bartlett.

Meyer N.L., and S. Parker-Simmons. In preparation for Torino 2006: Dietary needs of winter sport athletes. *SCAN's PULSE* 25(1):1–6.

Murray, R. 1995. Fluid needs in hot and cold environments. *International Journal of Sport Nutrition* 5: S62–S73.

Nelson Steen, S. 1998. Eating on the road: Where are the carbohydrates? *Sports Science Exchange* 11(4):1–5.

Nieman, D.C. 1998. Immunity in athletes: Current issues. *Sports Science Exchange* 11(2):1–6.

Noakes T. 2003. Fluid replacement during marathon running. *Clinical Journal of Sport Medicine* 13(5):309–18.

Otis, C.L., and R. Goldingay. 2000. *The athletic woman's survival guide: How to win the battle against eating disorders, amenorrhea, and osteoporosis.* Champaign, IL: Human Kinetics.

Otis, C.L., B. Drinkwater, M. Johnson, A. Loucks, and J. Wilmore. 1997. American College of Sports Medicine position stand: The female athlete triad. *Medicine and Science in Sports and Exercise* 29(5):i–v.

Putukian, M., and C. Potera. 1997. Don't miss gastrointestinal disorders in athletes. *The Physician and Sportsmedicine* 25:80–94.

Probiotics: Are enough in your diet? 2005. *Consumer Reports*, July, 34–35.

Rawson, E.S., and P. Clarkson. 2003. Scientifically debatable: Is creatine worth its weight? *Sports Science Exchange* 16(4):1–4.

Rehrer, N.J. 2001. Fluid and electrolyte balance in ultra-endurance sport. *Sports Medicine* 31(10):701–15.

Reid, S. et al. 2005. Consensus statement of the first international exercise-associated hyponatremia consensus development conference, Cape Town, South Africa. *Clinical Journal of Sports Medicine* 15:208–13.

Saunders, M.J., M. Kane, and M.K. Todd. 2004. Effects of a carbohydrate-protein beverage on cycling endurance and muscle damage. *Medicine and Science in Sports and Exercise* 36:1233–38.

SCAN. 2006. *Sports nutrition—a practice manual for professionals*, ed. M. Dunford. Chicago: American Dietetics Association.

SCAN's (Sports, Cardiovascular and Wellness Nutritionists) 22nd Annual Symposium. 2006. Striving for balance: Professional approaches for improvement in weight, body image and disordered eating.

Shephard, R.J. 1993. Metabolic adaptations to exercise in the cold. *Sports Medicine* 16(4) 266–289.

Slater, G.J. et al. 2005. Body-mass management of Australian lightweight rowers prior to and during competition. *Medicine and Science in Sports and Exercise* 37(5):860–6.

Soles, C. 2002. *Climbing: Training for peak performance.* Seattle: The Mountaineers.

Sykora, C., C.M. Grilo, D.E. Wilfley, and K.D. Brownell. 1993. Eating, weight, and dieting disturbances in male and female lightweight and heavyweight rowers. *International Journal of Eating Disorders* 14:203–211.

Tarnopolsky, M. 2004. Protein requirements for endurance athletes. *Nutrition* 20:662–68.

Torstveit, M.K., and J. Sundgot-Borgen. The female athlete triad. *Medicine and Science in Sports and Exercise* 37:184–193.

Tribole, E. 2003. *Eating on the run.* 3rd edition. Champaign, IL: Human Kinetics.

Tribole, E., and E. Resch. 2003. *Intuitive eating—a revolutionary program that works.* New York: St. Martin's Griffen.

von Dullivard, S.P. et al. 2004. Fluids and hydration in prolonged endurance performance. *Nutrition* 20:651–656.

Wagner, D.R. 1999. Hyperhydrating with glycerol: Implications for athletic performance. *Journal of the American Dietetic Association* 99(2):207–212.

Yeo, S.E. et al. 2005. Caffeine increases exogenous carbohydrate oxidation during exercise. *Journal of Applied Physiology* 99(3):844–850.

INDEX

Note: The italicized *f* and *t* following page numbers refer to figures and tables, respectively.

$V̇O_2max$

ABOUT THE AUTHOR

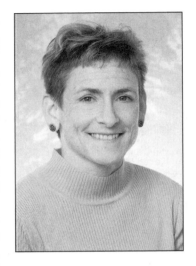

Suzanne Girard Eberle, MS, RD, is a sports dietitian who practices what she teaches. As a multisport athlete, Girard Eberle has 30 years of competitive endeavors under her belt. As a USA Track & Field 5,000-meter champion and member of three national teams, she has raced in countries around the world. Today, she runs 50 miles per week, is an avid cyclist, and enjoys hiking and climbing (rock and alpine). She has reached the summits of Mount Blanc, the highest mountain in the Alps, and Mount Kilimanjaro, the highest mountain in Africa.

She has served as contributing editor for *Running Times* and her nutrition advice has been featured in *USA Today*, *Newsweek*, *Runner's World*, *Men's Fitness*, *SELF*, *SHAPE*, and *Marathon & Beyond*. The founder of Eat, Drink, Win!, Girard Eberle holds a master's degree in clinical nutrition from Boston University. She is a longtime member of the American College of Sports Medicine (ACSM), the American Dietetic Association (ADA), and SCAN: Sports, Cardiovascular and Wellness Nutritionists. She lives and plays outside in Portland, Oregon, with her husband, John, and whippet, Asa Babu.